MODERN PROFESSIONAL NURSING

NEW AND REVISED EDITION

General Editor

MILDRED HAINSWORTH

R.R.C., D.N., S.R.N.

Sister Tutor, Queen Elizabeth Hospital for Children, Banstead, Surrey; Examiner for the General Nursing Council for England and Wales. Formerly Sister Tutor, Poplar Hospital, London; Sister Tutor, Hospital for Sick Children, Great Ormond Street, London; Out-Patients' and Casualty Sister, Bolingbroke Hospital; Gynaecological, Surgical and Accident Ward Sister, Miller General Hospital; Gynaecological, Surgical and Ophthalmic Sister, Royal Free Hospital; Sister Tutor, London Temperance Hospital, Royal Surrey County Hospital and Lord Mayor Trelaor Hospital and College Alton, Hants.

COMPILED IN COLLABORATION WITH THE
CONTRIBUTORS MENTIONED OVERLEAF

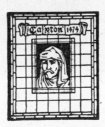

VOLUME TWO

THE CAXTON PUBLISHING CO. LTD.

CLUN HOUSE, SURREY STREET, LONDON, W.C.2

EDITOR FOR MEDICAL PUBLICATIONS : DOUGLAS HAY SCOTT, M.B., CH.B.

FIRST PUBLISHED .	.	April 1936
SECOND EDITION .	.	January 1949
REPRINTED .	.	October 1949
REPRINTED .	.	June 1950

Printed in the Netherlands by
Mouton & Co., The Hague
N. 8a

LIST OF CONTRIBUTORS

TO

MODERN PROFESSIONAL NURSING

(arranged alphabetically)

UNA W. DALDORPH, D.N., S.R.N., Sister Tutor Diploma (King's College Household and Social Science); Senior Sister Tutor, Royal Salop Infirmary, Shrewsbury; Examiner for the General Nursing Council for England and Wales.

FLORENCE DILLISTONE, S.R.N., R.S.C.N., S.C.M., Senior Dietician, The Hospital for Sick Children, Great Ormond Street, London. Formerly Ward and Departmental Sister, The London Hospital.

ANNE FORD, D.N., S.R.N., S.C.M., Registered Sister Tutor, Housekeeping Certificate, Tuberculosis Association Certificate; Sister Tutor Royal Halifax Infirmary, Halifax; Examiner for the General Nursing Council for England and Wales.

MARY E. FORD, D.N., S.R.N., S.C.M., Sister Tutor's Certificate, King's College, London; Sister Tutor, County Hospital, Lincoln; Examiner for the General Nursing Council for England and Wales.

MILDRED HAINSWORTH, Sister Tutor, Queen Elizabeth Hospital for Children, Banstead, Surrey. (For further qualifications see title page.)

L. B. HENDERSON, D.N., S.R.N., S.C.M. Matron, Noble's Hospital, Douglas, I.O.M.

DOROTHY LEWIS, S.R.N., M.C.S.P., M.S.R., M.E., L.E.T. Formerly Sister in Charge, Physiotherapy Dept., The Hospital for Sick Children, Great Ormond Street, London.

ETHEL MURIEL LEWIS, S.R.N., R.S.C.N., S.C.M., Assistant Sister Tutor, The Hospital for Sick Children, Great Ormond Street, London.

ELIZABETH M. B. LOCKHART, S.R.N., R.S.C.N., S.C.M., H.V., Health Visitor, Stirling County Council; Formerly Medical Ward Sister, Royal Hospital for Sick Children, Glasgow, Sister Tutor, Greenock Royal Infirmary and Larkfield Hospital, Greenock, Lecturer to Civil Nursing Reserve.

PHYLLIS M. PIPER, D.N., S.R.N., S.C.M. Formerly Sister Tutor, Hove Hospital, Hove, Sussex. Examiner for the General Nursing Council for England and Wales.

MILDRED MARY SLATER, S.R.N., S.C.M., Sister Tutor's Certificate, University of Manchester; Sister Tutor, North Lonsdale Hospital, Barrow-in-Furness; Examiner for the General Nursing Council for England and Wales.

HARRIETT WARD, D.N., S.R.N., S.C.M., Sister Tutor, Lewisham Hospital, London; Examiner for the General Nursing Council for England and Wales.

CONTENTS OF VOLUME II

SECTION III

HYGIENE

CONTENTS

CHAPTER 9

CHAPTER 10

CHAPTER 11

CHAPTER 12

SECTION IV

BACTERIOLOGY AND CLINICAL PATHOLOGY

CHAPTER 1

CHAPTER 2

CHAPTER 3

CHAPTER 4

CHAPTER 5

CHAPTER 6

CHAPTER 8

CHAPTER 9

CHAPTER 10

CHAPTER 11

CHAPTER 12

LIST OF PLATES

VOLUME II

COLOUR PLATES

BLACK-AND-WHITE PLATES

MODERN
PROFESSIONAL NURSING

VOLUME II

SECTION III

HYGIENE

CHAPTER I

THE LAWS OF HEALTH

WHAT IS MEANT BY HYGIENE. IMPORTANCE OF DISEASE
ORGANISMS. DEFINITION OF INFECTION. NATURE OF
INFECTION. INFECTING AGENTS. THE INFECTIVE PRO-
CESS. SOURCES OF INFECTION. MODES OF TRANSMISSION.

ALL of us have a right to the heritage of health. The very
process of living life to the full connotes the dual alliance of the
healthy mind and the healthy body. It is true that some are
luckier than others and possess in full measure every quality
which results in the happy achievement of every purpose for
which our ends may be shaped. But generally speaking we are all
endowed with sufficient power to make our existence a pleasurable
one, free from abnormal handicaps and untrammelled by disease
or defect which might force us to alter our route in the country
over which we have to travel. If it so happens that illness or
injury comes to limit our activities, we may have to be content
with a modified programme, but there is a meaning for everything, and the contribution of an individual to life as a whole,
unimportant as it may seem to be and insignificant as it may
appear, is nevertheless of value in the gradual evolution of the
human race towards that ideal which we all strive for and keep
ever in front of us.

What is Meant by Hygiene

Health means happiness and although Nature never intended
us to limit our outlets, she has postulated certain essentials, the
non-acceptance of which inevitably leads to an unhappy state.
These elementary laws of health are simple, natural and easy to

obey; they are all incorporated in the code of the science of hygiene which governs not only the individual but also the community. Hygiene shows us how to preserve health and prevent disease; its commonsense tenets appeal to everyone able to understand justice and they are a basis for all the regulations made by man to maintain his life at its maximum degree of efficiency.

A nurse must understand to the full how every hygienic law is applied and how she can rectify matters when the law has been broken. While she has a duty as a trained citizen to the community, and therefore by her labours can add her portion to the general hygienic improvement, she is more concerned with the individual side of hygiene. The State has set up machinery for dealing with the health of the people as a whole and our public health services are highly efficient in coping with the problems of our congested cities, our sanitation, our housing, our infant welfare, our fevers, our food and drink and numerous other matters demanding State supervision. Marked progress has been made under child welfare schemes for pre-school children, established before World War II. Of recent years the health of the school child and adolescent has been widely catered for. Youth hostels and camps have sprung into being throughout the country, and are taken advantage of by young and old alike.

As mentioned above, however, the nurse is concerned with the more detailed and more intimate aspects of hygiene; she may have to concentrate on ante-natal welfare, infant feeding, the dieting of dyspeptics, the principles of disinfection, the heating of the sickroom or the stamping out of disease before it has a chance to become established. She practises personal hygiene, which contributes to the work of the more comprehensive communal hygiene, and therefore she is a very important wheel in the machine.

With welfare as her aim, a nurse can do work which is not only good from a physical point of view but which is invaluable on the educative side by teaching the " science of health and its maintenance." By her action and example, she can sow seeds of hygienic principle in many places where they are bound to grow and so she is instrumental in assisting the public towards that complete knowledge of the rules of health which makes for the perfect creature. Prevention is better than cure; while it is no doubt impossible completely to stamp out disease, it is certain that much suffering and many disabilities can be avoided by the adoption of a code which, if adhered to, ensures the proper functioning of every organ, the perfect balance of every system, and the complete coordination of every part of the body. This is the state of health.

Importance of Disease Organisms

To understand the spread of disease completely is to master at least the half of medical knowledge and therefore no attempt is made in this section to do more than give the main structure of the subject. In the present chapter, the matter is carefully kept within the compass of hygiene as applied to nursing. For fuller information, reference should be made to subsequent sections of this work which deal with this matter. In all branches of nursing the application of hygiene is of paramount importance.

Definition of Infection.—For many centuries the spread of plagues and fevers was not understood. Epidemics of great severity swept countries and affected whole races, leaving an enormous mortality list and puzzling the earlier workers in medical research. The discovery of the microscope (in the latter part of the seventeenth century) which could magnify things to previously unthought of dimensions, and the work of Pasteur and the subsequent army of his followers (in the nineteenth century), made things very clear for us with regard to the causation of infectious disease. As time has gone on, the meaning of infection has been considerably enlarged. Today it stands for any process which involves the passage of certain living parasitic organisms of very primitive structure (usually unicellular) from one situation outside the individual to one in the individual. Transmission is very rapid, so that large numbers of individuals can be affected at the same time, and the methods of reaching the body may be direct or indirect. For example, a person may touch the clothing of a scarlet fever patient, or prick his finger with a knife containing germs from an abscess—this is direct infection; on the other hand the causative organisms may reach the human being by passing from the rat to the flea and from the flea to the human being—this occurs in bubonic plague and is indirect infection. When infection occurs, the result is a definite train of symptoms and signs known to be associated with the particular microbe transmitted. In time the person who is markedly infected by a certain group of organisms is a radiating centre for the dissemination of the disease, and is styled infectious.

Nature of Infection

There are several ways of looking at the infective process. It is essentially a condition in which there are present in large numbers certain rapidly multiplying groups of primitive organisms, but these organisms are of numerous types and varieties of type. It is almost possible to say that each person has his own peculiar reaction to a particular specimen of infecting agent.

Infecting Agents.—Much remains to be discovered about the organisms which are foreign to the human body; in many cases, we are forced to judge their characters by the effect of their activities. In the lowest part of the scale, many infecting agents cannot be either collected or seen by the most delicate instruments, therefore we have to judge them by the diseases they cause. We can classify the organisms into the following 4 groups: metazoa, protozoa, bacteria, viruses.

Of the above classification, the metazoa are discussed later on. The protozoa are in many respects like the bacteria, while the viruses are possibly very minute bacteria, therefore it is convenient to study the whole of the infective process by taking the example of the bacteria themselves. This is known as the science of bacteriology (see Sect. 4).

The Infective Process.—All we are concerned with in this chapter is the general effect of bacterial invasion. The questions of reaction of the defensive mechanism of the body, immunity, serum and vaccine therapy, bacterial cultivation and destruction and individual diseases are fully discussed elsewhere, as already mentioned.

If we take as an example of the infective process one of the common infectious fevers, we find that the first act in the drama is the gathering of a swarm or colony of microbes, which rapidly multiply in the body. The individual attacked is referred to as the host. For the first few days these germs show little or no evidence of their presence. If it were possible, however, to see the cells of the protoplasm, a considerable amount of active work would be found going on, indeed the whole process might amount to a hand to hand struggle between the germs and the body defences, represented by the leucocytes. Ultimately, after a certain fixed period during which the invading organisms undoubtedly become elaborated and increased numerically, the first signs of the disease are shown, possibly by a rash. The period which elapses between the arrival of the first batch of germs in the tissues and the appearance of the first signs of the specific fever is called the incubation period. This period is fairly well defined for all the well known infective fevers, and indicates the number of days spent by the invaders in preparing their forces, in becoming acclimatized to the host, in overcoming the primary resistance of the tissues and in gaining the complete ascendancy over the defence. Some people in this period are able to repel the enemy and so they do not become victims to the disease; it is impossible to say how often this goes on in a healthy person's life—probably every day. Generally there is some evidence of debility whether the person is going to go through the full effects of the attack or not. Especially is this so in measles, where pallor and irritability—" sickening for measles "—are characteristic.

The second period of a bacterial attack is called the stage of invasion. The microbes are ubiquitous and all the secondary counter measures of the body are required to deal with them. During this time, the signs and symptoms peculiar to the infection are evident—fever, rash, pains, cough, weakness and so on—and the more prominent these symptoms are, the greater is the effort of the body to overcome the invasion. In most cases this is accomplished by the production of antidotes in the tissue to the germs, so that the latter are quickly overcome; thus the patient is left to begin the convalescent stage, weak in muscle but strong in blood.

The stage of convalescence is characterized by rapid return to the *status quo* so far as the general health is concerned, but actually the individual has benefited considerably by being left with a huge store of antidotes which give him protection for many months to come against a particular, or several, germs. Even a very mild attack of an infectious disease produces a protective quality in the tissues.

Sources of Infection

Most germs like moisture, many cannot live in air, all dislike direct sun. The ideal source for bacteria is therefore a poorly lit, damp, close atmosphere. Many can stand cold well, but heating at any temperature above the boiling point of water will kill them. They thrive best at body heat. They abound in all excrement and in rotting animal and vegetable matter. They are known to remain on clothing and on any household fabrics. They may live comfortably in the intestines and in the lungs ot those who are chronically afflicted with enteritis or consumption.

In enumerating the sources of direct and indirect infection, therefore, we include all infected tissues (animal or human) and the ordinary excretions of the bowel, bladder or skin. Another factor is the discharge of any abnormal matter, such as the pus from a wound, the phlegm from the lungs or throat, the saliva in mumps and the secretion from the nose in diphtheria. Grease, dirt and decaying matter are full of all kinds of germs and there-fore a perpetual source of danger in slum areas. The cultivated soil may contain numbers of active tetanus bacilli which soon cause widespread effects in the human being. The bite of a dog with hydrophobia may give rise to rabies in the human being. Many more examples might be given. Our daily food would be a never ending source of disease if it were not protected by hygienic defences.

Modes of Transmission

How does the microbe reach the human body?   This is easy
to answer in some cases and difficult in others.   The simplest
way is by direct inoculation, as when a cut finger meets with a
group of septic organisms.   Nurses often have fingers poisoned
when working in the out patient department, as they may prick
their fingers with a pin or scissors, and in handling dressings
become affected with a group of septic germs which soon cause
an abscess.   Venereal disease is usually a matter of direct contact, and tetanus is often contracted in street accidents, where
the organisms, lying in the street dust, gain direct access to the
wounds.

Droplet infection is a very common way to spread germs.   The
exhaled breath or the expectorated sputum may disseminate in
the air tiny droplets of vapour or sputum, full of the germs of
phthisis, coryza, measles or other air borne infections.   Another
method is spread by dust; in this case the dust particles, attached
to which are numerous microbes, rise up in a cloud when dust
is disturbed and so pollute the air in the vicinity.   Persons who
may pass through, or who live constantly in, an atmosphere
charged with these droplets or dust particles, run the risk of
becoming infected in the air passages by breathing the tainted
air and indeed in many cases this is how consumption is spread.

Food may be the vehicle which transfers organisms to the
intestines.   The acid of the stomach is normally an antidote to
all intestinal poisons, but occasionally the microbes are so powerful that they are unaffected, and as soon as they reach the intestines they set up inflammation.   In summer more than at any
other season it is important to keep watch over our food, especially highly concentrated meats, which not only attract germs, but
are an ideal medium for multiplication; in a few hours a piece
of meat may become a teeming mass of bacteria.   These germs
almost invariably irritate the bowel and may set up enteric fever,
dysentery, infantile diarrhoea, tuberculosis and similar types of
illness.   The importance of purity of milk has already been
stressed.   Water may spread cholera.

Lastly infection may be indirectly carried by animals, like the
rat flea already mentioned.   The chief offenders in this matter
are, however, insects like the common house fly, the mosquito
(which spreads malaria) and the tsetse fly (the carrier of sleeping
sickness).

It is quite evident that the possibilities of infection from food,
clothing, insects, dust, the air and the surroundings of the sick
person are inestimable.   Nurses should therefore remember that
everything connected with the sickroom should be scrupulously

clean. Every item in the dietary should pass hygienic tests, and every precaution should be taken to prevent the breeding of germs from taking place. At the same time the communal side must not be forgotten. In an infectious case, it is necessary to ensure that all the clothing and utensils in contact with the patient should be carefully treated as described later. The bedclothes, garments, fabrics of the room, crockery, books and toilet articles may all be powerful mediums for the spread of disease. The nurse must never lose sight of the fact that she herself may be the intermediary in the spread of the disease, and she must also bear in mind that she is constantly running the risk of becoming infected herself.

CHAPTER 2

AIR

COMPOSITION OF THE AIR. PURE AIR. IMPURITIES OF
THE AIR. THE EFFECT OF RESPIRATION ON THE AIR.
HOW COMBUSTION AFFECTS THE AIR. CARBONIC ACID GAS
AND CARBON MONOXIDE. INDUSTRIAL EFFLUENTS AND
AIR POLLUTION. ORGANIC DECOMPOSITION. HUMIDITY.
VENTILATION. DEFINITION OF VENTILATION. NATURAL
VENTILATION. DIFFUSION. PROPULSION. CONVECTION.
PERFLATION. ASPIRATION. ARTIFICIAL VENTILATION.
THE PLENUM OR PROPULSION METHOD. THE EXTRACTION
OR VACUUM SYSTEM. THE BALANCE SYSTEM. ESSENTIALS
OF EFFICIENT VENTILATION. THE AMOUNT OF AIR
REQUIRED. HOW TO CALCULATE AIR ALLOWANCE.
STANDARDS OF AIR SUPPLY FOR VARIOUS BUILDINGS.
PRACTICAL APPLICATION OF VENTILATION TO HOUSES AND
HOSPITALS. VENTILATION OF A ROOM. ADJUNCTS TO
NATURAL VENTILATION. WINDOW APPLIANCES. WALL
VENTILATORS. ROOF VENTILATORS. METHODS OF ARTI-
FICIAL VENTILATION. HOW VENTILATION METHODS ARE
EMPLOYED. DUST AND THE HEALTHY HOUSE.

THE atmosphere which surrounds the earth, and in which we
live, consists of a mixture of gases known as air. Air is essential
to life.

Composition of the Air

The chief constituents of the air are oxygen and nitrogen, with
minute quantities of other substances, including argon, carbonic
acid gas, ozone, water vapour, nitric acid, ammonia and mineral
dust. Air varies so much according to locality that it is difficult
to say where the normal specimen is to be found. Undoubtedly
the purest air is mountain air whereas the most polluted specimens are obtained from the atmosphere of the large towns,
in which sulphurous acid, sulphuretted hydrogen, soot, dust,
microbes, fine particles of animal excreta, complex gases associated with various manufactories and many other factors all
add to the impurity

Pure Air.—The most perfect specimen of air roughly consists of the following:

Oxygen	21	per cent
Nitrogen	78	,,
Carbonic acid gas . . .	·04	,,
Argon and other constituents .	·96	,,

The essential constituent of the air is oxygen, which roughly takes up one-fifth of the total volume; it is generally agreed that the nitrogen and other gases of the air act as diluting agents, since oxygen in its pure state could not be breathed by the lungs. The small amount of carbonic acid gas is used by plants in the daytime, when they take it up and give up oxygen. Water vapour is the most variable constituent of the air, being influenced by climate and other factors. The presence of this vapour gives the quality of humidity to the air, which is a danger to health in certain places e.g. New York. Evaporation from moist or water surfaces produces water vapour. It is breathed into the air from the lungs of both men and animals. Saturation point is said to be reached when the air at any given temperature holds as much water as possible. In the United Kingdom, the average amount of water vapour is $1\frac{1}{2}$ per cent. Oxygen is in greatest concentration near to the surface of the earth. Ascents in aircraft to high altitudes have proved that as we rise in the atmosphere, the more does the percentage of oxygen diminish, necessitating the provision of a portable supply. This is one of the main problems of present day aviation. It is also a well known fact that those who climb high mountains become sickened owing to even a very slight deficiency of the volume of oxygen.

Impurities of the Air

Vitiation of the air may happen in several ways among which are those of respiration, combustion, industrial effluence and organic decomposition. These 4 sources account for most of the abnormal constituents mentioned above.

The Effect of Respiration on the Air.—In the chapter dealing with the physiology of breathing (Vol. I, pp. 190–194), we learned that 500 cubic centimetres of tidal air are inhaled at each inspiration, the proportion of gases being as stated above. Exhaled air shows that in the process of respiration, the oxygen has diminished by about 4 per cent whereas the carbonic acid gas has increased by about 4 per cent. There is also an increase of temperature and of water vapour. Occasionally there is a slight increase in the nitrogen. It is clear that the air around us must be continually increasing in its content of carbonic acid gas; Nature, however, sees to it that the surplus is used up by plants so that the poisonous gas is always kept at a constant level of about ·04 per cent.

Special consideration has to be made of a comparatively restricted air space such as is associated with a room or a ward containing 20 persons. Assuming that there is plenty of inlet and outlet for the respiratory gases, the atmosphere of the room may be kept very nearly normal. If for some reason fresh air were kept out and the room sealed up, we should find that the percentage of carbonic acid gas would rise rapidly until it became as high as that of the expired air viz. 4 per cent. Further pollution of the atmosphere would occur owing to the increase in the expired water vapour, the evaporation of sweat from the skin, the breathing out of germs and the fine powder rising from clothing and from human bodies. The smell of the stuffy, overheated, underventilated room is well known to all; such conditions give the occupants a feeling of relaxation, sleepiness, mental lassitude and often headache, but as a rule the effect is so overpowering that those in the vitiated air are not aware of the dangers they are running from a weakened defence against increased armies of microbes, especially the bacillus tuberculosis, commonly known as " T.B." While the percentage of carbonic acid gas (CO_2) is an index of the air impurity, however, it is not actually the cause of the symptoms. Careful research has shown conclusively that diminution in the heat loss of the body is the real danger. In a stuffy room we are dealing with excess of moisture, which prevents evaporation from the body; with rise of temperature, which does not allow the usual regular cooling process of the skin to operate; and with absence of air currents normally instrumental in keeping the skin at a steady temperature. Fundamentally, therefore, it is the cooling power of the air which is the all important factor; the more an atmosphere can absorb the surplus heat constantly being produced in our bodies, the better is its cooling power and the less do we experience all the discomforts of a foul environment. Whether or not the increased heat of the body prepares a better soil for germs is undecided; all we know is that conditions described above are ideal for the spread of T.B., influenza, measles, whooping cough, scarlet fever, diphtheria and the common cold.

How Combustion Affects the Air.—In a town every house has one or two chimneys steadily adding to the impurity of the atmosphere by sending up columns of smoke to increase the pall over the congested areas. The smoke of factories is also detrimental to the purity of the air, but many laws have been framed to control industrial emanations and a grave menace to health has been thus removed. In dealing with combustion we are concerned with carbon, which is represented chiefly by paper, firewood and coal; chemical fumes are in a different class and are discussed below. Coal is, above all, the important factor in the formation of smoke, which fills the air with soot and sulphur. We have not reached the stage of complete smoke prevention, but we are gradually moving towards a state of hygienic perfection in which the domestic fire will be abolished and its place universally taken by gas stove, electric fire or steam radiator, and the industrial smoke will be utilized for some purpose in which its by-products will be completely absorbed. Meanwhile large cities have to suffer in several ways because of the smoke cloud overhead. First, the sun's rays are filtered—the vital ultra-violet emanations are prevented from reaching the individual and this leads to rickets in children and to other signs of sunlight deficiency in adults. Secondly, a smoky atmosphere leads to fogs, because the increased moisture of the air clings to the small particles of soot and forms the characteristic density of the air. Thirdly, smoke is the cause of many bronchial troubles, the substance of the lung being irritated by the chemicals constituting the smoke. Tons of smoke fall in London every minute, making everything very dirty; this is a waste of good by-products, among which are ammonia, tar, oils, benzol and bitumen.

Carbonic Acid Gas and Carbon Monoxide.—CO_2 and its ally (carbon monoxide) are both well known products of combustion; the former has already been discussed. Carbon monoxide is a most dangerous gas which may quickly cause death without any warning. It is the gas which is given off when coke, charcoal or anthracite is burned in a closed stove, and it is present in domestic gas. Accident or suicide is responsible for many deaths from this substance; as explained by the physiology of respiration, CO_2 combines with the haemoglobin of the blood to form a cherry red compound; it has an immediate or delayed fatal effect, therefore it is doubly dangerous. Those who are exposed for any length of time to the smallest percentage of carbon monoxide in their environment are apt to develop a form of anaemia. Faulty stoves and leakages from motor exhaust pipes have led to many unexpected deaths from carbon monoxide poisoning.

Industrial Effluents and Air Pollution.—Although legal restrictions control the production of chemical waste products other than smoke, it is still found that city air contains many complex substances formed in the manufacture of the various articles of the industrial world. Fumes of acids, sulphuretted hydrogen, carbon dioxide, petrol and the like reduce the purity of the atmosphere, and in many of the busy thoroughfares of London on a hot sultry day it is quite apparent that the individuals of the crowded streets are affected by the pollution, especially when traffic jams pack the highway with motor cars, each adding its exhaust gas to an already stuffy air channel.

Organic Decomposition.—Included in this type of air pollution is that of bacterial invasion, fermentation, bad odours and the general emanations of inhabited places. When a glass slide is exposed on a window sill of a London house for about an hour and then examined by the microscope, we generally find a surprising collection of particles, consisting of brick, soot, seeds, grit from the street, animal excrement, microbes, spores and organic debris. The most dangerous thing is the microbe, and undoubtedly the congested areas fill the air with millions of organisms, since people cough and spit and generally exhale microbes as a routine habit. The use of a paper handkerchief or the rigid prosecution of those who spit on the pavement is not yet established, and so the air continues to receive its daily quota of bacteria. A bad smell usually indicates something harmful to the individual but not always so. The converse may also be true; for example the smell of manure may not be unpleasant to some, yet it may be teeming with harmful organisms. Local health authorities exercise the strictest supervision over piggeries, cowsheds and stables, and conduct campaigns against flies.

Country air or sea air is freer than any other from bacteria, which collect in greatest numbers in closed and congested areas. This is one of the reasons why a holiday is so beneficial to the town dweller. A dry atmosphere is not suitable for germs; they prefer a slight layer of moisture on surfaces, and this is why they are so constantly trapped by the mucous membranes of the respiratory passages in both inspiration and expiration. It is unwise to stir up old dust which has become very dry; a damp cloth collects all the organisms and we can then dispose of them by burning.

Humidity.—Humidity is not a chemical but a physical condition of the air; in excess it is considered as an abnormal condition and is therefore dealt with at this point. We know that the moisture in the air varies according to districts and to the type of weather we are experiencing. Thus humidity may be irksome to us, especially when the air is raw and damp or when the type of weather is referred to as " close." We become clammy and sticky and generally uncomfortable owing to the absence of fresh air and of sweat loss from the pores. People become used to certain regions, and this accounts for the discomfort initially felt for example by those who suddenly go to live in the south west of England after they have been brought up in the north of Scotland. Not only in the outside air is humidity important however. In certain industries, in factories, workshops and mills, it has to be carefully controlled otherwise the health of the worker suffers.

Regulations are in force to ensure that only a certain amount of moisture is permitted in any workshop. Even the use of an electric fan makes a difference to the humidity. The instrument which is the guide to the amount of humidity is the hygrometer or wet and dry bulb thermometer. We know that there are two types of ordinary barometer, one consisting of two columns of mercury and the other—the aneroid barometer—consisting of a sensitive metal drum; both indicate by pointers on a circular scale the weight of the atmosphere, and thus give warnings of approaching depressions. The wet and dry thermometer, however, allows us to estimate the moisture of a room, and helps us to obviate excessive humidity. As shown in the illustration (Fig. 1), there is one ordinary mercury thermometer placed beside another whose bulb is wrapped up in wet calico dipping into a small vessel of water so that it never becomes dry. The science of physics tells us that when there is evaporation the area from which the evaporation has taken place is cooled, therefore if the air is dry and the moisture is rapidly being taken up, the reading of the wet bulb will be less than that of the dry bulb. The optimum state is reached when a constant reading of wet bulb 56° F., dry bulb 60° F. is given. If the readings are the same, it means that the air is saturated with moisture. The most satisfactory condition of any room or workshop is ensured when there is present about 75 per cent of the possible saturation with water vapour. It is often found that gas fires and closed stoves using anthracite or coke dry the air of a room, making it uncomfortable and causing its inhabitants to become irritable. The remedy is the placing of a small bowl of water near the fire; this is a thing that should never be forgotten in the sickroom. When a room is damp, we can dry the air quickly by lighting the fire and opening a top window. The moisture is quickly driven out by the ascending hot air.

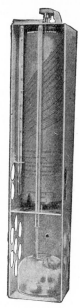

FIG. 1.—WET AND DRY BULB HYGROMETER (" HYGROVISOR ").

The advantages of this instrument are that it gives a direct reading of the humidity on the special scale provided, and that by a simple adjustment of the drum, the air temperature changes can be allowed for.

(By courtesy of Messrs. Negretti and Zambra, London.)

Ventilation

In the open air there is always a fresh supply of oxygen for our needs and normally the proportion of the gases is kept constant. This is accomplished naturally in several ways. The plants make use of most of the surplus carbonic acid gas by day and give up oxygen; the various currents in the air and the prevailing winds drive away the impure air and provide fresh air in its place; rain periodically washes out the particles from the atmosphere.

Definition of Ventilation.—Ventilation has been defined as " the exchange of impure for fresh air without causing draughts." It is easily divided into two categories: 1. Natural ventilation; 2. Artificial ventilation.

Natural Ventilation.—The first thing to keep in mind is that when air is heated it rises to the top of the room, leaving a blank space below which quickly fills up with fresh cool air. This is the underlying principle of all the methods used in changing the atmosphere of a closed space by natural means.

These methods vary. They are simply different ways of employing the ordinary forces intrinsic to the atmosphere which are the fundamental powers in natural ventilation.

1. *Diffusion.*—If two gases are poured into a glass jar, their particles will mix; in other words, we say that diffusion occurs. The same thing happens in a room. Although we cover our walls with paper or paint, there is always a certain amount of natural diffusion of fresh air and impure air through the porous bricks of the house. The smell of cooking is a diffusion from the kitchen to the other parts of the house, and the smell of fire or tobacco is brought to us by the same method. Diffusion is of little importance in practical ventilation, however.

2. *Propulsion.*—In this method the good air simply drives the bad air from the room and occupies the space left. On an ordinary quiet day, the opening of the front door or of the lower part of a sash window will cause this action to occur.

3. *Convection.*—This depends to a certain extent upon the above method of propulsion. After the latter has occurred, the fresh air particles take the place of a certain number of the impure ones, so that the impurity is diluted. In this process, currents pass between the unequally heated volumes of air, and these, known as convection currents, occur in any room in which hot air is constantly rising to the roof and cold air coming in to take its place. In the outside atmosphere the warm currents of air from the equator rising above the cold air from the poles become concentrated and intensified into winds.

4. *Perflation.*—We take advantage of winds by opening the windows and doors and allowing perflation to occur (the blowing of a stream of air through a room). This does not conform to the stipulation that all ventilation should not cause discomfort to the occupants, but it is a quick and efficient method of aerating

a room which is empty, and it is thus often employed. It would obviously be disastrous to try this system for instance in a library in which an author was piecing together the loose leaves of his manuscript. This method is also known as flushing, and is of great importance in the nursing routine.

5. *Aspiration.*—This is but another method of using winds. We all know how fires roar up the chimney when a gale is active. The reason for this is that the velocity of the wind sucks out the column of air at the top of the chimney and the air of the room rushes up the fireplace to fill the gap.

Artificial Ventilation.—Natural ventilation is not sufficient for large rooms such as halls, schools or works. The change of air has to be effected by mechanical means. There are 3 ways of doing this: 1. by forcing air into the space by fans; 2. by sucking out the bad air; 3. by using a combination of these methods.

1. *The Plenum or Propulsion Method.*—This system utilizes mechanical power at the beginning in order to bring fresh air to the building. It is usual to purify and warm the air first, and occasionally to moisten it (" conditioning "). Generally speaking, the air is first collected by a funnel situated at least 10 feet above the ground and covered with fine wire gauze which traps any dirt or dust before the air passes to the next filter which is finer still, consisting of a fibre screen kept wet by a constant stream of water. The air, filtered and moistened, passes over a series of hot pipes, and now at a temperature a little above the normal it is driven into the rooms by special air conductors. It is essential to have windows and doors closed, however, since the pressure of the incoming air is greater than that in the room and the outlets are so arranged that they can collect the vitiated air at the most convenient places. The only drawback to this method is that dust collects in the shafts of the air tubes, despite the fact that the incoming air is almost dust free, and in time it becomes a marked impurity of the atmosphere. Extra labour is involved in keeping the tubes clear.

2. *The Extraction or Vacuum System.*—In contrast to the above method, the system of sucking out bad air utilizes mechanical force at the end. The vacuum system is founded on the principles of the fireplace. All the vitiated air of the room is led to an outlet shaft. Wind at the top of the chimney is imitated by the use of an electric fan; the fire in the hearth may be represented by some form of heat at the bottom of the shaft. By these two methods, the bad air is drawn out to the external atmosphere. Use is made of this method in foundries and factories where dangerous dusts and fumes endanger health. Fans are more popular than heating methods; the latter may take the form of ordinary coal fires, hot pipes, a gas jet or a spray of steam.

3. *The Balance System.*—This is a combination of 1 and 2.

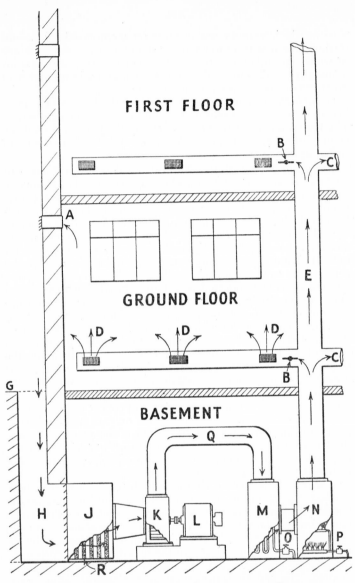

FIRST FLOOR

B

C

A

GROUND FLOOR

D   D   D

C

B

E

G

BASEMENT

Q

H   J   K   L   M   N

O   P

R

FIG. 2.—DIAGRAM OF SIMPLE AIR-CONDITIONING PLANT.

a, Air Outlet. *b*, Damper. *c*, Branch Ducts. *d*, Air Distributors. *e*, Main Air-distributing Duct. *g*, Ground Level. *h*, Air Intake. *j*, Air Filter. *k*, Fan. *l*, Electric Motor. *m*, Heating (or Cooling) Coils. *n*, Humidifying Chamber. *o*, Steam or Hot Water Valve. *p*, Water Supply. *q*, Trunking. *r*, Dust Collecting Screens. *(By courtesy of the British Electrical Development Association.)*

16

The principle is that of admitting warmed air into the rooms just above the heads of those standing in it, while the bad air is drawn off through holes in the ceiling. It is satisfactory for large buildings such as cinemas, but it means that windows and doors must be kept shut. The ventilation can be regulated so many times per hour by adjusting the two systems of fans; hence the use of the term, balanced.

Essentials of Efficient Ventilation.—When we enter an occupied room, certain immediate impressions are made on us. First we probably experience a hot current of air; secondly the smell of tobacco or of a pungent scent may assail our nostrils; thirdly we are aware of the peculiar odour associated with human beings. The whole three may convey the sensation of a stuffy atmosphere, and we frequently remark on it although the occupants may be quite unaware of it. Opening the door and window for a few minutes may put everything all right. But the question naturally arises: How are we to determine the correct amount of air necessary for perfect health?

First of all we must study the physical factors that are outstanding in a perfect air supply. The temperature should be as low as possible, but it must not result in actual coldness, which causes discomfort. If on the other hand the air is too hot, it cannot accept the surplus heat from our bodies. We perspire freely, which although it means we are cooled by evaporation of sweat nevertheless is not a comfortable process. It has been stressed by all research workers that the factor which is of greatest importance in air supply is a steady absorption of our body heat by the air in which we live. Another essential is that the humidity should not be excessive; the ideal is that which allows our mucous membranes to remain pleasantly moist but which is capable of taking up the moisture exhaled by the lungs and skin. Lastly movement of the air to a limited degree must be in operation, otherwise the atmosphere becomes clammy and overheated. There is a great difference between a pleasant current of air and an objectionable draught.

The Amount of Air Required.—One thousand cubic feet of air per hour per person is sufficient (Thresh). Many authorities, however, still stick to the older views that in an average living room (1,000 cubic feet), 3,000 cubic feet of fresh air per hour is necessary for one person. Now if two persons were sitting in the room for an hour, this would mean changing the air six times during that period, which is almost impossible without discomfort. In airing a room attention must be paid to the inlet. If the latter is small the air rushes in, creating a draught. The ideal inlet is found to be one which permits air to enter at a rate of about 3 feet per second for normal persons, but for invalids, 2 feet per second is to be preferred, because it ensures that there is not any

shock when the cold air reaches the patient's skin.   Nurses must
always make a point of careful supervision of sickrooms.   The commonest track for a draught is between a window and the fireplace
or a window and a door; if it should be found impossible to put the
bed out of this line the window or door should be screened.

How to Calculate the Air Allowance.—Although it is known that
the amount of CO_2 in the air is a subsidiary factor in bad ventilation, it is still used as an indicator of the state of the air.   By
passing a certain amount of air through a quantity of potassium
hydroxide and testing the solution afterwards, it is found that
even if the air contains ·06 per cent of CO_2 it is not toxic.   This
is referred to as the Ideal Allowable Limit, but as we said above
human beings can tolerate much greater amounts of carbonic
acid gas.   " CO_2 excess has nothing to do with the symptoms
produced by ordinary air vitiation " (Currie).   Brewers work in
an atmosphere of CO_2 which may be as high as 2 per cent yet
their health is quite good.   In establishing a standard, therefore,
we are faced with certain controversial factors.   Indeed, ventilation of a room often resolves itself into a consideration of the comfort of the inhabitants, and those who travel in railway carriages
know that opinions are distinctly varied.   Normally, however,
the available air per person in a room can be estimated by
measuring the room and calculating the cubic content.   If there
is an allowance of 1,000 cubic feet of space for each person and
a supply of fresh air for each amounting to 2,000 cubic feet an
hour, there should be ample to provide for a comfortable inter-
change of good and bad air all the time without discomfort or
danger to health.

STANDARDS OF AIR SPACE FOR VARIOUS BUILDINGS

1. General hospital ward . 1,800 cubic feet per head
2. Infectious disease ward . 1,400 ,, ,,
3. General hospital . . 1,200 ,, ,,
4. Bedrooms . . . 800 ,, ,,
5. Lodging-houses . . 360 ,, ,,
6. Factories, workrooms . 250 ,, ,,
7. Schools . . . 80 ,, ,,

Children under 10 years of age require about half as much air
space as do adults.   The ideal of 300 cubic feet of space per
person for living rooms is very difficult to attain in slum areas.

Practical Application of Ventilation to Houses and Hospitals

Generally speaking, the rooms of a house are ventilated by
natural methods while hospitals and large buildings have a com-

bination of both natural and artificial ventilation. The various systems and appliances are discussed below.

Ventilation of a Room.—Three openings— the window, the door and the fireplace—are the common provisions for ventilation in an ordinary room, and since much of a nurse's life may be spent there, she must know how to use these to the best advantage hygienically. The lighting of a fire causes the air in the chimney to rise because it is heated, therefore a current of air passes up the chimney from the room. Some of the air of the room, however, is heated, and rises to the roof. Now it is essential to admit a certain amount of new air without causing a draught. All incoming air should if possible enter the room above the heads of the occupants; as the cold fresh air enters, it mixes with the warm air of the upper layers and then gradually falls, to be taken away by the chimney. In this way a good system of ventilation is assured, especially if there is a breeze outside inducing aspiration in the chimney. On a very windy day, it may be impossible to open a window, and an uncomfortable draught is caused along the floor by air sucked in through the bottom of the doorway. The remedy

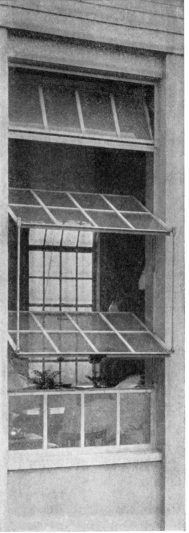

FIG. 3.—BALANCE WINDOWS WITH SIDE ARMS. A MODERN EXAMPLE OF HOSPITAL VENTILATION.
(By courtesy of The Crittall Manufacturing Co., Ltd.)

for this is to open the door wide, a screen being put round the opening. Windows may be used in several ways; many people use a sash window by opening it at the top and bottom, thus creating a free circulation, but efficient ventilation can be ensured by pulling down the upper sash of the window when the wind is quiet, so that the hot air flows out steadily without causing undue disturbance.   If the patient can be removed temporarily from the sickroom, the method of perflation or flushing can be employed, and it is eminently useful, since it is possible to clear the air in a few seconds by opening the window wide and also the door opposite it.   This is called cross ventilation, and is of great use when the room is empty, but naturally it is too vigorous to be tolerated by an invalid.

In addition to the 3 openings mentioned above, some large rooms have grids fitted, which act as both inlets and outlets

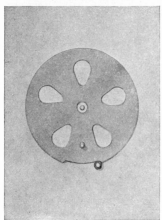 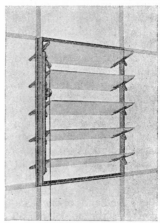

FIG. 4.   FIG. 5.

ILLUSTRATING TWO COMMON, SIMPLE AND EFFICIENT METHODS OF VENTILA-
TION. THE FIRST SHOWS COOPER'S DISC, THE SECOND THE LOUVRE METHOD.
(By courtesy of H. W. Cooper and Co., Ltd., London.)

These can be seen on inspection of the outer walls of any large house.   The inlet grid should be about 5 feet above floor level, and should direct the air currents upwards.   The outlet must be as near the ceiling as possible.

Adjuncts to Natural Ventilation.—In certain cases it is advisable to use some additional appliances in order to make sure of successful ventilation.   These may take the form of window appliances, wall ventilators and roof ventilators and may be either inlets or outlets.

Window Appliances.—1. Perhaps the commonest in this group is Hinckes-Bird's Window Device.   This consists of a batten of wood, 6 inches high and about 2 inches wide, fitted carefully below the lower, inner sash of an ordinary window.   When the lower sash is down, it allows air to pass from without inwards and upwards to the ceiling (Fig. 7), and it does not create a draught.

2. One pane of the window may be louvered, the air being directed also up to the top of the room; top panes are always used for this purpose (Fig. 5).

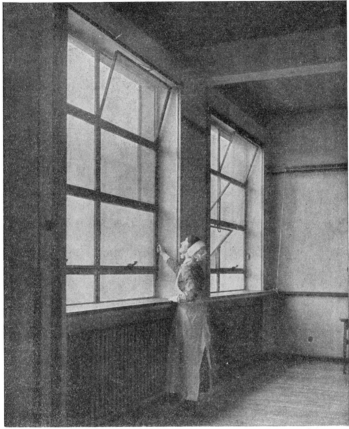

FIG. 6.—HOW UP TO DATE HOSPITAL ROOMS ARE FITTED WITH WINDOWS EASILY OPERATED SINGLE-HANDEDLY BY A NURSE. ALL DEGREES OF VENTILATION CAN BE SECURED.
(By courtesy of the Crittall Manufacturing Co., Ltd.)

3. Cooper's Disc is a familiar thing on high windows (Fig. 4). It consists of a disc of fairly thick glass perforated with holes or slots; this is fitted by a central pin to the window, which is also perforated in a similar manner, so that by turning the disc to make the slots coincide, air is allowed to pass in. The advantage

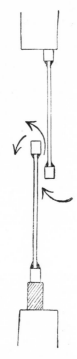

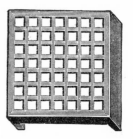

FIG. 8.—EXAMPLE OF A MODERN
SQUARE GRID FOR NATURAL
VENTILATION OF BUILDINGS.
(*By courtesy of Comyn, Ching & Co.,
London.*)

FIG. 7.—HINCKES-
BIRD WINDOW.

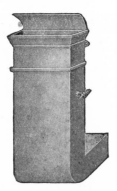

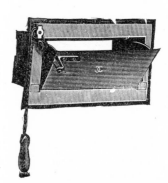

FIG. 9.—TOBIN'S TUBE.
(*By courtesy of Comyn, Ching &
Co., London.*)

FIG. 10.—SHERINGHAM'S VALVE.
(*By courtesy of Comyn, Ching & Co.,
London.*)

of this system is that the volume of air can be controlled to the finest degree.

4. Another common window opening is the Hopper Sashlight (Fig. 6), which is made by putting a hinge on the lower part of the window and allowing it to open inwards to about 45°. In this system the air enters about the middle of the room and is directed upwards. (see also p. 118, Fig. 51).

Wall Ventilators.—1. The simplest method of wall inlet is the square iron ventilating grid (Fig. 8), which is commonly seen on the outside walls of houses. Ordinary bricks may be bored so that a funnel-shaped channel is made with the apex outwards, allowing for the even diffusion of air after it passes through the brick. These are known as Ellison's conical bricks, which are used in farm buildings e.g. cowsheds and stables, also in school gymnasia.

2. Tobin's Tube is not so common as it used to be, but it is a very useful form of ventilation. It consists of a wooden or metal conductor, usually rectangular in section, and often measuring 3 feet by 1 foot; it stands very like a mantelpiece without fire-place on an outer wall of a room, about 6 feet high. Another tube feeds this ventilator at the floor level, receiving its supply of air through perforated bricks or an iron grid in the wall (Fig. 9). The incoming air can be both filtered and moistened by passing it through water and cotton-wool.

3. Sheringham's Valve can be used as an outlet as well as an inlet, since it is placed high up on the wall close to the cornice. It works on the same principle as the window sashlight mentioned above, except that it has a casing at each side and it is fed through perforated plates in the wall (Fig. 10).

Roof Ventilators.—Many devices, known as cowls, which revolve with the wind, and which are supposed to improve the draught in chimneys, are in vogue; illustration is unnecessary, as a perfect exhibition can be provided by looking over the roofs of any town. Many revolving cowls are unsatisfactory, but those on small halls and on railway carriages do their work well. Boyle's Ventilator is an example of an ornamental cowl used on buildings (Fig. 11).

Methods of Artificial Ventilation.—In addition to the propulsion and vacuum methods already discussed, there are simpler methods of artificial ventilation.

1. The effect of a briskly burning fire must not be left out of consideration. By this method we can remove with the average fireplace about 12,000 cubic feet of air every hour.

2. Many systems depend upon the burning of a small gas jet below a central roof ventilator. In the days of massive chande-liers it was a simple matter to ventilate a hall, especially as the chandeliers were placed high up in the roof. The most popular form of roof ventilator is McKinnel's. In this type, two tubes

are placed one within the other. The outer tube is like a chimney; within it is the smaller tube, projecting well above it, and usually covered with a cowl. The lower part of the inner

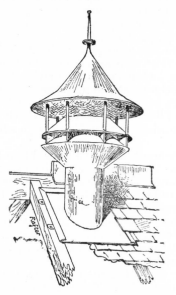

FIG. 11.—ROOF VENTILATION (BOYLE'S).
(*By courtesy of Halliday Boilers, Ltd., London.*)

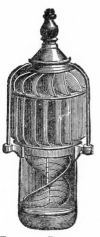

FIG. 12.—REVOLVING VENTILATOR.
(*By courtesy of Comyn Ching & Co., London.*)

tube expands into a funnel, the sides of which are parallel with the roof. Air enters by the passage left between the inner and outer tubes. A gas jet burns below the inner tube; this causes the air to rise and pass out by the cowl.

3. Mica Valve. In this contrivance, which as a rule is not very satisfactory, small mica sheets cover an opening on the wall leading into the chimney, but they are allowed to open only into the chimney. When the pressure in the chimney is less than that in the room, the valves open and allow air up the chimney. The idea is sound, but as with many other mica valves, the performance is not always according to programme, and soot and smoke find their way into wards and sickrooms now and then, to the discomfort of both patient and nurse.

How Ventilation Methods are Employed.—While it is possible to combine both artificial and natural methods of ventilation, one system usually defeats the other and, in the larger buildings, modern architecture provides for artificial methods. This means that all windows and doors must be kept shut, which may have a bad mental effect on the inmates, especially in schools, hospitals and institutions. In smaller buildings, it is found that natural methods are quite satisfactory when some of the adjuncts mentioned above are put into use, but in industrial works, textile mills and other places where dust is rife, it is obviously essential to use a forcible method of taking away the dust and the fumes.

Dust and the Healthy House

We have already learned that dust pollutes the air, especially in cities and congested areas; but in the household dust is a special menace, because it has a more placid atmosphere in which to collect and it is added to by the presence of so many textile fabrics. We can assume that the dust in an ordinary living room, used by people going in and out of the house frequently, will contain particles of soot, coal grit, ashes, wool, jute, cotton, flax, pollen, animal and vegetable scales, minerals, dirt from the street, grease and bacteria. These particles do not belong properly to the air, but it is almost impossible to eliminate them. The annual orgy of spring cleaning stirs up much dormant dust, but removes a certain amount of accumulated debris. To be efficient, however, removal of dust should be a daily routine and nothing is better than the use of an electric vacuum cleaner which is efficient, clean and sanitary.

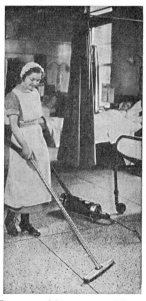

FIG. 13.—METHOD OF WARD CLEANING AS USED IN A LARGE LONDON HOSPITAL.

The benefits are (1) absence of noise, (2) cleanliness, (3) sterilization of the air passing through. In the model shown, there is also a device for polishing the floor and finally spraying it with an insecticide.

(*By courtesy of Electrolux, Ltd.*)

All dust is potentially harmful, in that it contains germs of disease, small particles which cause irritating coughs and a large surface of absorption for the moisture of the air.

We can overcome the dust of a house by making the outside air clean, which is difficult, even with the most up to date sanitary system; by filtering the air before it goes to a room, now commonly done; by avoiding furniture and hangings which attract or manufacture dust—a principle of hospital construction; and by keeping the rooms scrupulously clean. The external ventilation is a matter for the public health authority, and all our modern smoke prevention, street washing, road tarring and country housing schemes are planned to make the outside air less dusty. In hospitals and similar institutions where health is the first consideration the corners of wall and ceiling and wall and floor are rounded so that it is impossible to leave any dust in cleaning. All cornices, picture rails and ledges are forbidden; the circular always replaces the square when possible. The walls are painted or distempered, but it is best to make certain of a smooth wall, and one easy to wash, by giving it a coat of the best enamel. Gas fires or electric fires replace coal fires, but central heating, by radiators of metal or of piping, is the most popular, since it can be regulated more easily. Curtains, table-cloths and all fabrics of a similar type are dispensed with if necessary, while the floors are polished smooth and covered with easily cleaned rugs.

The nurse should get into the habit of using the vacuum cleaner daily in the sickroom, but the sound occasionally upsets the patient, and if so the only alternative is to use a damp duster and cleanse every article thoroughly. In sweeping a wax-polished floor, some wet material e.g. sawdust or tea leaves, is necessary, as the particles attract the dust, which would otherwise fly about and settle elsewhere. All refuse should be burned. The only things that should be found in a dustbin are ashes and incinerated crockery and metal.

CHAPTER 3

WATER

SOURCES OF WATER. RAINFALL. RAIN WATER. UPLAND
SURFACE WATER. SPRINGS. WELLS. SHALLOW OR SUR-
FACE WELLS. DEEP WELLS. ARTESIAN WELLS. RIVERS.
HARD AND SOFT WATER. HARD WATER. TESTS FOR
HARD WATER. THE DOMESTIC WATER SUPPLY. THE
ESSENTIALS OF PURITY IN WATER. THE DAILY SUPPLY.
HOW WATER IS PURIFIED AND DELIVERED. TREATING
HARDNESS. METHODS OF PURIFICATION ON A LARGE
SCALE. DOMESTIC PURIFICATION. WATER MAINS AND
PIPES. RELATION OF IMPURE WATER TO THE SPREAD OF
DISEASE.

WATER is one of the primary necessities of life. It exists everywhere, and without it both animal and vegetable kingdoms
would soon vanish. Even in the most solid looking article some
water exists, and it is well known that in chemical analysis a
most intricate and highly specialized apparatus is required to
get rid of the small amount of water that is present in many
substances. Many green vegetables, roots and fruits are almost
entirely composed of water; our own flesh depends upon it for
three-quarters of its bulk, and the sensation of thirst keeps us
informed of the slightest deviation from the normal so that
Nature ensures we make good the smallest loss. Such an important fluid is of supreme hygienic importance and demands
the nurse's most careful study.

Sources of Water

The great water reservoir of the earth is the sea. We cannot
use sea water as such, however, because it is full of sodium
chloride. The sun comes to our help. It sends its hot rays on
the ocean and from the surface there arises a fine mist or vapour
free of salt and all other minerals—the process of evaporation.
Being light, the vapour quickly rises, and meeting with cooling
winds it becomes condensed. Clouds are formed which are
driven by the winds over the land; the clouds become weighty
with ever increasing drops, and rain descends to fill our springs,
our streams, our rivers and our lakes, all of which provide our

supply and ultimately pour their surplus once more into the sea. Water is therefore always in abundance; it is our constant supply of an essential to life.   Our first study must be of the various ways in which fresh water is dealt with after it comes from the clouds. Rain falls evenly but its way back to the sea may be by different routes; in reality about one-third of the rain is evaporated from the earth's surface.   The other two-thirds either flow from the surface of the earth into ditches, drains, culverts or tributaries of rivers, or sink deeply into the earth itself to form springs or wells.

Rainfall.—It is well known that some places are rainier than others.   The western side of the United Kingdom has a climate which is not nearly so dry as that of the east coast.   This is explained by the fact that the warm winds from the Atlantic Ocean spend themselves with considerable force against the hills forming the backbone of the country, so that the warm air rises, is condensed and ends in rain of a very " soft " character.   When colder conditions prevail, the water is frozen and falls as snow, hail or sleet.   Whatever its form, however, water does not vary in chemical composition; it consists of two of the commonest gases, which are colourless and clear viz. oxygen and hydrogen, represented by the familiar formula, H_2O.   The amount of rain which falls during a given time is estimated by a rain gauge, an ingenious method of collection of rain in a large bottle by a funnel the collecting area of which is determined carefully.   By measuring the amount in the bottle after a certain period and making a simple calculation, we can express the rainfall in inches, which means that if all the rain which has fallen in a district in a day or a month or a year (whatever the period under review may be) were to be retained on the surface, its depth would be the number of inches given as a result of the calculation.

Rain Water.—The finest water supply is rain which falls in the country districts or in the hill areas.   The atmosphere is almost pure, pollution does not occur and therefore we may say that it is a perfect sample of the hydrogen-oxygen compound, similar to the distilled water sold for use in batteries and other appliances.   Country rain water is always saved for washing purposes because it lathers well and is " soft " in character; it can be used for drinking, but since it lacks many useful minerals and salts it is rather insipid.

In towns quite a different state of affairs exists.   In the previous chapter, it was explained that the air over any large and congested area is always polluted to a certain extent, indeed rain acts as a washing agent.   When it reaches the ground, therefore, it is full of impurities derived from the atmosphere viz. acids, soot, sulphur, bacteria and gases.   If it is essential to use the rain water (e.g. when the ordinary drinking water is very hard) it is collected from roofs by gutters and drain pipes which empty their contents into barrels. There is an ingenious device known as " Robert's Separator," which collects the first two or three gallons and automatically empties them into a drain, as they are always soiled by the dirt on the roof. It is not much in use in towns, where a municipal supply is nearly always in service, but in the country it is very satisfactory, especially when rain water used for drinking requires to be stored. The method ensures that the water which enters the underground cement storage cistern is satisfactorily pure and likely to remain unpolluted.

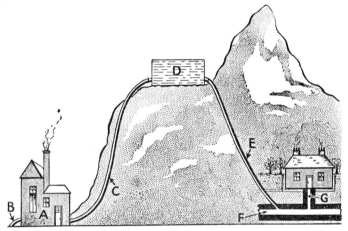

FIG. 14.—TOWN WATER SUPPLY.

a, Power House with Pump. *b*, Pipe from river or artesian well. *c*, Pipe going to reservoir (*d*) on top of hill. *e*, Delivery pipe to main. *f*, Water main on road. *g*, Branch delivery pipe to cottage.

Upland Surface Water.—This is the commonest way of supplying large communities. If there is a hollow at the foot of some hills or a flat upland valley, it is generally formed into a lake or loch by the rain which runs down the sides of the adjoining hills. The hill or mountain sides are known as the catchment area. Many rivers in Scotland begin in lochs which are fed all round by trickling streams, the channels of the surface water from the mountain side. In some cases, huge reservoirs or dams are created by a simple method of building a wall at the outlet and making a stream into a lake. For instance, the city of Glasgow is supplied by Loch Katrine, which pours its waters steadily into large mains running many miles to the area of supply. Upland surface water is an improvement on rain water in that it has a better taste. It collects a certain amount of acid from the peat, moss and vegetation through which it passes and is soft, as it has not sunk deep enough into the earth to dissolve the salts found there, but if it comes from a chalky area it contains lime, and is very " hard." Usually, however, it is soft and acid, which makes it capable of dissolving small quantities of lead from the pipes, and lead poisoning must be guarded against. There is very little risk of pollution. Usually the authorities direct that the reservoir should be carefully protected by fencing and the public are warned against fouling the supply. The area of collection is generally a lonely one and the excretions of the few inhabitants or of the cattle and sheep may be neglected. In any case, modern methods of purification and standardization are arranged for in addition to filtration.

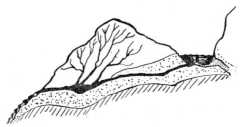

FIG. 15.—ORIGIN OF SPRING WATER.
Showing how a spring may collect water from an upland lake through a channel in an impermeable layer, and from the surface. It finally issues from the side of the hill, at a point at which the impermeable layer becomes bare.

Springs.—Quite the best water comes from springs, and the joy of drinking the crystal clear, ice cold water from a gushing source in the hills must be an experience remembered by everybody. The explanation of the existence of a spring is a geological one. On the surface of the earth there is first the soil, then broken rock mixed with soil, then a stratum of rock or slate or other hard impervious matter. When rain falls, it easily penetrates through the soil and loose stones, but soon it comes to the hard impermeable layer of the geological stratum. As more collects, the water becomes under pressure, and seeks to find an outlet. It burrows along until it comes to a break in the stratum, usually bursting out on a hill side. Some springs dry up in summer but most are permanent and provide an excellent supply which is not only cool and fresh, but which, in filtering through the earth, has collected a certain amount of dissolved mineral matter. Many medicated springs occur in various parts of the country e.g. Harrogate, Strathpeffer, Buxton, Droitwich and so on, and they have curative properties on account of the large percentage of iron or sulphur or other minerals and salts they may contain. The only time when there is danger in spring water is when the latter comes from a small bed; for instance if the geological stratum is close to the surface and occupies only 100 square yards, it is liable to pollution from various sources in the soil above. In most cases, however, a spring, to be established as a useful water supply, must be permanent and copious, therefore the water comes from a deep and wide bed and is safe to drink (Fig. 15).

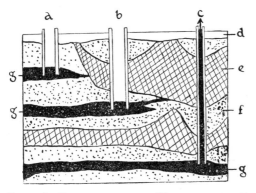

Fig. 16.—Semidiagrammatic Way of showing Three Types of Well.

a and *b* are both deep wells. *c* is an artesian well. *e* is a porous layer. *f* is an impervious layer. *g*, water. *d*, surface layer of earth.

Wells.—Wells are closely allied to springs; their origin is the same bed, but their distinctive characteristic is that they require an artificial outlet viz. a vertical shaft sunk into the ground. The illustration (Fig. 16) shows how the crust of the earth is divided into layers, the first impermeable layer having underneath it a porous layer, and the succeeding strata alternating between permeable and impermeable rock. Now there are 3 kinds of well, according to the depth of the bed. Shallow wells are formed by collections of " subsoil " or " ground " water above the first impermeable layer; deep wells occur above the second impermeable layer; artesian wells are not reached until we pass through two layers of impermeable rock.

Shallow or Surface Wells.—These are the simplest forms of well, obtaining their water from the subsoil water which has collected above the first impermeable layer. The village pump is a familiar sign of the presence of a shallow well, and its importance is obvious when we consider it is the centre of many rural activities. Water from this source runs the risk of surface pollution, but if it is collected from a depth of about 50 feet it is fairly safe and is pure, clear and pleasant to drink. In building a well, precautions are always taken to avoid any possibility of pollution of the supply by sinking a cylindrical shaft of specially made bricks cemented so that the well is watertight for the first 30 feet. Once the shaft has reached the area immediately above the impermeable layer of rock it is safe to allow the water to percolate through, because we can be reasonably sure that by the time the ground water has reached this level, it is purified mechanically and by the organisms it has encountered. The great necessity in the tops of shallow wells is protection from surface flooding or from sewage areas or manure heaps. The cylinder of brick and concrete is therefore continued for a few feet above the ground, and it is protected by concrete all round with culverts for the drainage of the surface water. Often a pump, almost sealed in by a closely fitting cover, is built in on the top, the old bucket and windlass being almost extinct (Fig. 17).

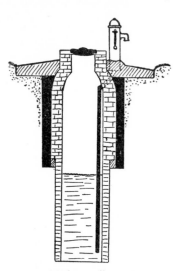

FIG. 17.—Modern well, carefully protected against pollution by concrete sides and coping. Note the closely fitted cover.

Deep Wells.—In a deep well, we have to penetrate the first impermeable layer (Fig. 16) until we come to the water lying just above the second impermeable layer. Here the water is very cold and often rich in mineral content; although hard it may be very pure. The water for this well may have filtered through a porous layer and may have collected from an area of several square miles, so it is rarely polluted. The same precautions must be taken in sinking the shaft for deep wells as are necessary for shallow wells; sometimes a depth of 100 feet is reached, thus there are difficulties in pumping and in keeping the shaft free from dangerous impurities.

Artesian Wells.—If we bore still further and reach a layer of water lying between the second and third impermeable layers, we come to a type of well which delivers its product without the need for any human or mechanical effort. This convenient phenomenon is the artesian well, which throws its water up as a spout several feet above the ground, and thus does not require any pump. The illustration explains the type of well clearly (Fig. 16). The water is under great pressure and so instead of bursting out of the side of a hill like a spring, it throws up a vertical column in the shaft which has been bored into its bed. There are many advantages in the discovery of a well like this. First the water is very pure owing to the fact that it may come from hundreds of feet below the surface; secondly it collects rain from a huge area—50 square miles or more; thirdly all that is required is an iron tube passed down the bore until it reaches the water, which taking advantage of the exit provided, shoots up to get rid of its pressure on the earth's surface.

Rivers.—While rivers may be fed from streams, springs, upland surface water and rain itself, the purity of the water is in doubt as soon as the river grows big enough to support towns and villages on its banks or to be used as a transport highway. Nevertheless, London is supplied mainly by the Thames and its tributaries at their lower reaches, where the water, although frankly polluted, is saved in special riverside reservoirs, carefully purified and delivered as one of the finest supplies in the world.

Hard and Soft Water

Generally speaking, water is of 2 types, 1, hard water and 2, soft water. Rain, which may be said to be free of minerals, lathers easily with soap and is the ideal soft water. At the other end of the scale is the water which contains so much chalk or other similar substance that a lather cannot be made; this is a typical hard water.

Hard Water.—The origin of the hardness of water is the soil and rock with which it has been for some time in contact. The commonest salts found are calcium carbonate and magnesium carbonate; when these are present they form bicarbonates which cause the condition of temporary hardness; this can be reduced partly by boiling or by adding lime. Permanent hardness is the result of contamination with calcium sulphate or magnesium sulphate, which are not deposited by boiling and which can be neutralized only by adding considerable amounts of sodium carbonate (washing soda).

In chalky areas, it is very difficult to eliminate lime and magnesia. Rain water penetrates the earth, absorbing oxygen and carbonic acid gas, and if it settles for instance in an area to be found in certain parts of Kent, it may lie for some time on a stratum of pure chalk dissolving the lime and transforming itself into a hard water. When we try to make a lather with this type of water, all that happens is the formation of a curdy precipitate, and we may have to go on and on, constantly adding more soap until the lime is neutralized. On account of this, hard water is very expensive; a pound bar of soap suffices for less than 2 ounces only of lime. As a beverage, hard water is quite palatable and the presence of a moderate quantity of lime does no harm; many people prefer the chalky water of certain areas to the rather mawkish and insipid varieties obtained straight from the hills. Food is altered to a certain extent by hard water, in both taste and digestibility. The effect of a hard water on pipes and utensils need not be described; everyone is familiar with the furring of kettles and the devices used to collect the lime from them, the universal demand for soap flakes and softening powders and for the numerous proprietary remedies for cleaning clothes, the "scaling" of boilers and the hard condition of the skin of the hands. Hard water has one important attribute however. It prevents lead poisoning by depositing a compound of lime and lead on the inside of pipes, thus ensuring that there is no further possibility of lead getting into the water in a dissolved state. On the other hand soft water, which is somewhat "oily," may act as a solvent on galvanised iron pipes, taking up the zinc; it also dissolves lead and thus may be the cause of lead poisoning.

Tests for Hard Water.—Chemical tests are carried out to ascertain how much hardness is present in water. These are simple, depending upon the amount of a standard soap solution required to turn a fixed quantity of water soft. After a permanent lather has been obtained the amount of solution used is measured. The unit of hardness is called the "degree"; 1 degree of hardness means that in every 100,000 parts of water, 1 part of chalk is dissolved; in soft water less than 10 degrees is the standard. A medium hardness is between 10 and 30 degrees, but above 30 degrees water is very hard, almost impossible to use without affecting tea, soup, clothing and the skin.

The Domestic Water Supply

Water is so much a fundamental thing in our daily lives that a very high standard of purity must be maintained. The first question we must answer is: "What is pure water?"

The Essentials of Purity in Water.—Water should always be clear. Occasionally a few air bubbles may be noticed in freshly drawn water. It must be safe to drink and pleasant to taste. Any tang or acidity should be regarded with suspicion, while turbidity means some abnormality, often dangerous and sometimes of bacterial origin. Water may thus require analysis from both a chemical and a bacteriological point of view.

Specimens can be collected in specially constructed bottles and are dealt with by the analyst to the local authority.

The Daily Supply.—The amount of water available per head per day varies according to the district, the capacity of the reservoirs and the climate. Nowadays we occasionally hear about temporary droughts, but in Great Britain, despite recent experiences, a real shortage of water is rare. Indeed we are so accustomed to a copious supply that we are apt to become prodigal and use water lavishly. Commonly 35 gallons are allotted for each individual per day. This is apportioned as follows:

Drinking and Cooking . .	1 gallon
Bathing	5 gallons
Washing	11 ,,
Sanitation . . .	5 ,,
Manufacturing . . .	5 ,,
Municipal Cleansing . .	5 ,,
Unavoidable Waste . . .	3 ,,
Total	35 ,,

This amount varies markedly and most large cities have a much bigger supply. Chicago allows 230 gallons per head; London, 37; Paisley, 83. Birmingham has an allowance of only 27 gallons. Most hospitals require about 50 gallons of water per day for each patient. Undoubtedly there is a great amount of avoidable waste of water. The watering of gardens makes a big demand on the supply during the summer. In an emergency, 5 gallons are quite sufficient as a daily allowance for each person.

How Water is Purified and Delivered

The easiest way to understand water purification and the treatment of water for domestic use, is to follow it from its origin to the tap from which it issues. We must frankly admit that water drunk straight from springs or wells or from other purely local supplies is taken at the risk of the consumer, but in the case of large municipal water distribution, the supply is carefully treated and tested, making the water both pure and palatable.

From the facts already presented, it is obvious that pollution may occur from hardness, both temporary and permanent; from the liquid and solid excretions of human beings and animals in the neighbourhood of the reservoir i.e. the village pump or the spring; from microbes such as the typhoid bacillus or the bacillus coli; from dissolved lead; from filthy storage tanks (e.g. when they harbour drowned mice or birds); from the soot and sulphur of the air; from sulphuric acid; and from certain minerals. The

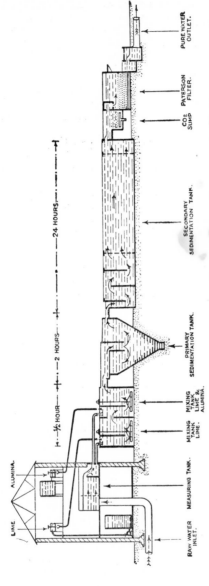

FIG. 18.—PATERSON WATER SOFTENING, FILTRATION AND STERILIZATION PLANT.

The illustration shows a diagrammatic section through a large installation of seven million gallons' daily capacity for the Southend Waterworks Company at Langford Works, where a hard, contaminated supply is converted into soft, hygienically safe, potable water, by chemical treatment, settlement, filtration and excess-lime sterilization. Similar principles are employed in cases in which filtration only is necessary for removal of suspended impurities and colour.

(By courtesy of the Paterson Engineering Co., Ltd., London.)

law states that water must be " pure and wholesome," and more than 30 grains of harmful minerals per gallon make it unfit for all uses. The medicated waters of spas and health resorts are in a different category, depending as they do for their special composition on curative salts peculiar to the neighbourhood in which they are found.

Treating Hardness.—Purification may be carried out in various ways. Reduction of hardness on a big scale is done by Clark's method. This is a simple process, depending upon the fact that the carbonic acid gas of the water takes up a certain amount of lime which is kept in solution. If we add more lime to the water, the CO_2 uses it up and forms calcium carbonate, which is deposited. A saturation of the water with freshly slaked lime therefore ensures that all the chalk will be thrown out. Afterwards the precipitate is treated by filtering; half a dozen methods are known. The general principle is to let the water remain in a settling tank until all the chalk is deposited, then the water above is drawn off. Occasionally filtration is done by using linen screens, wood wool and various other similar agents and appliances.

Methods of Purification on a Large Scale.—Ordinary storage is often sufficient to clear the water of most of its impurities. In a reservoir, the colour is improved, the ammonia is freed and bacteria are destroyed. If for instance typhoid organisms are present in a reservoir, they will die off in less than a fortnight.

Slow sand filtration is still very common, although it was devised over a hundred years ago. Many of the huge tanks can be seen along the side of the River Thames. As one is filled another is drained and cleared. The tanks are walled in by powerful watertight concrete. The water to be filtered passes through a valve at the upper part of the tank, and slowly filters through layers of fine sand, coarse sand, gravel, small stones and finally larger stones until it reaches a gathering drain, in which it is conveyed to another smaller tank from which it finds exit in an outlet pipe. The usual amount of water is about 3 feet in depth above the upper sand level, while the depth of the filter bed itself is about 4 feet; variations occur according to the district. The primary effect of this type of filtration is a trapping of the numerous primitive unicellular plant organisms, which may deposit a distinct layer of green sludge over the bed. This is one of the greatest benefits of the scheme, since this natural filter thus formed traps at least 99 per cent of the microbes, many of them harmful and existing in the water. For the first 3 days the filtration is imperfect; after that it does its maximum work for about a month, when the increasing film of algae impedes the water passing through.   The tank is then emptied and the scum raked into heaps; the sand is washed and the tank " set " again.   Many of these tanks cover several acres.

Mechanical filtration by machinery is the modern method; in this a substance known as filter alum is used.   Pressure or gravity

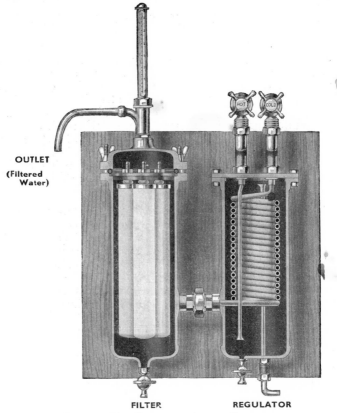

OUTLET

(Filtered Water)

FILTER   REGULATOR

FIG. 19.—THE BERKEFELD ASEPTIC IRRIGATOR.

By means of this apparatus, an abundant supply of filtered water is available for use in hospitals, regulated to the required temperature.

(By courtesy of Berkefeld Filter Co., Ltd., London.)

may be taken advantage of in passing the water through.   Two good points to note about these appliances is that they occupy very little space and the water is pure in less than 2 days. The most modern plant is illustrated in Fig. 18.

Chlorination of water i.e. the perfusion of the water by

chlorine gas, is used very commonly to sterilize water. The gas may be introduced direct or by adding bleaching powder, which liberates chlorine in the presence of water. In big undertakings, the gas is the established medium, this being delivered to the water from steel cylinders under pressure (see Fig. 22). Sometimes the taste of chlorine is noticed (or of one of its derivatives) but usually all possibility of any residual evidence is destroyed by careful neutralization. As in filtration, 99 per cent of the bacteria are destroyed. London water is stored first, filtered

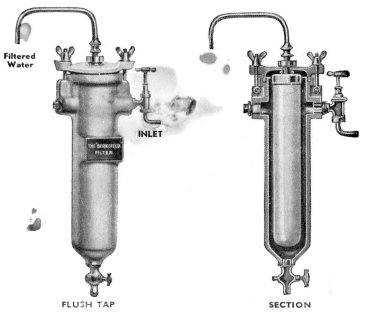

Filtered Water

INLET

THE BERKEFELD FILTER

FLUSH TAP

SECTION

Fig. 20.—Elevation and Section of a Suitable Water Filter for a House.

(By courtesy of Berkefeld Filter Co., Ltd., London.)

second and chlorinated last; this method is followed in many of the lesser areas, with excellent results.

Occasionally ultra-violet ray treatment and introduction of ozone have been proved successful, especially in America.

Domestic Purification.—There are two aspects of this form of treatment. The first is that certain regions do not have the benefit of a controlled supply, the second that many people believe in introducing private apparatus to ensure that the water is quite safe before they use it.

Boiling of water makes it absolutely free from microbic dangers.

Many people do this in hot weather, and then allow the water to cool in ice. Hardness is reduced, but taste is affected, because many gases are driven off. Ice seems to lessen the insipidness. A domestic method in common use is to pour the water through a sterilized hair sieve, which breaks it up into fine droplets; as these fall through the air they collect more oxygen. It is simply a homely method of cascading, which is used in many systems to aerate water on a large scale.

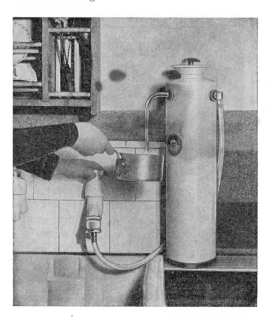

Fig. 21.—Ensuring a supply of soft water for cooking and other purposes by attaching a simple apparatus to the cold water tap.

(By courtesy of Electrolux, Ltd., London.)

Chlorination by bleaching powder may be used in houses, and indeed is employed in the regimental water carts of the armed forces. Tablets are sold which are carefully weighed to provide the correct amount for so many gallons. If the chlorine should be in excess, the water will be unpleasant, but by adding sodium sulphite all traces disappear. This method is quick and efficient, the water being ready for use in about a quarter of an hour. Roughly a teaspoonful of bleaching powder is carefully mixed with 4 teacupfuls of ordinary water. This is the first solution. To every 2 gallons of the water to be drunk must be added 1

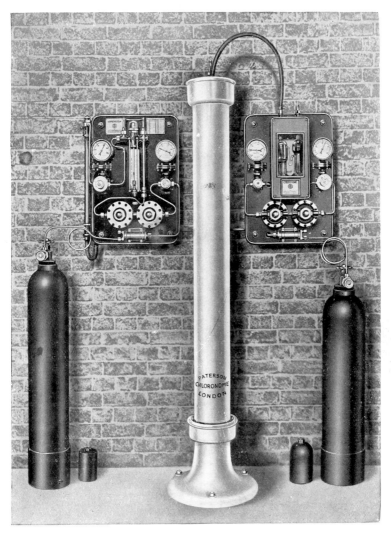

FIG 22.—PATERSON CHLORONOME AND GASEOUS AMMONIATOR FOR STERILIZATION OF DRINKING WATER SUPPLIES AND THE WATER IN SWIMMING POOLS.

(By courtesy of the Paterson Engineering Co., Ltd., London.)

teaspoonful of the first solution, making a concentration of about 1 part in 2,000,000. This is a very quick and useful method and should be understood by nurses who may have to decide upon water purification in a country house.

Small mechanical filters adaptable to the domestic taps are features of all housing exhibitions, and their popularity is becoming more and more marked. Two well-established varieties are of proved value: 1. the Pasteur-Chamberland filter; 2. the Berkefeld filter (Figs. 19 and 20). The principle is the attachment of a candle or bougie of porcelain to the water tap. This is done by fitting the hollow candle inside a metal casing which is tightly screwed to the top. The water flows round the candle, slowly passes through to the hollow core and in so doing gets rid of all its bacteria. The candles must be cleaned every 3 days, otherwise the water is in danger of being more than usually impure owing to retained deposits. Some modern filters combine their function with water softening. Domestic softening is often done by using permutite or similar substances. A modern form of water softener is illustrated in Figs. 21 and 23.

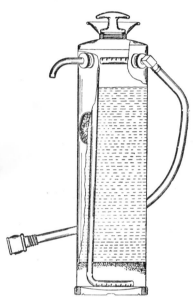

FIG. 23.—HOW THE WATER SOFTENER OPERATES.

The ordinary tap water passes through a layer of granular substance which removes the hardness. The softened water is withdrawn (as shown in Fig. 21) from the pipe which collects the water after it has passed through the filter layer. In this type, simple percolation with brine "regenerates" the softener in a few minutes.

(By courtesy of Electrolux, Ltd., London.)

Water Mains and Pipes.—The mains conveying the water from the reservoir to the distributing area are usually made of cast iron; in some cases a man can stand upright in one of them. They are very carefully jointed and protected from frost. They are lined with a special resistant material. Sometimes the mains are buried to prevent frost from doing any damage. Just as the aorta divides up into fine arteries, so these mains end in the supply pipe going to each house. After the inlet pipe reaches the house, cast iron gives place to lead, since the latter can be bent so easily and fitted to all parts of the house. Copper lining or copper itself may be used.

There are various ways of storing water in a house, depending chiefly upon the system adopted by the local authority for distribution. In the ideal and now almost universal constant system, the water is unlimited, being kept at a constant pressure. In the intermittent system, the water is supplied for a certain period every day and during this time storage cisterns must be filled up. These cisterns are a constant source of infection and of pollution, as already mentioned elsewhere, and fortunately they are passing out of use. Where they exist, they should be carefully covered, inspected frequently and cleaned regularly. One further method must be mentioned, that of the dual supply system. In this there is a certain amount of water supplied which is for drinking and a certain amount for washing and various other purposes. Dangers are apt to be encountered if mistakes are made in the type of water used or if by accident the supplies become mixed.

Relation of Impure Water to the Spread of Disease

Cholera and typhoid fever are the commonest infectious diseases caused by tainted water. Typhoid fever occasionally occurs in sudden and localized epidemics, and the source is often found to be a well or a spring which has been soiled. It is almost needless to remind nurses how much care must be taken with the stools of those suffering from diarrhoea, enteritis, dysentery or typhoid fever. Incineration is the best preventive of spread when water carriage is imperfect. In summer various bacteria irritative to the intestinal tract may gain access to the intestines through bad water. If there is any suspicion of infective processes at work—and indeed as a routine in infantile illnesses—it is well to boil the water before using it, even for washing.

Parasites may be spread by water—threadworms, hookworms, roundworms and tapeworms, and it must never be forgotten that stagnant water is the breeding ground of the mosquito, which may give rise to malaria or to yellow fever. Often vegetable matter such as cress is the vehicle which transfers the parasite from the water to the host.

The presence of certain minerals in water, and occasionally the absence of others, may lead to constitutional diseases. Regarding the former, the common ailments are lead poisoning, and to a lesser extent, copper, arsenic and zinc poisoning, which usually are due to faulty pipes or to the drinking of water which has been standing in lead or copper cisterns and only intended for the hot water supply; it is interesting to note that many housewives use the hot water tap for the supply of cooking water; this is an unwise thing to do. Goitre occurs in certain districts where lack of iodine is a feature; too little chalk in the water has been blamed for contributing to the condition of rickets. Whether cancer depends upon the condition of the water or not is still a very moot point.

Finally it is known that when a person is transferred from a soft water district to a hard water district, he may suffer from gastric and intestinal irritation, accompanied by diarrhoea, for a few days. This is due to the presence of the extra minerals, including sometimes clay; the person soon becomes acclimatized to the new conditions and the symptoms pass off, but this possibility must always be borne in mind when patients are transferred from one area to another.

CHAPTER 4

DISPOSAL OF REFUSE

In any large community there is inevitably an accumulation of
waste matter which is generally referred to as refuse. It is difficult to classify this material, which may accumulate from trades,
shops, public buildings, houses, open spaces, streets, stables, cowsheds and so on; which may be made up of dry refuse or liquid
refuse; which may consist of solid and liquid excretions; which
may be of a special nature destroyed only by special processes;
or which may be of such a type that its disposal may present a
peculiar problem for the local community. From a hygienic
point of view, the efficient treatment of the waste products of an
area involves a perfect system of removal of material the existence
of which is a menace to the general health of the district, and
while the nurse is especially concerned with the domestic side
of refuse disposal, it is nevertheless essential that she should have
an outline of all the branches of this most important department
of public health.

Various Methods in Use

Taking the average dustbin, we might find in it ashes, household dust (including sweepings from carpets, linen, cotton and
wool fabrics), broken crockery, bottles, tins, paper, worn out
kitchen utensils of aluminium, iron or enamel, and the vegetables,
tea leaves and other oddments discarded by the cook. In recent
years, however, sanitary education has become so much a

popular study and domestic heating furnaces so common, that a new school of destruction by incineration has become established and most housewives contrive to dispose of all their refuse by fire, leaving only the ashes, the charred tins and the metalware and crockery for the dustman. This is a most important step in sanitation, and it benefits the housewife in two ways. First she removes all possibility of germ activity and secondly she utilizes every source of heat in the refuse burned.

Unfortunately we are not all at the most advanced stage of hygienic enlightenment and it is necessary to arrange for the communal disposal of all types of waste from house and street. In country districts there still linger many primitive customs and there is great scope for improvement in sanitation. Many of the methods are defined by the situation and conditions of the village or country community. What is suitable to one house or group of dwellings may not be suitable to another, and the rural medical officers of health are constantly faced with new and difficult problems. The means of disposal adopted is often determined by trial and error. So far as the country is concerned, both solid and liquid excreta may be found in the domestic ashpit, or an earth closet or removable buckets may be in use. Each system is discussed in detail below. In the towns, the excreta are removed by special water carriage, while the dry refuse is almost invariably stored in bins and removed at frequent intervals. Ashpits are rapidly disappearing from town areas.

The Dustbin System.—Examining the ideal conditions of well organized towns, we find that the bin system is very popular. These receptacles vary in size; sometimes they are specially provided by the corporation in order to ensure uniform type. Usually, however, they are cylindrical, watertight and made of galvanized iron, with a tightly fitting lid. The last is most important; it is disturbing to see how often these lids are either left off, or lost or placed half over the open top. The very reason for their careful construction is that they will always be kept in position to prevent spread of disease by flies and other carriers of disease and every nurse should use her special knowledge in explaining to people why the lid of the bin should always be kept securely in position. Generally a town council cleansing department arranges for the emptying of these bins up to 3 times a week —sometimes in fact every day, which is the ideal. Housewives should see that the dustbin is disinfected once a week by using a little strong lysol or potassium permanganate or chloride of lime. Dustcarts are used to remove the contents of these bins, which are tipped into a cart with high sides and a hinged lid, so that the refuse cannot blow about or otherwise pollute the neighbourhood. In some cases the dustbins are removed and emptied away from the town, but this is rather a cumbersome method.

How Town Refuse is Dealt With.—Assuming that all liquid refuse is taken away by water carriage, we must learn what is done with the solid waste. Various systems are in operation, each one with its undoubted merits. It is well to keep in mind that a thousand people produce a ton of refuse per day.

1. *By Making a Dump.*—Dumping (or tipping) of refuse is still carried out fairly extensively. In some cases the town refuse makes excellent manure and is eagerly sought by farmers. Usually, however, some old quarry half filled with water, or the side of a river, may be used. For example, the city of Dundee has reclaimed several hundred acres from the Firth of Tay by running out a protection wall and slowly filling up the space left. The advantage is that at high tide the water rises almost as high as the dump, and at low water a few feet of water are left in the "dock" constructed. In this system, owing to the abundant supply of clinker from factories and foundries, the system of " regulated tipping " can be carried out i.e. as the dump is added to, the loads are covered by a foot or so of mineral ash or earth, thus ensuring a sanitary condition. This system of " regulated tipping " gets rid of the old objection to tipping without covering, in which there was great danger (from flies and microbes) to the health of the people living in the neighbourhood. Formerly, when wind blew, the papers flew in all directions and rats became a plague when food refuse was left bare. It should be mentioned here that " made ground " must not be used for building.

2. *By Sea Disposal.*—When the town is close to the sea it may be possible to carry the refuse out a considerable distance from the shore and tip it into the sea. Special barges are used, with machinery for quick tipping. In this method, it is well to make sure that the tide is not on the flow otherwise the shore may become littered.

3. *By Incineration.*—Undoubtedly this is the best method of refuse disposal; it may be represented by a corporation undertaking on a huge scale, a small communal incinerator for a group of houses (as used in the Army) or the domestic furnace for the hot water supply. The ashes resulting from this process are very useful, being hard and dense and forming clinker which can be used for making foundations for roads or, when pulverized, for adding to cement. Two types of incinerator are in use—the high-temperature destructor and the low-temperature destructor. Special precautions are adopted in order to prevent any offensive odours arising from the chimneys. This is a most economical method, because it is well known that a certain proportion of the cinders from a household is not properly burnt when put in the dustbin, and this material keeps the incinerator going. The heat is utilized for various purposes. In the small brick

incinerators, solid excrement can also be burned, so that there is complete destruction of every source of disease.

Other Methods.—Pulverization is used in some parts of London. The refuse is broken up into a fine dust and used as manure. Separation, or special sorting, is a system in which the refuse is passed through sieves. The residue is then transferred to a moving platform, from which, by various devices, the solid constituents are collected according to their material composition and sold as scrap.

Removal of Excreta in Towns.—A water carriage sewage system exists in most towns i.e. the solid and liquid human excreta are carried away in drains to sewers, and so to a river, to the sea or to sewage beds. These sewers also take away the waste from bathrooms, sinks and kitchens. Rain falling on the roof is collected in gutters and empties straight into the main drain pipe running to the sewer, which is also fed by gullies draining the water from the streets. A main sewer usually runs at a fairly deep level along the course of a street, being fed from the collecting drains of the houses on either side. It is obvious that this method is unassailably the best of all disposal systems, especially when there is a copious supply of domestic water. There are 3 main varieties of sewage disposal. The first is called the Combined System, and is described above. The second is known as the Separate System, which excludes rain; it is not common in towns and need only be mentioned. The third is also a country method. It is known as the Conservancy System, and is used in conditions in which water is not in sufficient quantity to provide a water carriage flow; the excreta is specially collected, the only materials drained being house water and rain water.

Removal of Refuse and Excrement in the Country.—As mentioned above, the country presents far more problems than the towns; and since nurses as often as not find themselves faced with problems of an acute type regarding the primitive sanitation in rural districts, they must know what to do about the disposal of both refuse and excrement there. One system frequently overlaps the other, but the following is a list of the principal varieties likely to be met with.

1. *Middens.*—The most elementary and the most insanitary type of disposal is by that ancient monument, the family midden, often with its omnivorous pig at one end, munching the vegetable refuse of the house, and at its other end the open outlet of the communal privy, unprotected by disinfectant or earth. Fortunately this dangerous breeding ground for disease is almost a thing of the past.

2. *Privies.*—These represent a stage further on in hygienic

progress. The old fashioned privy consisted of a seat built round a wooden receptacle which was fixed but which could be occasionally cleaned out. The next stage in development is the earth closet; in this the excreta are covered with sand or earth and in time the faeces are completely dissolved.

3. *Pail Closets.*—Undoubtedly this type of privy is the best in the circumstances. The essentials are a well ventilated brick shed with a lean-to roof, absolutely watertight, with a window above the doorway for light and air. The floor should be concreted, with a slight slope towards the doorway. A very closely fitted wooden seat with lid set so that it falls when the closet is not in use is built round the space at the back of the privy. This space contains a bucket which is movable and which is of such a size that it almost touches the seat with its rim. It can either be removed through a trapdoor at the back of the privy or extracted by lifting up the seat. This is such a common and useful method in the country that its properties should be understood fully. The slightest defect of function may cause disease. The excreta can be received into crude tar, cresol, lysol, potassium permanganate or lime, and usually sand, earth or ashes are provided to cover each motion. The liquid excrement of the house should not be emptied into the bucket. The ideal system is the emptying of the bucket every day, but this is possible only in rare cases, once a week being quite a common frequency. Most authorities on public health recommend that the privy should be as far away from the house as possible, and set so that when the buckets are being removed they do not have to be taken through the house. Usually it is placed at the far end of the garden. It must not be within 6 feet of the house or within 40 feet of the water supply.

4. *Deep Trench Latrines.*—Although this is an Army method, it is often employed on camping sites and in places in which temporary dwellings exist. The deeper the trench the better. Over it is built a seat. If the trench is deep enough, it will allow the contents to become sterile in time, but earth and disinfectant can also be poured in. The trench is filled in after the camp is closed down. Sometimes caustic soda is used in these trenches. Chloride of lime is also commonly employed.

5. *Refuse Disposal in Country Areas.*—In many agricultural areas, the house refuse goes into cattle courts or into nearby dumps where it is removed periodically as manure. Ashpits, which were at one time common in towns, still exist in the country, but they are often over-filled; many country people make heaps of their refuse and leave it to disintegrate in the fresh air. In some cases, private incinerators burn up all the dry refuse of the house, and now and then a more sanitary minded inhabitant will bury his refuse at periods, but the disposal of refuse is a matter that

is left to the individual in country places, and in non-congested areas there is not much to fear if refuse is far away from the house. Most people nowadays have learned to burn their refuse, however.

Destruction of Excreta in Town and Country

All local authorities make provision for the destruction of excreta in some way. In a town with water carriage systems, the collecting sewers deliver the excreta into the sea—an ideal method—or into rivers, which have their restrictions, or into special sewage beds in which scientific methods are employed to disintegrate the excreta. In the country the drains of houses may open into cesspools or a conservancy system may be in operation which treats the material by incineration or deep trenching. These methods may now be considered individually.

Sewers.—We have already mentioned how sewers collect the contents of the house drainage, and now it is appropriate to study the structure of sewers a little more fully. The size of a sewer depends upon the amount of work it has to do; as the system is like that of a river with tributaries, we can imagine that the terminal pipes must be fairly large. The largest ones are now made of reinforced concrete, but iron, steel and glazed earthenware are also employed, and sometimes brick. The great essentials are that the sewer should be watertight and have an easy flow. The introduction of a trap, whilst effectually cutting off sewer air, tends to obstruct the flow of sewage. Some are therefore made so that they are egg-shaped on section, and many have a double wall. A common size is 2 feet diameter. There should not be any sharp turns in the sewer, and where drains join it they should do so obliquely.

In flat country, various devices employing suction, compressed air and special flushing are used to expedite the flow of the sewage, but in towns which are situated on a hill, especially those on the sea coast, the disposal of the sewage is very simple. Ventilation is one of the most important aspects of sewage conductors. The contents of sewers are offensive and in a decomposing state give off gases which may collect in great volume. To overcome this, it is usual to have a manhole in the streets every 60 yards or so. This is familiar to everyone; it is a shaft with a square iron grid fixed over it, flush with the roadway; this allows easy inspection and a continuous supply of fresh air. In certain congested areas with narrow streets it is sometimes necessary to carry the ventilating shaft above the houses by a chimney-like pipe. Ordinarily the dangerous gases (sulphuretted hydrogen, coal gas, benzene, carbonic acid gas and so on) are freely dispelled by the air, but now and then an old sewer gives trouble and causes temporary poisoning of the men who have to keep it in working order, and it may cause general debility, with bloodlessness and intestinal irritation, in those who are constantly subjected to the fumes coming in through their windows. Nevertheless sewer air is more offensive than harmful. House drain air is actually more dangerous to health than sewer air.

Sewage Disposal.—The aims of sewage disposal are 1. removal of suspended solids; 2. conversion of organic compounds, by oxidation, into substances which will not putrefy further. Large cities which are situated on the sea or on the banks of a wide river mouth with tidal water are very lucky, because the clearance of the sewers is automatic. The only thing that has to be allowed for is the rise of the tide above the sewer outlet. This might cause back-flooding of the sewer if some adjustment were not made. The difficulty is overcome by having a flap-valve at the end of the sewer, so that it allows the sewer to empty when the water is low, but is automatically closed when the tide is high. This also serves to carry the sewage well out to sea on the ebb tide. This method of sewage disposal is called direct disposal. Some preliminary treatment may be necessary, when the sewage is from a large and populous district viz. screening out of solid matters and erection of storage tanks. In some instances storage tanks are fixed near the outlet so that there is no possibility of damming back the matter in the sewer itself; as soon as the tide turns, the flap operates and discharges the pent up sewage.

Inland Disposal.—When there is no sea to make use of, local authorities lead the sewers to special areas, where it is dealt with. If there are any manufacturing works or chemical processes in the neighbourhood, the sewage from them may present special problems. Rivers may be said to be universally banned from a sewage point of view as they are easily polluted and it is dangerous to those living on the banks, and perhaps using the water, to make rivers into receptacles for sewage outflow. It must be remembered that by the time sewage has reached its outflow it is a mixture of solid and liquid nitrogenous and carbonaceous matter, with some sodium chloride, sand, oddments of mineral origin and above all bacteria. The bacillus coli is prevalent and is dangerous to health. In addition to this there is the possibility of certain waste matter peculiar to the trade of the area.

Inland Sewage Treatment.—In some cases it is arranged that the sewage will, after " cleansing," be discharged into a river or stream. Under the Rivers Pollution Prevention Act of 1876, it is illegal to empty untreated sewage into a river. The degree of purification therefore must be determined by the final disposal of the sewage. The following are the common systems in use.

1. *Screening.*—The first process at a sewage works (which is situated usually on the outskirts of a town, some distance away from all habitation) is screening. This is a simple matter of placing a grid with vertical iron bars over the sewer at its end so that all the odd paper, cloth, large faeces and other matter can be stopped, collected, taken away and buried. The grid is constantly raked to keep it clear. About 10 per cent of the gross matter is stopped in this way.

2. *Collection in Tanks.*—The next stage in purification is the settling of the screened sewage in tanks. These vary according to the amount of sewage to be treated, and to the system adopted by the authorities, but in general they are in duplicate, so that while one is being cleaned, the other is doing its work. They are built of concrete, and, known as detritus tanks, allow the grit and other heavy material to settle; occasionally lime is added to hasten the action. This is known as chemical precipitation, and is adopted to hasten the settling of suspended matter and the clarification of sewage. Sulphate of iron, or a combination of alum and iron (aluma ferric) are also used.

A more extensive method provides a large enough tank to allow for the sedimentation of sewage over a period of about 8 hours. This tank is made like a swimming bath with a deep end and a shallow end. At the deep end the screened and degritted sewage passes in slowly and the flow is so much retarded that there is time for about 50 per cent further sedimentation. The deposit, called sludge, sinks to the bottom, collecting especially at the deep end, at which there are traps from which it can be collected into a well. Now and then these tanks are emptied and thoroughly cleansed, the sloping bottom aiding the work considerably. The overflow of this tank is a weir, which takes the water from the top layers of the tank and passes it on.

The so-called septic tank is still in use here and there, but it is now out of date as it is not so efficient as the above. It consists of a tank which is covered over and which can retain the sewage for 24 hours if necessary. A very thick, tough scum forms on the top, and one of the principles of the process is that this should not be disturbed, since the microbes which are at work below it (anaerobes) do their work in the absence of oxygen by splitting up the harmful materials and turning much of the semi-solid into liquid matter. The inlet and outlet pipes are thus arranged to open just below this important layer. It is found that the gases (ammonia and carbon dioxide) produced frequently disturb the essential quietude of the tank, while sludge settles to the bottom. The effluent liquid is also impure, so the septic tank, while good enough for a small private domestic system, is not successful in big schemes.

The above methods are known as the preliminary processes.

Completing processes are concerned with further dissolving of the impurities and final collection of the remaining particles, prior to the passage of the cleansed effluent into a convenient stream or river.

3. *Land Treatment.*—The effluent is now at a stage at which it is almost free from gross constituents, but it is still dense with very finely divided particles of an organic nature and there is a very high percentage of bacteria. To get rid of these, various methods are employed, the first being land treatment which itself has several subdivisions. The fundamental in this form of sewage disposal is that both the bacteria of the soil and those of the effluent work together to break up the fine particles of organic matter, the products of which are transformed by oxidation into rich nitrates for the soil. Much of the ammonia in the excreta is utilized in this way. Irrigation may be on the surface, just under the soil, or as a filtration process, and if the soil is light loam or sand, the results are excellent. Occasionally vegetation can be grown, especially foodstuffs for cattle.

The " sewage farm " method of broad, or surface, irrigation is one of distribution of the effluent by open ditches containing concrete open drains. The fluid is thus led to absorbent rect-angles of soil, which rapidly suck up the moisture and its con-tained particles. In the soil the chemical actions go on, filtration occurs and the cleansed liquid drains through to a set of agricul-tural drain pipes placed about 6 feet below the soil, all of which run to a main drainage system emptying into a stream. The benefit of this method is that it allows the cultivation of foodstuffs for cattle, but its disadvantage is that one acre is required for every 100 of the population. Sometimes this land becomes " sewage-sick," and requires a rest.

In the land filtration method no vegetation is grown; the plots are sandy and employed mainly as filter beds. The action should be intermittent, 6 hours of flow of effluent being followed by 18 hours' rest. This system has the advantage that it can deal with 1,000 people per acre. When the surface of the plot becomes choked it may require to be ploughed over. Drains are gener-ally laid about 5 feet below the surface to take away the water.

A third and more scientific method of effluent purification is that of filtering the liquid by allowing it to percolate slowly over a bed of broken stone, clinker or ashes. Various patterns are made. The principle is the biological one of nitrification by special organisms, while oxidation also occurs freely. These artificial filters are quite commonly used as they occupy a minimum of space, and they are familiar and of interest to many who discover their existence, generally on the outskirts of the town or village. Sometimes the outline is circular, sometimes rectangular, but the same construction is to be found: a chamber

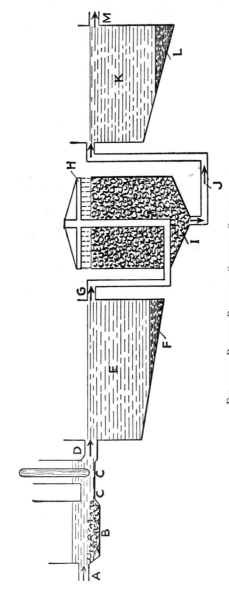

FIG. 24.—ROUGH PLAN OF SEWAGE SYSTEM.

a, Sewage entering grit pit (*b*) and being screened at *c* and *c*. *d*, Screened sewage passing to sedimentation tank (*e*).
f, Sludge deposited. *g*, Effluent from tank passing into sprinkler (*h*). *i*, Percolation filter with effluent passing through to
(*j*) (filter effluent pipe). *k*, Humus tank with deposited humus (*l*). *m*, Clear water in pipe on way to river.

is made, about 6 feet deep, by building a wall of brick; this chamber is filled with graduated stone or clinker, the top layers being of cinders about $\frac{1}{2}$ inch in diameter. The effluent pours over the bed; in the rotatory sprinkler it is fed from a central pipe into arms which are studded with perforations. As the " wheel " slowly goes round, we can see the gentle trickling of the effluent, which is quickly absorbed. In the rectangular method, the sprinklers pass to and fro like a street watercart. The floor of this chamber is of concrete and watertight, but drains are constructed below to take away the treated effluent. Some distributors (e.g. the Candy Distributor) have a diameter of 75 yards, but they can be made in any size. As in water purification, the film of jelly like material collects on the surface, and this is the medium which reduces the constituents of the effluent. The two main essentials are a plentiful supply of fresh air, and a periodic rest for the beds in order to allow the micro-organisms and the oxygen to do their work properly. In badly working filters, hydrogen sulphide (H_2S), a well known and very offensive gas, usually collects and soon advertises its presence. Flushing out of the beds is done at periods in order to collect the "humus," which is the name given to the products manufactured. It is claimed that this type of filter reduces the number of germs by 95 per cent, but even that leaves a great number behind. It is sufficient purification to make the effluent clean enough to be led into a stream, however.

4. *Disposal of the Sludge.*—So far we have followed the purification system as applied to the effluent; now we must consider briefly how the sludge is dealt with. Even after the most perfect screening and tank collection, sludge is nine-tenths water, and if there are any harmful chemicals they may make the value of the sludge negative as farm manure, so the problems attached to its disposal are many. In some cases, the sludge is run into special beds, where it dries in time and can be lifted with a spade. This is called lagooning. A similar process is that of flooding; in other methods the dried sludge is ploughed in, but at all times sludge is offensive because it creates a smell that may clearly come within the category of " nuisance," and farmers are lukewarm in their attitude towards it. In certain districts, the water is pressed out by a machine and the resultant mass of solid matter is either burned or given away for manurial purposes. Many of the large cities take the sludge out in barges to the sea or to the estuaries of rivers. London, Glasgow and Manchester dispose of their sludge in this way.

5. *The " Activated Sludge," or Bioaeration Treatment.*—This is the most modern development in sewage treatment. It is successfully established in Manchester, Sheffield and elsewhere. Various mechanical devices are used to carry out the principles

of the treatment, but it is not necessary to discuss them in this work. The principle of the activated sludge method is that when sewage free from detritus is " bubbled " with compressed air, it forms particles which are important centres of activity—leaven for the whole mass, so to speak—for any further sewage which is passed through. The sewage is run into tanks on the floor of which are many pipes sending in columns of fresh air; the whole liquid becomes agitated, the flakes develop and they settle out in a few hours after being delivered in " settlement tanks." The process of purification is thus shortened very much, since the effluent from these tanks is as pure as that from the longer processes. The only difficulty is the disposal of the activated sludge; a small quantity is retained to set the new sewage going, but the remainder consists of more than 99 per cent of water, and it rots very quickly. Sometimes it is sprayed over the ground and then ploughed in. So far it has resisted all attempts at rapid drying and it is generally taken out to sea when possible.

6. *Sterilization of Sewage.*—Several tests have been made with chlorine, and in samples of sewage so treated sterilization has been proved; but the Royal Commission on Sewage Disposal considered that the additional expense would not be worth while, nor would sterilization of the sewage alone clear the pollution from the rivers. In Great Britain, therefore, sterilization is not done on any large scale.

General Arrangements of House and Hospital Drainage

It may seem that this part of the chapter is out of place, and indeed it might have been dealt with before the study of sewage disposal was taken up. Since, however, internal sanitary arrangements are of supreme importance to the nurse, it is considered that this subject should be left to the last part of the chapter, as with a knowledge of all the other aspects of refuse disposal, the domestic side of drainage may be more easily followed. This includes the carriage to the main sewer of the liquid and solid excreta of the house, the waste water from baths and taps and the rain water from the roof. In cases of non-provision of water carriage of excrement already dealt with— never to be found in hospitals and rarer and rarer in houses nowadays—the only effluent from a house is the sink water, because generally the rain water is saved.

The Ideal Water Carriage System.—In a modern house or hospital, an abundant supply of water is provided by the local authority or other approved service board. Water closets amply flushed from cisterns, ample baths, sinks and lavatories, and other methods of rapid disposal of waste, can thus be established. The pipes, traps and other appliances which lead to the sewer are universally known as drains. The individual constituents are dealt with in order below.

Water Closets.
—In the course of evolution, many types have been devised, but today the most perfect and most sanitary water closet is the Short Hopper, or Washdown Closet (Fig. 25). The others are now only of historical interest. All closets should be made of glazed earthenware or stoneware, and should be of pedestal

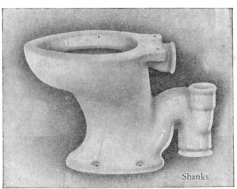

FIG. 25.—MODERN PATTERN OF WASHDOWN CLOSET.
(By courtesy of Messrs. Shanks & Co., Ltd., Barrhead.)

type. The following points should be carefully noted. The flushing water should be operated by a cistern with ball-cock which is liberated by pulling a plug. This cistern should belong to the closet alone, should be filled automatically from the house tank, and may be placed a few feet above or in a box immediately above the seat. It should allow for the liberation of at least $2\frac{1}{2}$ gallons of water through an iron delivery pipe about 2 inches wide, which terminates by flooding a rim flush running under the brim of the closet. All water closets are made with the pan and the trap below it in one piece (Fig. 26). The trap must be of the siphon type and the water seal should be $2\frac{1}{2}$ inches in depth. The back of the pan is vertical, while there is a slight slope of the other sides leading to a circular water seal. The seat of the average water closet is 15 inches above the floor level. It is advisable to have the floor below laid with glazed tiles or with rubber, so that it cannot become soiled. The seat should be of stout wood, smoothed by sandpapering or enamelled with good paint, and

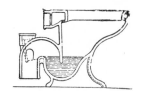

FIG. 26.—SECTION OF THE W.C. SHOWN ON FIG. 25.

should have a covering lid, both being hinged so that they can be raised clear of the closet. In certain institutions and public lavatories, the seats are dispensed with, small wooden rims being fitted above the rim of the closet. This ensures cleanliness. In

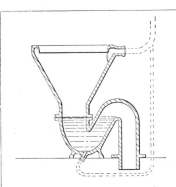

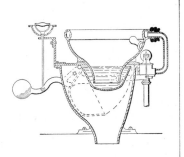

CARMICHAEL CLOSET

THE EARLIEST ATTEMPT TO MAKE A SIPHON-JET CLOSET WITH AN ORDINARY HOPPER AND TRAP.

DESIGNED BY A GLASGOW DOCTOR NAMED CARMICHAEL ABOUT 1860. THE FLUSHING WATER, FROM EITHER A CISTERN OR A VALVE, IS DIVIDED; THE MAJOR PORTION GOING TO THE RIM, AND AN AUXILIARY PIPE LEADING TO THE BOTTOM OF THE TRAP WHICH INDUCES SIPHONIC DISCHARGE.

PAN CLOSET

A TYPE OF CLOSET LARGELY USED IN THE SIXTIES AND SEVENTIES OF THE NINETEENTH CENTURY. ITS OBJECTIONABLE FEATURES ARE WELL KNOWN. EVERY TIME THE HANDLE WAS LIFTED THERE WAS OPEN CONNECTION TO THE SOILPIPE, AND THE RECEIVER VERY SOON BECAME FOUL AND INSANITARY.

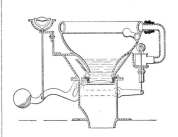

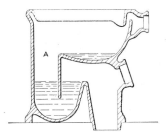

VALVE CLOSET

A TYPE OF CLOSET LARGELY USED IN THE NINETEENTH CENTURY – AND SOME PEOPLE STILL PREFER IT BECAUSE OF ITS QUIETNESS IN ACTION.

THE OBJECTIONS TO IT ARE: (FIRSTLY) THE VALVE OFTEN LEAKED AND LEFT THE BASIN DRY: (SECONDLY) DISCHARGE OF CLOSET OPENED CONNECTION TO THE SOILPIPE.

WASHOUT CLOSET

A TYPE OF CLOSET LARGELY USED IN THE NINETEENTH CENTURY – AND WHICH, IN SOME COUNTRIES, IS STILL LARGELY USED.

THE CHIEF OBJECTION WAS THAT THE FRONT PORTION (MARKED 'A') BECAME SOILED AND FOUL, SO THIS FORM HAS BEEN ABANDONED IN GREAT BRITAIN AND IN AMERICA.

FIG. 27.—TYPES OF WATER CLOSET.

(By courtesy of Messrs. Shanks & Co., Ltd., Barrhead.)

all rooms containing water closets, whether they be separate
chambers or contain a bath and washhand basin, there must be
ample ventilation by a window at least 2 feet square.   The water
closet must have a properly constructed door and fastenings, and
it should not open into a room in which people work or live.
There must be one outside wall; the ideal system is that in which
the closet is fixed to this wall, but this is not always practicable.
The nearer the exit pipe from the closet is to the outside drain
running down to the sewer, the better.

Other Types of Water Closet.—As the nurse may encounter
now and then examples of old fashioned water closets, a brief
summary is given below of the main properties of each of the
best known types.

The Long Hopper Closet is conical, and much deeper than the
washdown closet.   It was the forerunner of the latter, but its
disadvantage is that it cannot be properly flushed and therefore
it becomes soiled with excreta, and offensive (Fig. 27).

The Pan Closet is rarely seen nowadays; in it a hinged pan
faces down and deposits its contents into a trap when a lever
is raised.   It is most insanitary as it is never free from excretal
clogging, and the very fact of its complex mechanism makes it
impossible to keep clean (Fig. 27).

The Valve Closet is a little better than the foregoing, but
although there is no pan, the circular valve is a menace to
health, since it often refuses to shut tightly and frequently
becomes choked and soiled with excreta (Fig. 27).

The Washout Closet is still in use here and there, although it
cannot bear comparison with the washdown type.   It has an
upper shallow pan, with a little seal of water, and while for certain reasons of comfort and in some cases of medical investigation
it has its uses, there is a great disadvantage in the fact that the
pan is not always properly cleansed by the imperfect flushing,
and the break in the fall of water does not make a complete
clearance in the water of the trap (Fig. 27).

Hospital Sanitary Appliances.—Where there is a constant demand
for disposal of excrement, special slop sinks and flushing pipes
are fitted in hospital lavatories.   These operate by turning on
taps which liberate water at great pressure (see Sect. 5 Figs. 74
and 75). All these fixtures are modern and thus perfectly sanitary.
They are trapped and led straight to the drains by soil pipes.
In some schools and institutions there is a common trough for a
series of closets, flushed at intervals, but it cannot be said that
this process is sanitarily perfect.

Plan of a House Drainage.—Before going any farther it may
be well to examine the plan of the drains in an ordinary house
or hospital.   If possible, all the drains should run on one side

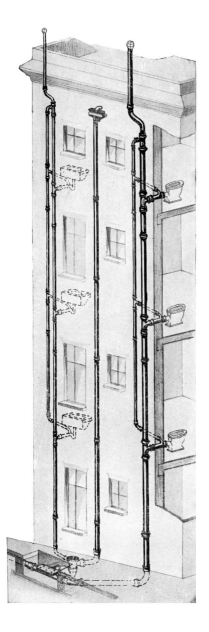

FIG. 28.—DRAINAGE.

This illustration shows how a building is drained. Note that the sinks are first trapped and then the waste water passes to a common drainpipe, which is not only provided with a caged air vent high above the roof, but it has also an anti-siphon pipe. Finally the waste water drain meets the rainwater pipe (middle) at a common accessible "box," and this passes more deeply by a U trap into the main drain leading to the sewer. The W.C. pipe is entirely distinct from the others, and passes through the manhole to the main drain. Manholes are usually fairly close to the sewer, and have ample facilities for inspection.

By courtesy of Burn Bros. (London), Ltd.)

of a house; they should never be seen at the front of the house, but they are better with a northern exposure rather than with a southern exposure. In the plan (Fig. 28), we see that pipes lead down to the house drains which run to a large inspection chamber and so to the sewer. The pipes to be seen on a house wall are 1. the rain water pipe, leading down from the roof; 2. the waste pipe from baths and sinks and 3. the soil pipe from the closets and urinals. These enter the drain pipe at various intervals, but the whole pipe slopes towards the inspection chamber, and the latter may be called the clearing house of the building which it serves. A preliminary study of the diagram will help considerably in the understanding of the various parts described below.

Traps.—All drains require two specially important provisions: 1. efficient supply of fresh air, and 2. means of prevention of foul smell from permeating the house. The latter is done by making certain bends in the piping called traps. In any house, traps will be seen below water closets, underneath sinks and wherever it is necessary to cut the underlying drain off from the pipe above by a water seal. There are various types of trap, according to the local need;

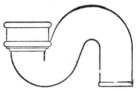

FIG. 29.—A simple illustration of the principle of S trap drainage.

(By courtesy of Burn Bros. (London), Ltd.)

they are simple, but one of the most important adjuncts of drainage. To be effective, a trap must contain water. Unsealing of the trap may be caused by disuse (in which case the water has evaporated) and also as a result of violent backward pressure or siphonage. If the trap is a good one, water evaporation should be checked as far as is possible. Repeated inspection of traps is necessary, as no traps are perfect.

If a double bend is made on a pipe, we get an S shaped trap (Fig. 29) in which (as shown in Fig. 26) each limb is full of water. The P trap is not so elaborate; the outlet is horizontal. The amount of water left in the double bend after the rest of the pipe is empty is called the " seal " of the trap; it is the amount of water necessary to keep back all offensive effluvia from drains. The seals are usually about 2 inches deep. A special form of trap for drains is U shaped; this is commonly found at a point just before the drain joins the sewer, and is known as the Buchan trap. It has a special fresh air inlet to provide a regular supply for the waste and soil pipes of the house, and also an inspection cap, which enables cleansing and investigation to be carried out easily. All traps should be well glazed inside and of hard materials so that there is no risk of causing dents which might result in soiling.

Soil Pipes.—These are the pipes which convey the excreta from the lavatories, water closets and other fittings to the drains. There is only one trap in a soil pipe viz. at its commencement, immediately below the water closet. In fact, as we have already noted, all water closets are supplied with the trap as part of the pedestal. This prevents leakage. Most closets have a lateral screw cap, for inspection of the trap if necessary. (The soil pipe itself should be of stout cast iron, very carefully jointed with lead and specially treated to make it proof against leakage or corrosion.) It discharges straight into the house drain without further trapping. When two or more closets empty into a common soil pipe, it is found that the seals of the water closets may be disturbed by the suction action of closets emptying from the top storey. This is due to a form of siphon action, sucking the water out. By a simple method of leading out a small pipe from the crown of the water seal either to the external air or to a common " anti-siphonage " pipe running vertically up the wall beyond the roof, this is prevented. The soil pipe, which is about 4 inches in diameter, is continued up well beyond the roof, where it acts as a ventilating shaft, thus serving two useful purposes. It is usual to fix a small wire cage to the tops of these and other pipes, so that birds cannot nest in them (see Fig. 28).

Waste Pipes.—These take away all the waste water from sinks, basins and baths, which are always trapped immediately below. It must be remembered that, especially in areas where there is hard water, curdy soap, grease and other material are constantly evacuated from these sources. Furthermore, grease may be dissolved when in boiling water, but it sets as a skin or precipitate when it touches the cold pipes. In the case of baths and washbasins, a screw cap is fitted at the lowest part of the bend of the trap so that any of the precipitated material can be removed. Waste pipes open into a separate or common gully, which is also trapped before it reaches the house drain, and which has a ribbed grid. By this trap air is prevented from reaching the house drain and effluvia from passing up the waste pipe. Most kitchens have a special grease trap provided. The hot grease passing into this trap is received into a glazed stone chamber, about 1 foot deep. As the fat solidifies it rises to the top, and when the next outflow occurs from the kitchen sink it sends the lumps of fatty matter into the drain. Theoretically this system is all right, but as a matter of practical experience it is often found that the traps become choked with fine pieces of grease and soap, and the curdy mass has to be removed by hand, fortunately a very simple matter. Most waste pipes are about

2 inches in diameter, and are made of lead until they reach the outside wall, when they are made of cast iron and are about 3 inches in diameter. They are also carried above the eaves like the soil pipe. Anti-siphonage systems are necessary in high buildings with many outlets e.g. hospitals and flats.

Rain Water Pipes.—The rain collected from the gutters running round the house should pass by a special down spout, or rain pipe of cast iron and of about 3 inches diameter, which leads into a P or S trap. Sometimes a gully is provided to collect the surface water at the same time. The rain water then passes into the drain.

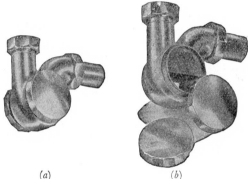

(a)   (b)

FIG. 30.—AN INGENIOUS TYPE OF ACCESS TRAP FOR SINKS.

The chromium plated disc nuts are screwed on either side of the trap when the latter is in use (a). To clean the trap, unscrew both nuts, as shown in (b), and rinse out with disinfectant.

(*By courtesy of Benham & Sons, Ltd., London.*)

Referring to the plan again (Fig. 28), we see that the drain thus receives 3 main tributaries—soil pipe, waste pipe and rain spout. The drain itself must now receive consideration.

The House Drain.—As the main connecting link between house and sewer, the house drain is of supreme importance. It may be made of glazed earthenware, stone or cast iron, with socketed joints sealed carefully with various materials. If possible, it should run parallel to the side of the house, but if it should have to pass through the house, it should be of iron, and should be sunk into a bed of concrete. Stoneware pipes are about 3 feet in length, but iron pipes are 6–9 feet long and about 6 inches in diameter. A certain amount of " fall " is allowed before the drain opens into the sewer.

Inspection Chamber and Manhole.—Lastly, just before the drain passes into the sewer, it may be trapped by a Buchan trap, as already mentioned, and this trap is usually in association with a manhole or inspection chamber (Fig. 28). This chamber, built of brick and cement, and about 2 feet square, gives free access to the drain, allows the Buchan trap to be cleared if necessary and provides for the passage of fresh air to the drain. It is covered by an iron top, but at one side there may be an opening through which air, sucked through a special mica valved inlet ventilator, passes into the chamber   This is the final defence of the house against smells, back-flow, rats and other anti-hygienic possibilities. In hospitals and large buildings extra drains may be allowed, all depending upon the amount of work to be done. Thus a rather more complicated system may be found, but in principle it is exactly the same as that described for a dwelling house.

Drainage in Areas where there is a Conservancy System.—The sump pits of the Army with their brushwood and straw represent the simplest method of dealing with waste water in country districts. Most houses have some sort of drainage leading away from the house, but as often as not it ends in a nearby ditch, which is a source of nuisance and disease. Often a simple soak pit may be constructed, but in communities where there are large houses, a private cesspool may be made. This is simply a miniature septic tank, and it should be very carefully constructed in a situation as far away from the house and water supply as possible, and certainly not less than 60 feet from either. On no account should its contents drain into any ground where children play or where wells are situated. It must be well covered in and capable of being emptied by pumping at intervals, since it is supposed to liquefy all its matter which cannot percolate through the bricks. It is a bad system, but inevitable in many parts of the country. It is interesting to see how cleverly some of the drainage obstacles are overcome in isolated places by taking advantage of the natural situation. In many instances, the houses are drained quite successfully by agricultural drains which are set in radiating lines from the houses and which spread out over the fields by the method of subsoil irrigation.

Testing of Drains

When drains have just been completed, and before they are covered in, a water test is carried out. This is done by filling up the various drains with water, and observing if they leak at any spot. Sometimes compressed air is used with a gauge fitted to the drain for comparison of the pressures every minute. In a perfect drain, the index should be stationary. In the smoke test we have the commonest example of test for old drains. A smoke machine, worked by bellows, is introduced at the fresh-air inlet of the Buchan trap; it should work its way up the soil pipes and waste pipes and be seen issuing from them at the top, but not from any other part of the system. It is difficult to find underground leaks by this method. In the smell test, strong aromatic oils, such as oil of peppermint, are used. A little is poured down the trap, followed by a bucket of boiling water; if there is a leak it will soon advertise itself. Drain testing is important, as a leaking or inefficient drain is a nuisance, and as such can be condemned by the Medical Officer of Health. This means that the defect must be remedied at once. It is recommended that all drains be inspected regularly by the sanitary inspector of the district.

PERSONAL HYGIENE

THE process of living, complicated as it is by the factors of age, youth, disease, occupation and the hundred-and-one circumstances which influence earthly existence, when analysed becomes plainly a search for health. For the most part, our studies up to this point have been on the side of communal health, but now we must turn to the individual aspect. We are all ruled, guided and advised by certain laws which have been evolved from long experience of trial and error. Every man is a law unto himself after a certain point. His personal health depends upon the application of his guiding principles as affecting his own peculiarities of mind and body. No two people are the same, and that is why the world is so complex. The science of personal hygiene is therefore intimate, specific to each member of the community and essentially applied to the individual in a manner most appropriate to the situation and having regard to every circumstance. Accordingly the rules laid down in the following pages are of a general nature, but fundamental in their framework. Their complete interpretation and ultimate application depend upon the sum of personal peculiarities which form the characteristics, say, of Mary Brown or of John Smith. The nurse, in studying the details of personal hygiene, must ever bear in mind that when she goes into practice and applies these principles to her patients, she must be ready to make allowances for local conditions, individual peculiarities and deviations from normality, all of which may demand a seasoning of the justice involved in the sentence of good health meted out to the patient, by a merciful interpretation of the many regulations of the hygienic code. In the following pages, therefore, while the instructions regarding habits, exercise, rest, recreation, cleanliness, clothing and parasites are somewhat strict and dogmatic, they must be regarded as the mere guiding lines of personal hygiene.

Habits

If we take the example of our body as a regulated piece of machinery we realize that routine is one of the most important factors in health. The heart never stops, pumping its blood steadily at an average in health of 72 beats a minute; the digestion goes on with ordered sequence, one dissolving process following on the heels of another; sleep automatically follows fatigue, resting body and mind. This is enough to warn us that any function over which we consciously have influence must be regularized. How often, however, do we transgress the law in this respect. Good habits seem to be so much more difficult to observe than bad habits, yet their observance is fundamental to the continuance of the full enjoyment of life which we call perfect health. Disease is the inevitable punishment of those who break the simple hygienic rules which govern the normal existence. These rules lay down a certain period for work, for play and for sleep, hours for eating and standards of food. They aim at producing the ideal conditions which will allow the activities of the body and mind to be exercised to their greatest extent, thus giving the organism every facility for progress and for development. In the daily round, we spend ordinarily 8 hours in bed, 8 hours at work and 8 hours at some sort of recreation, yet these are not in any way hard and fast rules. It may be that for some a few hours' hard work may require more time off spent either in sleep or at play; again work may be, as in a nurse's life, a matter of being on duty for a certain number of hours during which it is a part of the routine to include recreation; brain workers may apparently trifle all day and sit down in the evening to consolidate their thoughts on a manuscript; for certain types e.g. bakers, work begins at a very early hour and ends correspondingly early in the afternoon; many other examples could be given of the varying routine of life as applicable to different trades and professions. Nature does not inflict the penalties of sickness on people who order their lives so that the rules as amended satisfy the code. It is when flagrant excesses and unnatural habits are in vogue that a crash occurs. We all break the laws of health now and then, and return to our routine with an added zest; constant late nights, too much excitement, excessive fatigue and broken sleep, however, are known to amount to a wearying of the flesh which must inevitably end in a breakdown and compulsory rest. When we do not have the good sense to limit our activities by our own will, Nature steps in and forces us to do so by upsetting some function and so leaving us no other course than that of submission.

A routine is a good thing for the mind and for the body, but it must be elastic, otherwise it is impracticable. Life becomes a drudgery when monotony is the rule. In this connexion, the work done by National Institute of Industrial Psychology is very important. This body has done much to improve working conditions by introducing variety into factories and workshops and by investigating the psychological aspects of labour. The result is easier work and brighter workers. Employers (including those of nurses) realize now that more efficient production is the natural outcome of increased consideration of ways of making work less of a drudge.

Generally speaking, the best time to work is when the sun is in the sky, whereas sleeping hours are the hours of darkness. The ideal day is that in which we rise after a normal healthy sleep and, with plenty of time to prepare ourselves for the work before us, dress and have an uninterrupted breakfast. The mid-day meal should come when we are ready for it, and should be a welcome break after several hours' labour. The work of the afternoon is less efficient, because we are beginning to get tired. By teatime, the mind and body require the soothing influences of recreation, which must be carefully distinguished from the degenerating process of pleasure seeking. Hobbies, whatever they may be—music, art, sport, the theatre, the cinema—are all beneficial in moderation. The real difficulty about recreation is to know exactly when it is in danger of taking toll of the tired mental and physical make-up. This is the reason why heavy meals, strenuous games, high revelry or other exciting things are so detrimental to health late at night. By eleven o'clock the body normally is in need of refreshing sleep, and it is wrong to deny the brain its rest. Of the other daily habits, regular evacuation of the bowels is of great importance. Today we have lost our inborn habits to some extent, and many are dependent on various lubricants and stimulants to produce the daily motion. In physiology, the reflexes of defaecation have already been referred to (Vol. I, p. 222). If we can make these reflexes function without medicine, so much the better. It is unwise to become a slave to a purgative or laxative, however convincing may be the slogan displayed on train, bus or hoarding. A diet of wholemeal bread, green vegetables and fresh fruit (raw and cooked) should leave enough " roughage " to stimulate the lower part of the bowel and prevent constipation, which is an abnormal condition of far greater toxic power than is generally realized by the public. Moderate exercise is also of great help; sedentary occupations invariably tend to cause constipation.

To sum up, habits of a beneficial type are essential to healthy life. By education and training, a state of body and mind is reached in which a certain routine is found to be most suitable to the realization of the fullest benefits of health. When this routine is upset by prolonged distractions, wellbeing is affected and illness of some kind, mental or physical, is the result. Good habit training should be started very early in life, as it greatly affects individual health and happiness in succeeding years.

Exercise

Presumably when Adam delved and Eve span, there was enough muscular and cerebral activity to keep the body in good condition. The savage ancestors of modern man were not puzzled to devise schemes for keeping fit. Roaming the woods and the valleys, they had to hunt for their own food, and having killed their prey, they cooked it lightly over a simple fire. With such simplicity of life, there was no chance of flabby muscle or torpid liver and recreation enough and to spare was provided by the hunt. The brain was not highly developed, however; with the increases of the activity of this organ, the mental as opposed to the physical power has gradually gained the ascendant, until we are now, in this so-called civilization, reaping the doubtful benefits of responding to the mental stimulations of a brain in which there has been evolved thousands of functions and activities in the gradual advance of the human race. One of the most prominent of these is the faculty of economizing in work. We are a race of work dodgers, striving with every muscle to avoid the use of our voluntary muscle power wherever possible. Thus we have surrounded ourselves with all sorts of devices to do the work we are supposed to do with our own limbs. Mechanical transport by train, tram, bus or other conveyance relieves us of the duty of walking; complex machinery manufactures our food, our clothing, our furniture; all we think of is how to do a job with the minimum of effort and all we want is the maximum leisure. In this unnatural existence the body, framed and devised by Nature as an animal structure, cannot keep fit for its normal functions, hence it either breaks down altogether or makes representations to its " consciousness " that something must be done to use up the idle muscles. Exercise of all kinds is therefore part and parcel of our modern life, whether it be in the form of strenuous athletics or mild bowling games on the country green.

Fortunately the present generation is alive to the need for

regular exercise, and the craze for life in the open must have far reaching effects on the future health of the race.   Walking is excellent exercise, as not only does it put into natural action many of the vital muscles of the body, but it also keeps the brain and mind active by changing constantly the environment and scenery.   Dancing and swimming are also beneficial; the latter is excellent in cases in which posture is poor.   The net result of exercise is a clearance of the waste material from the body and an increase in the metabolic activity of the protoplasm.   There is a saying that hard work never killed anybody, but today mechanization has taken the place of hard muscular effort and therefore the mass of the people must have some amount of extra work for the muscles apart from that demanded by occupation, if fitness is to be maintained.   The obvious solution is adoption of some form of athletics in the evenings, on Saturdays and Sundays, or at other odd times.   Life for most people thus becomes a period of brain work and a period of muscular work, one carefully balanced by the other ; although circumstances of life have changed, the body, which has undergone almost imperceptible changes, maintains all its original functions by arranging its supply of stimulation in an altered way.

The man or woman who deliberately leads a sedentary and slovenly life soon discovers that weak flesh quickly reacts on the spirit.   Muscles which are allowed to wilt become thin, flabby and degenerate; as a proof of this the weak condition of the body after a long illness and the need for re-education of muscles by manipulation and exercise are ever present in the nurse's mind.

There is the danger, however, of over development of certain muscles, which may upset the rhythm of the coordinated action of the whole muscle system and thus make a person unbalanced. Professional athletes tend to suffer from this condition, and a state of what is termed staleness is the result often of over stimulation of one group of muscles to the detriment of the others. The great aim should be not only to develop the normal powers of every muscle but to employ at the same time a certain amount of brain activity.   In most games, therefore, the mind as well as the body must be exercised; this is provided for amply by the competitive element in sport and the setting up of high standards of achievement and refinement.   The effect of moderate athletics, even although they may be specialized, is to improve muscle tone, which depends upon the integrity of the nerve-muscle communications all over the body.   Training for an event is simply a matter of allowing the heart and lungs and other organs to become accustomed to respond immediately to brief but extraordinary demands on their resources.   In time these vital organs gain a reserve which is of maximum benefit to the individual in his ordinary life.   The erect carriage, the square shoulders, the prominent chest and the flat abdomen of the man or woman of good muscular tone compare markedly with the drooping head and shoulders, the hollow chest and the prominent abdomen of the person whose physique has low tonal value.

Lastly, exercise should never become a duty. There are those who plod round a golf course simply and solely because their doctor told them to do it. And there are armies of people who do their daily exercises because they are actually afraid of ill health. Doubtless they succeed in escaping disease, but they are reaping only a fraction of the possible wellbeing associated with recreative exercise in the fresh air. To each must be granted the privilege of selecting what suits him best; the old man may feel fit by hoeing his herbaceous border, the vigorous young lady may not be completely satisfied unless she appears on the centre court at Wimbledon. So long as recreation succeeds in promoting the maximum efficiency of the heart, the lungs, the kidneys and the digestive system, and ensures the complete elimination by kidneys, bowels and skin of the refuse of the body, it is completely justified. The only objection to it arises when it is carried to excess and produces pain, fatigue and disharmony of the whole system because of excessive amount of work.

Rest

Despite training, the work of the body cannot go on for ever. Rest is essential, either at frequent intervals or for a long spell after a certain amount of work. The heart and lungs require a period of time in which to recuperate, depending upon type of work, age, sex and physical build. Cramp in certain muscles (cf. writer's cramp) may occur if the constant demand on their output has been too prolonged. The fundamental element in this condition is collection of waste products in the muscle cells as a result of flagging activity of the blood supply. With rest, the blood takes up plenty of oxygen and soon drives out all the accumulated bad gases and other harmful residues. Fatigue brings with it a lack of interest in work, a desire to rest the muscles and an urgent signal from the brain that sleep is required.

Sleep.—The mechanism of sleep is difficult to explain. We have already dealt with the physiology of sleep (Vol. I, p. 269) and it was said there that certain functions are depressed, but the reasons are not clear. What we do know, however, is that sleep is one of the greatest refreshments known; it is the only remedy for tired muscles and weary brains, and in illness it does far more good towards a cure than any drug. It is essential for the physical worker as well as the brain worker, because each suffers from fatigue of the brain, but in a different way. Insomnia is

a grave condition, too little appreciated by those who are easy
sleepers. The result of a broken night or of too little time for
sleep is inevitably mental dullness which makes the brain inefficient as a directing organ; thus every organ of the body
suffers and general debility is the result. This is especially
marked in nervous children and in highly strung individuals of
an imaginative nature. The so-called night terrors in children
are often the warning symptom of a brain that has been too much
excited and should be regarded as evidence of unnatural cerebral
pressure. The time most suitable for sleep is from 10 p.m. until
7 a.m. This does not necessarily mean that all this period should
be occupied in sleep; the ideal amount of sleep is 8 hours, but
very few adults require as much as this and many intellectual
people can do with but a few hours. The great essential about
sleep is that when it is in possession of a person it should be absolutely profound. Children require about 10 hours normally,
but again individuals differ and it is unwise to worry a child
about being " sleepyheaded."

Unfortunately modern conditions of life are such that in the
brain there frequently develops such a high pitch of activity
during the day that it is only with difficulty that the brain can
be put out of action at bedtime. Late hours, and especially late
meals, do not help this condition. All kinds of soporifics may
be tried, from the hop pillow to the hot drink (alcoholic or otherwise), from reading of a light novel to the taking of a hypnotic
drug, the last a habit far too common these days. But nothing
is so good for inducing sleep as a clear mind and a tired physical
frame and it is only a matter of habit to get into the way of
relaxation of all muscles and clarification of the compartments
of the brain. Nurses often have the trying task of looking after
patients with insomnia. These unfortunate persons must be
sympathetically dealt with and understood. Sleeplessness is one
of the outstanding problem diseases of this age; its cure is not
by drugs but by the elucidation of the pathological processes at
work in the mind and the nurse must make it her duty to try to
help to the best of her ability.

Adjuncts to Sleep.—Putting a sleepless patient to bed must
be a calm routine, with every element of excitement or dis-
quietude avoided. The nurse should see that the windows are
opened at the top and bottom sufficiently to allow a gentle
current of air to pass during the night. If there is any danger
of the room becoming cold, a gas fire should be left burning low.
The bed should be made inviting, with the sheets tightly drawn,
the pillows set so that the head is held easily and comfortably,
the blankets and quilt as light as possible but sufficient to retain
the heat. The patient should never have to complain of the
weight of the clothes. A hot water bag gives its maximum

benefit when it is put into the bed several hours before the patient retires. It is unwise to hurry the patient over undressing, and the night attire, pyjamas or nightgown, should be loose and easy, not of material that will cause the patient to perspire, but porous and yet warm. A hair mattress with spiral springs below is the best inducement to sleep. Feather beds are often stuffy and the weakly patient sinks too much into them, putting a strain on the muscles and spine. The blinds should be carefully drawn after the patient has been comfortably settled in bed. It is not wise to give the impression that a hasty departure of the nurse is contemplated. Often conversation may be kept up with advantage for 15 minutes, or the nurse may, by the simple expedient of holding the patient's hand, give the confidence and support that allows the passage from consciousness to sleep to be accomplished without hitch, and thus tide over a very critical period of muscular relaxation which precedes sleep and which is so often interrupted in cases of insomnia by active worries.

In some cases, a short sleep in the afternoon is good for people, especially babies and old persons. In healthy people it is not to be advised, but conscious relaxation for half an hour after lunch in those who lead a very active life is good for the mind, which may benefit from the release from routine activity.

Recreation

We have already mentioned recreation in a general way in connexion with exercise. Recreation, however, need not demand physical work. Most indoor games are mental exercises, employing and diverting the mind into side channels by functions which are the converse of the usual daily round. The ideal is to be found when mental and physical recreation are combined, as in some hobbies. Thoughts are thus distracted from the strain of serious brain work, and the cerebral cells are benefited by the change of circumstances.

Physical recreation implies an added zest owing to some mental stimulus, possibly a competitive one. It is distinct from "physical jerks" or routine development exercise which is the plain unvarnished method of improving the muscular tissue in a very uninspiring way. A game keeps all the qualities of mind and body on the *qui vive*. It stimulates people to accomplish something new, whether it be the lowering of a standard record or the winning of a team trophy, and in the achievement there is a natural satisfaction of the mind which is of the greatest utility in promoting happiness and mental welfare. All recreation should have this type of moral uplift, otherwise it belies its name, is a form of perversion and full of harm. It is the sporting spirit which makes for the consummation of the sound mind and the sound body.

Recreation for Invalids.—Even patients who are seriously ill require some form of recreation. It is a very important part of a nurse's skill that she should be able to devise entertainment for her patient suitable to the trouble. But the real benefit of games is apparent when the invalid has turned the corner and is hurrying towards convalescence; this is a critical period during which the nurse has to prevent the mind from dwelling too soon on the more serious things of life. Jigsaw puzzles, crossword puzzles, games of cards, patience, little odd jobs, rearrangement of furniture, flowers, pictures and hangings, wireless concerts, music of the right type (not, for example, the riotous competition of 3 raucous gramophones) and light reading, will help to spin out the day in easy stages. When convalescence comes gentle walking exercise may be followed by croquet, clock golf and so on, until a holiday may be arranged to complete the cure. Holidays should be completely free from worries about home or business, and the most important point is that all treatment should be at an end before they are begun. Routine should be abolished as much as possible, so that there is no curb on the natural bent of the holidaymaker. Those who do physical work may benefit by a quiet rest at the seaside, reading novels; those whose life is one round of mental activity will probably benefit most by fishing in the Scottish Highlands. A real holiday should mean a complete change of environment and action. The man who goes on holiday must go in the holiday spirit, otherwise it is of no use. Nurses may take these words to heart; when off duty, they should always try to leave every trace of their profession in the sickroom and make the most of their leisure, so that they return to their patient fresh and keen for further progressive work.

Amusements.—The lighter form of recreation is entertainment, which usually affects the risible qualities in us and makes us see the humorous side of life. The theatre, the cinema, sports, dancing and many other forms of amusement are of great value to a tired brain. The great thing to avoid is overdoing our pleasures. There comes a time when we are in danger of letting the film or the football hero interfere with our work, or dancing may be carried to excess, depriving us of sleep and bringing fatigue to our bodies which lasts until the next day. Moderate allowances of fun never do any harm; too much is a danger.

Hobbies, too, are of great importance, especially in neurasthenic or mild mental cases. Many pleasant and curative hours can be spent by a mentally tired lawyer in the garden, while engineers may occupy their sagging brains with problems of canary breeding. The essential principles of a successful hobby are that it is engrossing and progressive, showing some result which has as much good effect on the brain as building a famous bridge or conducting in a difficult case in a court of law.

Cleanliness

In the present age cleanliness has become so much a cult that it seems superfluous to discuss it, but there are degrees of being clean, and very often the thing that seems clean on the surface is dirty from a hygienic point of view. Dirt is very often hidden by colour, therefore the nurse must have a knowledge of how to look for it and how to deal with it if she is to be successful in keeping down disease and preventing sepsis. She should remember that so far as the body is concerned the inside as well as the outside should be kept in a state of cleanliness. Further, cleanliness is real beauty; no one will deny that the fresh complexion of the country girl is something of great artistic quality. Even the tramp knows that he feels a better man after his hot bath; the moral effect is of great tonic value; indeed if he had it oftener he would not be a tramp.

Surgical cleanliness is the ideal condition in which the microbes are either killed off or absent altogether. This perfect state is most difficult to reach, and the endeavours to reach it are responsible for all the complex manoeuvres of the aseptic and antiseptic treatment of the sick. Every nurse is expected to know the routine of the various systems in force; these are fully dealt with in subsequent sections of this work.

Normally, it is a standard of cleanliness of a house that all the dust, the superficial grease and any of the other non-fixed particles should be removed. Living conditions are at their best when the air of the room is fresh and " smells " clean and when the combined efforts of housewife, scrubbing brush, soda, soap and water have been fully successful.

The Skin.—Turning to personal hygiene proper, we deal first with the skin, which, above all other tissues, receives most attention from a cleansing point of view. Remembering that the skin is naturally covered with a greasy layer exuded from the sebaceous glands, that the sweat from the pores dries and leaves salts behind, that the hairs of the skin collect all kinds of grit and dirt, that germs revel in the thin fatty layer of the surface and that much of our skin is nowadays exposed to the outside air, we need no further evidence that cleanliness of the protective layer of our bodies is absolutely essential to health. If dirt is allowed to accumulate, the pores and the sweat glands become congested, the microbes multiply and inflammation of the skin (dermatitis) may result. We all know the unpleasant odour of the rancid sweat on an unwashed body and we also understand how easy it is for the armpits, the groins, the perineal regions and the webs of the toes to become dirty and irritated when they are not regularly washed.

Bathing and Washing.—In order to remove the ever accumulating film of greasy dirt which gathers on the skin, we use soap and water, reinforced by sponges, nailbrushes, flesh gloves, loofahs and similar toilet articles. Washing is a mechanical and chemical action, involving the dissolution of the fine fatty globules by the alkaline soap. In a good soap, the concentration of alkali is such that however long it is in contact with the skin, nothing but the grease is dissolved. Washing soda crystals, which are usually the main constituents of bath salts, are stronger and if used in great enough concentration will make the skin rough, tender and irritable, owing to epidermal erosion. In dealing with patients, therefore, nurses should always be very careful to see that the skin is not damaged in the daily cleansing. In this connexion, nurses may also be reminded that disinfectants, especially the lysol group, should always be tested first on a patient to see how the skin reacts. No two people are the same; some can stand strong soaps and disinfectants, others are upset by the finest soaps. Generally olive oil or palm oil is incorporated in the best soaps, so that when the grease is removed a fresh layer of very fine vegetable oil is left to take its place. Hard water is naturally more severe on the skin than soft water; the scrubbing involved in using a hard water is not good for the tenderest skins. It is well known that when the hands have remained for any length of time in water they become dry and shrivelled; this is due to temporary fluid loss from the skin and is soon put right. It is wrong to say that certain types of soaps dry the skin. This is not so; frequently they remove completely the grease from the epidermis, which feels dry, but if the normal exudation of sebum is going on, the skin will soon become greasy and smooth again. This is especially important in the scalp region. When the scalp is dry, it is not the fault of the shampoo, but usually of the individual, whose hair follicles and sweat glands are not working at proper flow.

Nothing is better for cleanliness than the daily bath. This is especially true in cities, and the pity is that there are not more facilities for town dwellers to have the whole of the skin washed once a day, or to enjoy the bathing rights of the ancient Greeks and Romans. It is possible to perform a toilet of the whole body by sponging all over, especially the folds of the skin, and everybody washes hands and face several times a day, but there is nothing to match immersion in a tepid bath, with an unlimited supply of soap and the scrubbing brush and sponge used to remove every particle of foreign matter from the skin. There are many opinions about the temperature of baths. Apart from the cleansing properties, the temperature is all important, since a cold bath stimulates the muscles and has a bracing effect on the system, whereas a hot bath opens the pores, dilates the superficial capillaries and allows the maximum activity of the skin for a certain time, ensuring efficient disposal of the waste products. The hot type of bath is ideally represented by the Turkish bath, while the cold bath is at its best in the cold spray so beloved of athletes, retired military men and other Spartans. The controversy rages over the pros and cons of hot and cold baths. A hot bath is pleasant, warming, relaxing, cleansing and soothing, but it may get rid of too much heat at a time, and may thus put a strain on the heart, besides causing shivering afterwards unless the person goes into a warm bed. A cold bath is stimulating, nerve activating and bracing to the muscles; its after effects are a glowing condition of the whole body, with tingling of the limbs and freshness of the mental outlook. The fact remains, however, that cold baths do not remove the dirt when the water is hard, and as hard water is very common in the most populous, and therefore the dirtiest, parts of England, they do not come within the category of practicability. It is recommended that a daily morning bath of a temperature of 90° F. should be taken, and if necessary, a cooling spray should follow. Everything depends upon the individual and the climate. It is impossible to dogmatize about the ideal temperature for the bath. It must be agreed that many of the so-called dangers of hot bathing are rarely experienced. In illness quite a different outlook must be taken; naturally the patient is in an abnormal state of health and the nurse must decide for herself what is most hygienic for her patient, having regard to all the circumstances of the case. Extremes should always be avoided.

While the full length bath is ample in the cleansing process, an additional spray is very comforting, especially in the cooling down process after a hot bath. Cheap rubber sprays, which can be fixed to both taps, and the temperature thus adjusted, can be purchased in all the large stores; they act as well as a fitted shower bath. In choosing a soap, some people like to have a carbolic, tarry or sphagnum moss soap; these serve different purposes and are all beneficial to the skin. After a bath, a brisk rub down with a large towel, special attention being paid to parts at which two skin surfaces are in apposition, and a final powdering of the folds of the skin with talcum are adjuncts which complete the cleansing process.

Toilet of the Hands and Feet.—One of the first things a nurse has to do when a patient comes into hospital is to cleanse his hands and feet. This process is of importance, and it is no light task which the nurse has to face. Often the skin of the hands and feet is hard and thick, corns abound, nails are long and full of dirt and in a fair number of cases the patient accepts his manicure and chiropody under protest. As a routine the hands should always be well scrubbed before a meal, the nails being cleaned with a blunt pointed pencil of solid bone. The "quick" of the nails should be carefully dealt with; if it grows too thick it may be trimmed, and by keeping it soft with fine oil any peeling can be avoided. The nails today are found in all degrees of culture from the vermilion claw to the shell-pink, neatly curved nail, with the cuticle carefully pruned to show the "half-moon" of the base. Many diseases can be carried by the nails, and a septic condition of the quick of the nail is most difficult to get rid of once it is established. In the toes, all hard skin should be cut away, corns should be softened and pared, and the nails cut as carefully as those of the hands. Cutting of the toenails horizontally has been found most beneficial in prevention of ingrowing toenail.

The Care of the Head.—Washing the face is a process demanding a certain amount of care, especially in frosty weather, as the skin may peel and show small sores. Every woman seeks a good complexion and has an excuse for the application of a delicate cream or lanoline product to the skin after washing, followed by a covering of good face powder of talcum or of orris root. It cannot be said that it is either healthy or necessary to paint the lily however. Those who adopt cosmetics on a lavish scale must stand up to the criticism of those who know that a woman with a good natural complexion is healthy and does not need to camouflage her face. Face washing, as we know from schoolday experience, is a matter of particular attention to the neck, the ears, the eye sockets and the nostrils. While every corner of the external ear should be cleansed, it is not wise to introduce too much water into the meatus as this may result in deafness and discomfort. The nostrils should be daily cleaned out with a pledget of fine gauze; city dwellers know that the nostrils need this attention badly. There is no need to use a douche, but vigorous blowing of the nose carried out morning and evening will have a splendid effect in clearing out all particles of dirt, soot and other foreign matter from the nasal passages.

The scalp receives far more attention today than formerly, and it must be admitted that from a hygienic point of view, short hair is better than long hair. Carrying out a routine shampoo of the scalp, either with soft soap or by using an alkaline and spirit lotion (dry shampooing) does the scalp much good. The tendency of the age is for the scalp to become easily congested and scaly with dandruff, which is simply a flaking of the layer of dirty grease from the surface of the head. If the hair is lifeless, lustreless and dry, it may be the result of lack of oil in the follicles or of defect of the sebaceous glands. A dry shampoo may clear the ducts and allow the flow to proceed, but sometimes it is necessary to rub in a little coconut oil. This, combined with careful brushing and combing twice daily, will stop itch in the scalp and prevent the tiresome knots and tangles so typical of bedridden patients. In children lice are a trouble sometimes, and they are not always the result of dirt; in fact a crop of lice may be found in a child obviously clean and well cared for. Generally, however, carelessness and sloth on the part of the mother are responsible for the condition, and the nurse may have a few hard days of fighting until the parasites are overcome. Parasites will not attack a head that is treated thoroughly with a fine comb twice daily (see p. 87).

Hygiene of the Mouth.—We should all brush the teeth twice daily, and some of us wash out the mouth and even gargle the throat as a routine measure. In the case of sick persons the toilet of the mouth is much more important, and it adds greatly to the comfort of the patient to have a clean mouth.

The Teeth.—These are of supreme importance. To ensure a perfect foundation of good teeth for the unborn child, all expectant mothers should have a daily diet rich in foods containing Vitamins A and D, and mineral salts, particularly calcium and phosphorus.

Breast feeding of the infant is best for teeth development, but if artificial feeding is resorted to, vitamin D, as contained in adexolin, halibut liver oil or cod liver oil, must be given.

For the everyday patient, the tooth brush should be used in all the corners, and the nurse should make sure that the dentifrice, which contains alkali, disinfectants and various other ingredients, gets right below the overlapping gums and between the teeth, where food may be held up and where microbes may breed. Septic teeth lead to caries, and many of the serious constitutional diseases can be traced to bad teeth. The organisms of pyorrhoea cause an inflammation with pus at the edge of the gums, and their toxins are very powerful when absorbed into the blood stream. The acids, derived especially from sugary and starchy foods which erode the enamel of the tooth, are neutralized by tooth pastes or by sodium bicarbonate, which acts equally well. On the back of the teeth it will be noticed that thin scales of yellowish black tartar may be found; these are derived from the saliva, and may require to be scraped at regular intervals by the dentist. It is a good plan to visit the dentist at least once every 6 months, since a routine inspection prevents either the onset of caries or the further advance of a septic process, which may be the starting point of a serious illness.

With certain people the care of the teeth is almost a fetish, but in some cases the teeth may bear evidence of rough usage. For instance, the hygienic enthusiast who believes in dealing with the teeth as a charwoman would deal with an office floor may score the enamel and wear it into tiny holes by rubbing in the gritty particles of a rough tooth paste.   Great care should be taken in selecting a moderately hard tooth brush with good bristles; when not in use it should be kept in a disinfectant solution.   In cleansing the teeth the movements should not be so much from side to side as up and down from the gum edges to the free margins; care should also be taken to clean the back of the teeth and the crowns of the bicuspids and molars.   Many dentists recommend the use of dental thread after each meal to clear out the debris which lodges between the teeth.   After the teeth have been cleaned a mouth wash may be used; this may contain thymol, sodium bicarbonate, potassium chlorate and other antiseptics and alkalis.   Detergent food e.g. apples, should be given last thing at night, especially to young children unable to use a tooth brush effectively.

The Throat.—Habitual gargling of the throat regularly is commonly carried out by those who spend their lives in a dusty or congested atmosphere.   By this process the back of the nose, the tonsils and the upper part of the pharynx are bathed in a disinfectant fluid, which thus mechanically and chemically removes disease producing particles and prevents the common cold, tonsillitis, pharyngitis, laryngeal congestion, influenza and many other ailments due to infection of this particular area.   Droplet infection is one of the chief sources of disease.   Handkerchief drill is now taught in schools, and children are trained to do all they can to prevent germs from passing from their mouths, noses or throats to the person or persons nearby.   Spitting in public places must be discouraged.

Internal Cleanliness.—Waste products are got rid of by internal methods in addition to those of the skin.   The solid excrement is discharged from the bowel; the liquid excretions collect in the kidney and pass out by the urethra; the lungs send out waste gases and surplus heat and moisture at each expiration.

Bowel Evacuation.—This should be a daily habit, although many cases have been recorded in which longer periods or shorter periods elapse without the slightest harm being done to the individual.   It is also impossible to lay down hard and fast rules regarding the time of the daily motion.   Patients should never be forced by the routine of the sickroom into having a motion at a given hour.   The reflexes of defaecation (already described in Vol. I, p. 222) must always act naturally and normally, and it may be very upsetting to a sick person to suffer the acknowledged discomforts of a bedpan motion when there is no desire to go to stool.   The subject of bowel regularity has already been treated.   A few remarks on constipation must be made now. Of all troubles affecting the civilized peoples, this is one of the worst, since it means the retention and decomposition of bacteria-laden matter in the lower part of the bowel. It is impossible to estimate how much of our present day illness starts from a sluggish colon; suffice it to say that a large percentage of the public apparently cannot exist without laxatives or purgatives, the constituents of which are sold by the ton. Constipation may cause acute symptoms, with pain, discomfort and sickness, and is soon dispelled by a brisk saline purge taken first thing in the morning. It is an experience of temporary disorganization common to all of us at one time or another. It is the chronic type of constipation which is the more serious, however; this produces in time a condition of sallow complexion, furred tongue, heavy breath, dull headache, lack of energy and general bodily and mental depression. These things are the forerunners of constitutional diseases such as rheumatism, gout, anaemia and so on, and they may be difficult to treat. For instance cases have been known in which there has been a partial daily evacuation, but the residue has done much harm. The aim must be to clear out the whole of the lower bowel.

Correct Breathing.—Deep breathing is often advised for health reasons, and it is beneficial to those who lead sedentary lives and do not have much exercise in the fresh air. The air going out and in should pass through the nostrils, as described already; this is the correct nasal breathing. Some people get into the habit of letting the air pass by the mouth (mouth breathing); this is often the result of nasal growths or of other obstructions, or, commonly in children, the natural sequence of adenoids, which block the back of the nasal passages and lead to all kinds of facial and constitutional changes owing to deficiency of normal air supply. Removal of tonsils and adenoids is of very little avail, unless the person, usually a child, is taught to breathe through the nasal passages.

Bladder Evacuation.—When the bladder reaches a certain state of distension, reflex action comes into play and urine is passed by the urethra until the organ is empty. Urinary regularity and normality are just as important to the patient as is bowel action. Frequency of passing urine varies very much; females can retain it longer than males, but cold weather, gravel, abnormal constituents and inflammation of the bladder and of the kidney may all affect the frequency, usually making it much greater. If there is any leakage or incontinence, the nurse must try to determine the cause by investigating the history of the case and finally having a specimen saved for examination by the doctor. Retention of urine is a very dangerous condition and it must never be allowed to continue for a moment longer than is necessary.

Clothing

The subject of dress has interests far reaching and complex; clothing has become for us a mixture of protection, screening, adornment, allurement and conventionality. It seems that we are naturally intended not to wear clothes at all i.e. if we compare ourselves with all the other animals. With enlightenment and education, the cultured human race appears to be slowly reverting to a condition of clothes restriction amounting in extreme cases to nudism. Much depends upon climate. Above a certain temperature, it is proved that we can comfortably and hygienically exist without clothes; below that temperature we need clothes, or at least we have to admit that we have not yet reached the measure of accommodation necessary to be able to react without harm to colder conditions of climate. There is undoubtedly an irrepressible tide flowing towards greater exposure of the skin to the sun; it is impossible to say how evolution will work in the future generations to affect the need or propriety of a covering for the body. The whole subject is intimately bound up in religion, tradition, custom and fashion, and any change will be made very gradually.

The physiology of heat regulation and the part played by the skin in heat loss (Vol. I, pp. 225 and 226) have already been discussed in full, and the student nurse is recommended to refresh her memory on these subjects before beginning the study of clothing dealt with below.

The Need for Clothing.—At certain temperatures heat loss from the body must be prevented; at others it must be increased. By putting coverings over the skin we conserve the heat; by removing them we allow the heat to diffuse: this is the simple rule of dress. Since we must maintain a very finely adjusted level of body temperature, whether we are in the heart of Africa or in the region of the North Pole, we are faced with two problems : 1. the question of the increase or limitation of the production of body heat (i.e. by work and food), and 2. the question of increase or decrease of surface loss of heat from the skin, from the breath and from the excretions. Of these the skin is far and away the most important structure involved, accounting for 80 per cent of heat loss (see Vol. I, p. 225). Rain, wind, direct rays from the sun and frost are all part of the heat regulating influences at work.

Clothing is also a shield against injury; boots protect our feet from the hard ground; our suits or dresses are worn to keep insects, plants, stones and furniture from damaging our skins.

Since the aspect of dress which comprises colour, design, decoration and propriety is essentially a cosmetic and not a hygienic matter, it can be left without further discussion. What is of more use to the nurse is a knowledge of the amount of clothing necessary and the texture and composition of the various fabrics.

Reasons for Clothing.—To understand fully why we wear silk or cotton or wool or linen next the skin, it is necessary to have a complete understanding of the way in which the heat rises from the body. We have learned of the insensible perspiration (Vol. I, p. 236) which constantly goes on normally. In conditions of nudity this is immediately absorbed into the air. When clothes are worn, much depends upon the type of clothing worn and the number of garments. Assuming that the perspiration becomes vapour and is absorbed into the air forming a layer close to the skin, it must be carried away. If our clothes are such that evaporation is checked (e.g. when we wear a rubber garment), the sweat collects and literally runs off our skins, making us uncomfortable and clammy. On the other hand, if the clothes are made of such calibre that they are absorbent and air holding, the moisture will gradually filter through as if it were in contact with blotting paper and so become lost in the outside air. This state of affairs would leave our skins dry and comfortable. It is a filtration process involving both conduction and radiation, because heat has a good deal to do with the sweat mechanism, which is increased on a hot day or in a hot room. What is most important, however, in the whole process, is the state of the fine layer of air next the skin. This must be kept dry and cool and therefore everything depends upon the fabric which lies over it. This is the reason why underclothing is of such fundamental importance to our general health. We have learned from history of the vagaries of fashion from decade to decade, we have seen the much beflannelled lady of the Victorian age give place to the scantily clad Diana of the present day, we have seen males shiver in greatcoats while females sweltered in flimsy garments, but all the time Nature has kept our normal bodily temperature at 98·4° F. The individual has adjusted the skin covering at all times to suit the need of the bodily heat regulation mechanism. While much depends upon early training, the Spartan upbringing and the like, it must be agreed that some people are like hothouse plants and influenced by the slightest change, whereas others are hardy trees, unaffected by the vagaries of weather. The mother who coddles her child with too many clothes and expects him to flourish when every limb is swaddled in tightly drawn napkins and binders, is much more primitive than the mother who turns her baby out for a sun bath with a small pair of pants round his middle. School children, too, are much better when their knees and their necks are bare. The wearing of a greatcoat by an active child may be as severe as a punishment to him. It is the fear of illness more than anything else that prompts the mother to overweight her child with extra garments. The great national movement for hiking in the open is a splendid one, since rational clothes are worn by thousands who less than 40 years ago might have been condemned for it. The benefit to health of the hiker's kit or of tropical wear is undeniably evident already; the race is likely to improve under its influence.

To sum up, clothing should be just sufficient to promote a comfortable warmth of the body and its weight must be adjusted accordingly. The more air there is in clothing the better.

Fabrics.—Generally speaking the most suitable fabric to wear next the skin is one which takes up moisture rapidly and which conducts heat badly. By this we are assured of conditions of maximum absorption and minimum heat loss. The best fabric is wool, manufactured from the sheep, camel or rabbit. Others are linen, made from flax specially treated by soaking of the fibres, silk from the silkworm, cotton (the fluffy material which is collected from the seed processes of the cotton plant), the modern artificial silk made by a chemical process and plastic yarns synthetically manufactured. The choice of fabric is governed by the nature of the garment. Comfortable clothes are not only light, warm and loose; they must also be free from irritating fibres which cause uncomfortable itching of the skin. Below are discussed the characteristics of each fabric, but it must be remembered that nowadays linen may be mixed with cotton, silk with wool and so on, depending upon the mood of the public for a certain type of garment.

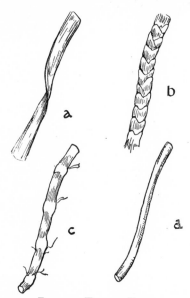

FIG. 31.—TEXTILE FIBRES.
a , Cotton. *b*, Wool. *c*, Linen. *d*, Silk.

Wool.—Wool is the warmest fabric. When a fibre of wool is examined under the microscope it appears to be scaly, with segments overlapping as shown in the illustration (Fig. 31). The sharp edges of these segments give the sawlike edge to wool which makes it intolerable to many with delicate skins. The natural grease of the hair is quite distinct in woollen fabrics, therefore for external garments it is protective against rain and for underwear it is warm. Further, although each fibre is slow to take up water owing to the coating of oil, woollen fabrics are openly woven, and thus water can be collected and held in the network until it is slowly absorbed by the outside air. Owing also to the fact that air is held in the meshes, wool is not a good conductor of heat, therefore taking all the properties into consideration, it is ideal for heat regulation of the body. The one disadvantage, well known to all housewives, is that woollen garments cannot be treated with boiling water or with washing soda, as they shrink owing to loss of the greasy elements. The fabric thus loses the most of its assets in this way; to prevent shrinking, rain water may be used in which to soak the woollen garments, which are afterwards washed in tepid water with a superfatted soap. The number of special soaps on the market for this purpose is sufficient evidence of its need.

Cotton.—The disadvantage of cotton is that its fibre (see Fig. 31) is like a sponge, absorbing water rapidly and getting rid of it as quickly. Since it is also a good conductor of heat it is not a suitable material for all weathers, as it is chilly to the skin. It is commonly combined with other fabrics, however, and its cheapness makes it very attractive to those with limited means. It is very satisfactory when used in the specially woven cellular form, in which the air is held by the net and cooling is not so rapid. In other forms cotton is used extensively for sheets, aprons, print dresses and many other garments. Its smooth surface makes it easily ironed and it always looks fresh; it is the most sanitary material for nurses' indoor dresses and aprons.

Flannelette.—Flannel is a form of woollen fabric; flannelette, however, is a type of entirely different composition. The materials are made from cotton, the fibres being left untrimmed so that a fluffy surface is presented. It is analogous to wool in its protectivity. Its combustible nature makes it dangerous, but it can be treated with 5 per cent alum solution and allowed to dry with this impregnation which makes it fireproof.

Linen.—Linen was formerly much in demand, but flax is so highly priced and so scarce that pure linen is regarded as a luxury. It is the " coldest " fabric of all, taking up water and heat quickly and as rapidly passing them on. It is used for tablecloths, sheets, napkins, handkerchiefs, but rarely for underwear, although certain firms manufacture linen in a mesh like cellular cotton. It is ideal for tropical suits and for dresses because it has a smooth surface and is glossy when starched, thus ensuring the minimum of dirt and all associated with it (Fig. 31).

Silk.—Silk is the most luxurious of all materials. The threads are spun by the silkworm, and when viewed under the micro-

scope they appear as very fine smooth fibres with very little tuft-
ing and very few " roots " (Fig. 31). Silk keeps in the heat but
does not take water up so well as does wool. Nevertheless it is
very pleasant on the skin, is light, does not shrink and is very
clean. Its high price is often value for the comfort and elegance
of the garment.

Artificial Silk.—Artificial silk has little in common with pure
silk, and is a poor substitute, except in appearance. It is manufactured by a special process of treating the cellulose of plants by
acids and it is produced on an enormous scale in Great Britain,
America and Japan. It is almost universally used for stockings
and underwear for ladies. It is not so good as silk, as it conducts
heat more quickly, and although its surface looks smooth and
silky, it has a hardness and heaviness which is not very agreeable
to those who have refined tastes in intimate garments. Nevertheless it has become established as an indispensable fabric for
those with a limited purse and has much to commend it.

Other Materials.—Other materials such as fur (which is warm
on account of the hair and skin of the animal being used and on
account of the ample supply of air), leather, felt, waterproof
material and similar examples are in a category which belongs
to the adjuncts of ordinary dress.

Plastic clothing may be summed up by saying that it is still
in the trial and error state.

Articles of Clothing.—Taking all the countries of the
world, the list of individual types of clothing is enormous and
our study must be limited to the dress of Great Britain. Boots
and shoes are made of stout prepared leather from the hides of
oxen or other animals; they are protective against the hardness
of the streets. Stockings may be made of wool or of artificial
silk for ordinary beings, but pure silk stockings are the per-
quisites of the rich. Outer garments may be made of wool in
different guises—serge, tweed and so on. It is better to avoid
any constriction at the waist or legs; for this reason tightly laced
corsets, which are less and less worn today, and garters, which
have given place to suspenders, are not to be recommended. All
clothing should hang from the shoulders if possible. This gives
freedom of circulation and muscular action. It should always
be borne in mind that efficient footgear, warm gloves and the
right kind of underwear should be *de rigueur* in winter, and
vanity must always be subordinated to health, for however un-
sightly a thick soled shoe and a rough woollen stocking may be
in comparison with a flimsy silk stocking and a high heeled shoe,
there is no doubt that the vagaries of the English winter demand
protection against wet feet. The danger of sitting in offices,
trams, buses or schools with thin soled shoes is very great and
leads to all sorts of debilitating troubles associated with the wet

and the cold. Another important hygienic point about dress is the need for careful fitting in footwear. Far too many people try to reduce their foot space to a minimum in the interests of neatness; this results in bunions, corns and foot deformity; properly a shoe should be fitted to a foot and tested by x-rays, which are installed in most big stores.

Undoubtedly, however, the most important articles of clothing are those collectively known as underwear. For the most part, they are worn next the skin, and as we have already learned, they must take up water quickly and lose heat slowly. In climates which do not have great extremes, the external clothing does not count so much as the underwear, which can be altered in texture, fabric and weight according to the season. Woollen material is the best, but the various examples of silk and wool, cotton and linen in cellular form, pure silk and artificial silk all have their adherents. It is certain that the open mesh linen and cotton fabrics are most comfortable and most useful from every point of view, and it is probable that they will yet go on to greater popularity. As in other matters, however, no two individuals are the same; dress may have certain fundamentals, but the superstructure may vary in thousands of ways to suit the wearer. Even the colour of clothes has an effect which is both physiological and psychological. Black absorbs heat and is sombre; white is coolest, and always looks clean and bright—this is one reason why it is the predominant colour in the medical world; green is soothing to the eyes, but certain forms of red are irritating.

Lastly the effect of a frequent change of clothing must be stressed. Clean clothing on a clean body has a remarkable moral effect which is most important from a mental point of view as well as from the physical aspect. Three days are normally sufficient for wearing an intimate garment, and if laundry expenses show a rising tendency they are amply compensated for by a sound mind and a sound body. To get into a change of clothing after work is over is especially beneficial to nurses. It removes all traces of the daily round and gives an air of newness and relaxation after the concentrated atmosphere of the day.

CHAPTER 6

PARASITES, INSECTS AND DISINFECTION

EXTERNAL PARASITES. LICE. THE HEAD LOUSE. THE
BODY LOUSE. THE PUBIC LOUSE. FLEAS. BUGS. THE
ACARUS. RINGWORM. INTERNAL PARASITES. CLASSI-
FICATION OF WORMS. CESTODES. NEMATODES. TREMA-
TODES. INSECTS. COCKROACHES. MOSQUITOES. THE
HOUSE FLY. THE TSETSE FLY. DISINFECTION. PRIN-
CIPLES. DISINFECTANTS. FUMIGANTS. INCINERATION.
BOILING. STEAMING. SICKROOM DISINFECTION.

A PARASITE is defined as a plant or an animal which lives on some
other plant or animal to the detriment of its host. In this
chapter the external parasites are dealt with first, then the
internal parasites (metazoa) and thirdly certain insects, which
although they are not, strictly speaking, parasites, are yet closely
associated with human beings and cause disease.

External Parasites

The common external parasites with which the nurse has to
deal in practice are lice, fleas, bugs, the acarus of scabies and the
ringworm organism, which is a vegetable parasite.

Lice.—On many occasions, when washing a newly admitted
hospital patient, a probationer nurse has become alarmed by
finding a small punctate rash all over the body. This may
resemble the rash of an infective disease but is well known as
evidence of the feeding ground of the body louse. Lice attack
three main regions—the head, the body and the pubic region,
and they vary in appearance according to their habitation.
They are usually associated with chronic dirt and low standards
of life, but they may attack very clean persons. They all have
the same dangerous and dirty habits and live solely on human
blood, to obtain which they have to bite the skin of the scalp
or body. In all wars they are the bane of the soldier and were
the cause of the spread of trench fever in World War I. They
have also been known to spread other fevers such as typhus fever
and relapsing fever, and they may also cause sepsis. The puncture of the skin causes great irritation (pediculosis) which results

86

in a form of nervous debility in children, chiefly the result of lack
of sleep. On examination, the skin is found to be covered with
these little spots and with angry looking scratches due to the
tearing of the epidermis. The whole condition is one of depression—the child looks pale, tired and generally " off-colour."
The poor constitutional condition does not help to overcome the
parasites and so a vicious cycle is frequently set up. Lice do not
breed from dirt, as many people imagine. The three types have
the individual characteristics described below.

1. *The Head Louse.*—This is a medium sized louse which
inhabits the hair of the head, sometimes including the eyebrows
(Fig. 32). The female of the species is about one-eighth of an
inch long and is slightly larger than the male. Her custom is
to crawl a short distance up the hairs and deposit a small egg
(known as a nit) on the surface of each, gumming it securely
with a special fixative made by the louse. If nits are left undisturbed, they will hatch out in 9 or 10 days' time. When many
nits are present, they are easily found as small
yellow-grey pinhead droplets on thin dry hair;
when the hairs are parted the parents are found
congregated below, usually closely fixed to the
scalp. Generally the scalp is covered with
small septic scabs. Cases may occur, however,
in perfectly clean persons in whom only one or
two lice and eggs are found, and often it is very
difficult to be sure of the diagnosis. The careful
use of a toothcomb may ultimately produce the
definite evidence sought for.

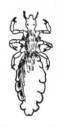

FIG. 32.—THE
HEAD LOUSE.

Lice can be avoided by adopting the following
rules of cleanliness:

1. Routine cleansing of the hair and body. A good disinfectant soap gives an effective shampoo.

2. Regular combing with a fine steel comb, and thorough
brushing should be carried out.

3. " Lethane Special," an effective hair oil, should be rubbed
in and left on the scalp for 10 days, when the hair is again
shampooed and tooth combed.

4. Regular daily inspection and combing should be carried
out.

In dealing with this type of louse, experience has proved that
close cropping of the hair is the only feasible remedy. Parents
and children object to this, but any temporization results in a
relapse. In all marked cases therefore the hair should be removed with the finest clippers, and it should be immediately
burned; the clippers are put into strong disinfectant or sterilized
by heat. The scalp should then be well shampooed with a lotion
containing a tarry disinfectant, washing soda, strong ammonia

and spirit.   When dry, it is advisable to put on for one night compresses of lint soaked in paraffin oil.   Next day the head is again shampooed and left dry, the child being kept out in the fresh air as much as possible.   It is usually necessary to destroy the headgear which has been worn.   The technical name of the head louse is *Pediculus capitis*.   Head lice may cause swelling of the lymphatic glands of the neck, also impetigo of the scalp, which is due to scratching followed by infection of the abrasions.

2.   *The Body Louse.*—The body louse, or *Pediculus corporis*, is bigger than the head louse, and usually lives in the area covered by the underclothing.   The eggs are laid in the folds and seams of the clothing, especially under the collar bands of shirts, and as in a fortnight one female louse can lay about 50 eggs, which hatch in 10 days, the multiplication is rapid.   The eggs are fixed to the fibres of the garment in the same way as the nits are attached to the hairs.   They are very resistant to the elements and can only be called safe when destroyed by fire or by great heat.   The young lice are hungry from the day of their birth and soon start sucking blood; they grow very rapidly to maturity, casting their skins several times in the 14 days before they reach the adult stage.

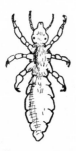

FIG. 33.—THE BODY LOUSE.

The small punctures (surrounded by a reddish ring which later is yellowish) are easily recognized, and when the seams of the underclothing are carefully searched, the eggs are visible.   The greatest difficulty may be experienced in clearing out body lice.   To detach the parents from the body is a matter of scrubbing vigorously all over with carbolic soap, but the nits require most complete destruction, otherwise disinfection fails.   In World War I special arrangements were made to delouse large numbers of men at a time, and the clothing was disinfected on a big scale, but usually the nurse has to deal with one or two only, and probably the best way to treat the condition is to bathe the patient as above and then to take the undergarments and iron the seams carefully with a hot iron.   The eggs are destroyed and the garment can be washed immediately afterwards.   Often it is an economy to destroy the clothing altogether.   In hospitals the usual methods are those of sterilization in an autoclave such as the Thresh disinfector.   There are various fumigants and sprays on the market, depending upon formalin, sulphur or paraffin for their disinfectant properties, but the louse is a parasite that does not succumb easily and it must be treated by drastic measures.   Many powders are on sale for the prevention of these pests; some contain ground camphor or menthol.   D.D.T. has been used in many ways, especially in the armed forces, and with success. The powder was one of the chief weapons adopted by the U.S. Army in the typhus epidemic in Naples; epidemic louse borne typhus is a fever markedly contagious and spread by the louse. For the disinfection of clothing and books, naphthalene is very good. Persons who are daily occupied in delousing patients can be protected against typhus by Cox's vaccine. It should be remembered that the body louse also transmits relapsing fever, trench fever and pustular dermatitis.

3. *The Pubic Louse.*—Known also as *Pediculus pubis*, or the crab louse, this parasite infests the hair of the pubic region, of the perineum, of the axilla and even of the eyebrows. It is the smallest louse of the three, being almost invisible. It causes a great deal of troublesome irritation, however. The best way to get rid of it is to shave off the hair completely and rub in mercury ointment for a day or two. Careful lathering of the affected regions with a tarry soap twice daily will be of great assistance.

The skin may be severely affected, as the scratching is often strong enough to draw blood; the appearance of the crab louse is the reason for its name (Fig. 34); it clings very tenaciously. On the eyebrows, the use of yellow oxide of mercury ointment is sufficient to kill the lice and their eggs. The pubic louse does not transmit any specific infection.

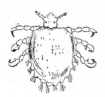

FIG. 34.—THE CRAB LOUSE.

Fleas.—While the flea, as compared with the louse, may be said to pay only a flying visit to the body, the damage done and the severity of the symptoms make it much more intolerable. Some people are more attractive to fleas than others. In very susceptible persons, a series of fleabites may be shown as a group of prominent wheals, with a small central depression to mark the bite. Two types of flea are known: 1. the human flea (*Pulex irritans*), and 2. the rat flea (*Pulex cheopis*). The latter is responsible for carrying many diseases, particularly from ships, and is known as the carrier of bubonic plague. The annual Rat Week is of great importance, especially concerning rats in harbours and docks, which are known to carry numerous rat fleas. These fleas normally live on the blood of rats. If one rat is stricken with plague bacilli, the flea swallows some of the blood and continues to live on the rat till the latter dies. But fleas do not like cold, and thus an infected flea may reach a human being and so inoculate the dangerous bacilli either by biting the skin or by rubbing in its faeces which are swarming with germs. The warning sign of an epidemic of bubonic plague among human beings is the discovery of numerous dead rats at

various ports.   The house rat does not spread bubonic plague.
Unlike the louse, the female flea does not fix her eggs to the
host.   They are deposited singly, often on the ground, and on
the bedclothes.   In a house in which dirty persons live the flea
has thus peace to breed; it is never
prosperous in the hygienic home.   The
eggs are variable in their incubation
period.   Some hatch in 72 hours, but
when the atmosphere is cold they may
be delayed for as long as 14 days.
There is a larva stage of another fortnight and a cocoon stage of a further
fortnight, at the end of which the young
flea begins his activities proper.   Fleas
are therefore more easily got rid of, since
by destroying all dust and dirt, there is

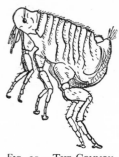

FIG. 35.—THE COMMON
FLEA.

a good chance of disposing of the
larvae.   Fumigation is most efficiently
done by using formalin, the room being
carefully sealed up and fumigated for 3 or 4 hours.   Another method involves the burning of sulphur, but in an average
room about 6 lb. of sulphur are required.   After fumigation, the
most extensive cleaning of the room must be done, in which the
boards are scrubbed with a disinfectant solution consisting of
1 in 1,000 perchloride of mercury, or of lysol in the strength of
one teaspoonful to the pint of hot water.   Sometimes it is advisable to spray the room for a few days with 5 per cent paraffin
solution in soft soap and water, or to spread naphthalene freely
over the floor and other wooden parts of the room, leaving the
latter shut up for a week.   In dealing with the flea, we must
keep in mind that it is elusive and resistant.   It can jump as
much as a foot, and has been known to exist for 3 months without
food; the larval and cocoon stages may also be extended up to
2 or 3 years.   If the flea itself cannot be found, the evidence of
the wheal or of the blood stained excrement on the garments or
bedclothes is a positive sign.

Bugs.—Known technically as *Cimex lectularius*, the bed bug
(Fig. 36) is flat and somewhat resembles a beetle.   It has a very
sharp, powerful beak, which it uses with effect on its victims,
sucking a considerable quantity of blood through its proboscis
at each stab.   This gives the body a brownish red tinge.   Bugs
prefer to remain hidden in corners all day, coming out from
behind wallpaper, skirting boards or mattresses to feed at night.
They are the cause of rapid deterioration of the houses affected.
Their presence is the index of the quality of housekeeping and
management.   Domestic cleanliness beats the bug in the long
run.   Infants are chiefly affected.   The presence of bugs may

be detected by a typical smell associated with them. When they bite, it is not the mild gnawing of the louse or the prick of a flea; it is something which is decidedly stabbing, and the pain remains in the wound for some time. There are not any known diseases conveyed by the bed bug. The female lays her eggs in cracks in the walls or between floorboards; about 150 are deposited. In about a week hatching takes place, and after a further 6 weeks the adult stage is reached. Bugs, like fleas, can go for a long time without nourishment; 6 months' starvation will not kill them. The disinfestation methods are much the same as those for fleas. Cleansing of the house with scrubber, soap and water, also use of oil of

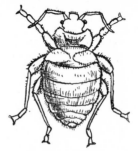

FIG. 36.—THE BED BUG.

pyrethrum and paraffin in an insect sprayer, are to be recommended. In addition, fumigation with hydrocyanic acid is advocated, but it must be carried out by trained sanitary officers, who are able to control its strong poisonous fumes.

The Acarus.—The itch mite, or *Acarus scabei*, is the organism which, by burrowing into the surface of the skin, causes the common itch, or scabies. It is very easily transferred from one person to another or from wood to the skin, and it does not necessarily have an association with dirty conditions. The full description of the disease and its treatment is given later on (Vol. III, Sect. 8 chapt. 16). The eggs are laid in the tunnel bored by the female, which is rather like a small spider, and just visible to the naked eye. The eggs hatch in a week, and by the end of another 3 weeks they are mature. One female may have about 4 broods, after which she dies. New females have taken her place, however, so that scabies is a progressive disease, associated with severe itching, worst at night when the person becomes warmed up in bed or when sitting at the fire. The sites chosen for the tunnels are usually the wrists, webs of the fingers, the buttocks, axillae and groins, and the palms of the hands in infants. Usually the great scratching produces septic spots and general dermatitis, a condition of inflammation of the skin with pustules. Skin ointments containing sulphur, sphagnum moss preparations and zinc oxide were formerly used. The most modern form of treatment is briefly as follows. The affected person should first of all have a hot

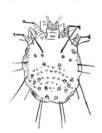

FIG. 37.—THE ACARUS OF SCABIES.

bath, followed by the application of benzyl benzoate emulsion, preferably applied with a fine brush. Twenty-four hours later, the patient should have another hot bath, and after thorough drying, should have a complete change of underwear.

Ringworm.—There are several varieties of the ringworm parasite, which is a vegetable and not an animal. The spores affect the cores of the hairs or their outer layers, resulting in the establishment of circular areas, forming the rings of the disease, in which the hairs are brittle and broken off, like a patch of long grass that has been roughly cut and trampled on. Both animals and human beings may be affected, and the trouble is most contagious, often occurring in several members of the family at one time.

Of especial interest is this disease in school children. The medical authorities usually undertake the treatment, since it demands careful supervision for several months, with isolation of the patients from other scholars. The x-ray treatment has proved of great value. The initial doses of x-rays cause the hair to fall out completely. This is followed by a luxuriant growth of new hair, which is often curly and quite different from the previous crop. By a special method of investigation, in which Wood's glass (a medium which shows up any infected hair as phosphorescent in appearance) is used, the arrest or progress of the disease can be determined. It is essential to go on with treatment as long as there is a single hair showing the presence of the parasites.

Internal Parasites

The metazoa represent a large and important class of internal parasites which are commonly called worms, and which are much more prevalent than is generally believed. About a dozen worms of various types are known to be prevalent in Great Britain, and many more exist in tropical countries, but the following table includes all the metazoa about which nurses should have some knowledge.

Classification of Worms.—
    (a) *Cestodes* (*Tapeworms*):
        1. Taenia solium (the tapeworm of pork).
        2. Taenia saginata (or mediocanellata) (the tapeworm of beef).
        3. Diphyllobothrium latum (dibothriocephalus latus) (the tapeworm of fish).
        4. Echinococcus granulosis (taenia echinococcus) (the hydatid tapeworm).
    b) *Nematodes* (*Roundworms*):
        1. Ascaris lumbricoides (the common roundworm).

2. Enterobius (oxyuris) vermicularis (the threadworm).
3. Anchylostoma duodenale (the hookworm).
4. Trichinella (trichina) spiralis (the muscleworm).
5. Filaria (the bloodworm).
6. Dracunculus medinensis (the guineaworm).
7. Trichuris trichiura (trichocephalus dispar) (the whip-worm).

(c) *Trematodes* (*Flukes*) :
1. Schistosoma haematobium (the bloodfluke).
2. Fasciola hepatica (the liverfluke).

Only those important to the nurse are fully dealt with in the following pages. The full classification is given on account of the fact that often nurses who go abroad may have to deal with a worm infection, and the table given above, together with the notes below, may be of assistance to her in an emergency.

Cestodes.—The general characteristics of tapeworms are flat, long, narrow ribbon-like formations consisting of a " head " and several hundred segments. There is no real mouth or alimentary canal, and each segment, or proglottis, contains rudimentary male and female sexual organs, so that the worm is a hermaphrodite. The cestodes exist by fixing themselves by suckers and hooks to the lining of the intestine of an animal. The upper segments are immature, but as we trace them down the length of the worm, we find that gradually they become mature, fertilized and full of eggs,until at the " tail " of the worm there are many ripe proglottides, ready to be cast off in the motions of the host (Fig. 38). Preventive measures may be summarized as follows:

1. Meat inspection carried out very thoroughly; 2. cold storage of meat; 3. salting of meat; 4. thorough cooking of all foods.

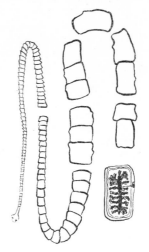

Fig. 38.—Tapeworm, show-ing essential segments springing successively from the minute head. A pro-glottis is shown in detail.

Taenia solium.—In the human being, this worm is usually found in the duodenum. When the adult is recovered intact it is found to consist of a bead like head, provided with 4 circular suckers, and 2 rows of hooklets with about 14 in each row, for fixing the minute head to the intestine. In colour it is dirty white or faint yellow.   Sometimes it reaches a total length of 10 feet, but 6–8 feet is quite common.   The proglottides vary from 500–1,000.   The existence of the worm depends upon its contact with the intestinal lining by the tiny headpiece.   The expelled mature segments are very resistant to the elements and may keep their eggs alive for many days.   Generally they are unaffected by damp grass or other herbage, and as they lie on the ground they may be eaten by a pig.   In this way the second stage of their career is ensured.   The eggs develop to a certain extent in the pig; the main point is that their capsules are dissolved by the gastric juice and the small embryos project themselves through the wall of the bowel, ultimately reaching the muscles of the pig by the blood stream.   In the muscles, they again become encysted, living as partly developed tapeworms, with head and neck only.   Pork which is badly infected with these embryos is said to be " measled."   When this meat is not properly cooked or when it is eaten in a semi-raw state, the embryos are transferred to the human intestine and begin to form their proglottides, so the whole routine starts all over again (Fig. 38).

In treating a patient for this trouble, we can be sure of stopping the irritation of the bowel, the colic, diarrhoea and the worry of the condition, if we concentrate on the removal of the all-important head.   This can be done in various ways, most of which are dependent upon the following system.   The principle is the emptying of the bowel first by purging and starvation, then the giving of a special antidote (e.g. liquid extract of male fern, carbon tetrachloride, oil of chenopodium), but the motions must be very carefully examined in order that the head may be discovered, and since it is about the size of a large pinhead it is better to have expert advice as to its identity.   It is hygienic to have all the segments disinfected in strong lysol, as they can infect the human being on occasion.   Special attention should be paid by the nurse to the cleansing of the hands after attending to a patient with tapeworm.

Taenia saginata.—This parasite occurs all over the world, but is the commonest tapeworm in Great Britain.   There is little or no difference in the life cycle of this worm from that of the T. solium, except that the beef tapeworm spends its intermediate stage in the flesh of the ox, commonly in the tongue, so that it is frequently transferred to the human intestine, where it behaves exactly as the T. solium.   In appearance the beef tapeworm is very like the pork worm.   It has no hooklets but has 4 suckers, and its length may reach over 20 feet, with 1,200–1,500 segments.

Diphyllobothrium latum.—This type is spread by fish, chiefly pike, perch, salmon and trout, and is common in Russia, Switzerland, Japan and Sweden, but occasionally reaches Great Britain.   It is the longest cestode, often reaching 30 feet and showing 4,000 segments. A rather severe type of anaemia may be caused by this parasite. In order to avoid it we should ensure that all fish are well cooked.

Echinococcus granulosis.—This cestode is very different from the above three. In the first place, it passes only its intermediate stage in man. Secondly, it is very small (about quarter of an inch) and has only 4 segments in all. Nevertheless it is easily the most virulent and dangerous of the group. The last segment contains the ova, and is about eighth of an inch long. The adult worm lives in the intestine of the dog or sheep. The head is fixed to the bowel lining by a headpiece with typical barbed hooklets and 4 suckers. When the dog passes the mature proglottis, the latter may reach the sheep by the grass, or be conveyed to man by water. The embryos burrow through the intestinal wall and ultimately reach some organ (very commonly the liver, but the lungs, kidney or brain may be the chosen site) and there cavities known as hydatid cysts are formed. The ova give rise to tiny embryos, each a headpiece provided with 6 barbed hooklets, and they live in a cystic fluid which is manufactured from the inner wall of the cyst. One cyst may bud from another until the organ is a mass of cavities as big as a golfball; the contents are swarming with undeveloped headpieces and sometimes sepsis occurs. If the dog eats offal of the sheep thus infected, he carries on the next stage of development. Dogs are therefore rigorously excluded from slaughterhouses. Hydatid disease in man is almost always fatal (Fig. 39).

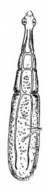

FIG. 39.—THE HYDATID WORM, *Echinococcus granulosis*, WITH ITS 4 SEGMENTS.

Nematodes.—In this group there is differentiation into male and female types, an alimentary canal exists, the worm is not segmented and it tapers usually at both ends. In many respects the nematodes resemble the earthworm. The female worm is slightly larger than the male.

Ascaris lumbricoides.—There is very little difference between this worm and the earthworm; it is rather lighter in colour. It may be found in the intestines of both man and the pig, but it is occasionally found in school children and is a worry to parents, although it may not give rise to serious symptoms. The worm may be about 10 inches long, usually 8 inches. The source of the eggs, which are laid by the female in the upper part of the intestine, are the vegetables or water they may reach (e.g. from sewage). In children the eggs may be transferred by the fingers or by clothing. When swallowed, the eggs lose their capsules in the usual way, and the larvae reach the lungs or liver by the blood stream. In the lungs, for instance, they pierce the alveolar wall, crawl through bronchioles, bronchi, trachea and larynx, and then may be swallowed again, to complete the cycle (Fig. 40).

The specific anthelmintic is santonin, usually given at night for 3 successive nights, followed by calomel.

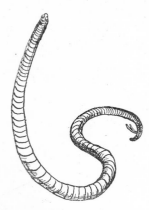

FIG. 40.—MALE ROUNDWORM. Note copulatory spicules in the curved tail.

Enterobius vermicularis.—No nurse can call herself experienced unless she has had to deal with a case of threadworms, and when a whole family of children is affected, the task of getting rid of these small parasites is no light one. The threadworm is the commonest form of intestinal parasite in Great Britain and it also infests children in all parts of the world. Thousands are yearly attacked, and the condition is usually well established before it is suspected. It is commonest between the ages of 2 years and 10 years, and is marked by great irritation of the anus, enteritis, nervousness of the child, dry skin, hollow eyes, voracious appetite which is never satisfied and a general appearance of debility which designates a " wormy " child. Hundreds of small white worms are found in the stools, like short broken cotton threads, $\frac{1}{8}$ inch to $\frac{1}{2}$ inch long. The female is about four times bigger than the male. The caecum and rectum are commonly infested. It is thought that the female lays her eggs round about the anus, from which they are transferred by children's nails to the stomach. The mature worm reaches the caecum in 2 weeks. The eggs are very much more resistant than is generally known, and they may reach the gallbladder, but usually they collect in the folds of the large intestine. Although a stool may show only one or two threadworms, it does not mean that the infection is a mild one; the eggs may be present in hundreds. There are various remedies, many of recent discovery and some too potent for the human being. Those now of proved efficiency are mercury (given internally and externally), quassia or common salt enema, gentian violet, hexylresorcinol and tetrachlorethylene. So far as drugs are concerned, the prescribing of these must be in the hands of the doctor, who will choose the remedy most suitable in the case. Scrupulous care must be taken with the child's hands and body. Gloves should be worn at night by all infested children. Calico linings should be worn both in the knickers and sleeping suits, and should be freshly laundered for each change—night or morning. The finger nails should be cut short.

Anchylostoma duodenale.—The hookworm is very common in tropical countries, especially in India, South America and Egypt. The female measures a little over half an inch, the male just under half an inch. They have strong hooked teeth with which they fix themselves to the jejunum; they are blood suckers, and may cause severe anaemia. The eggs are passed out in the faeces, and rapidly hatch out into a larval stage which may persist for several months. In this state they reach the intestines again either by being ingested with food or drink, or by the devious route through the skin. The latter is worth our study. In certain places (e.g. in tunnels) in the damp parts of mines or in the tropical plantations, the larvae become fixed to the skin of the hands or the feet. The disease is known as tunnel disease or coolie ground itch. The latter title is due to the fact that the barefooted coolies of the tropics pick up these larvae in the webs of their feet and become affected with a very itchy condition of the skin, like scabies. The larvae pass through the skin, into the lymph vessels, then into the inferior vena cava, the right side of the heart, pulmonary capillaries, alveoli, bronchioles, bronchi, larynx, mouth and so back to the intestine: a very long journey, and bound to be debilitating to the host. The symptoms are due to the itch and to the severe anaemia. Preventive measures are adopted in most districts.

Trichinella spiralis.—Once again the pig is responsible for the transmission of a worm to man, but the rat also harbours the trichinella. There is thus the possibility of a double source of infection, since rats inhabit piggeries. This worm is rare in Great Britain. The female lays about 1,000 eggs, which are in the form of tiny embryos. The latter pierce the wall of the bowel, reach the muscles and form little cysts, in which they curl up like spirals, and they may remain in this larval state for many months. The muscles become dotted with these small white points. If semi-raw pork is eaten, the embryos develop in the human being, and a similar condition of the muscles arises, only the human being suffers acutely from fever and severe cramp-like pain in the muscles, which may show many calcified cysts. Advanced cases may show millions of small cysts. The remedy is the cooking of all pork thoroughly.

Filaria.—The filaria group contains several types, the most important of which is the *Wuchereria bancrofti*, very common in the tropics, but unknown in Great Britain. The female is about 3 inches long. Mosquitoes are responsible for the transmission of the filaria, which normally breeds in the lymphatic glands of the human being and which may be so numerous that the lymph channels become blocked, and the condition of elephantiasis is produced. The hatched embryos live in the lung capillaries by day, but come into the peripheral vessels by night. This is interesting, since it is a night mosquito which takes some of them away when it bites a sufferer from filariasis.

Dracunculus medinensis.—This worm is unknown in Great Britain, but in India it is found in water carriers, and it also occurs in other tropical parts. The female guineaworm is about 3 feet long and only 2 millimetres broad, so it is like a thick thread. The female can crawl through the body until she emerges from the skin, usually at a limb, where she can be sure of contact with water. This having been achieved, she liberates her eggs, which are taken from the water by a crustacean, which in turn is swallowed by man and so the embryo finds its way back to the subcutaneous tissues.

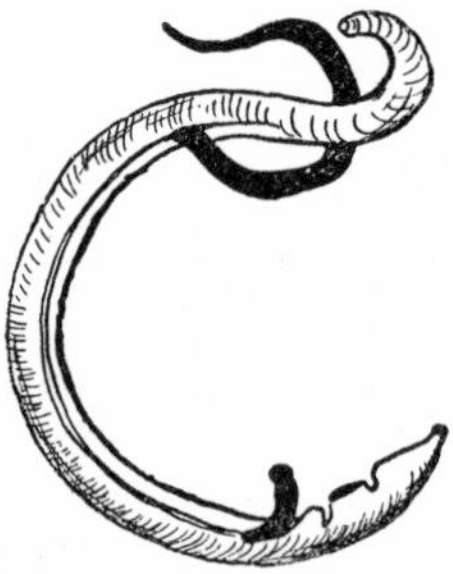

FIG. 41.—BLOODFLUKES
(MALE AND FEMALE).
The black female is lying in the gynaecophoric canal of the male.

Trichuris trichiura.—This worm is about 2 inches long, and inhabits the large intestine of man. It is supposed to resemble the lash of a whip. It seems to do no harm, as it does not produce any symptomatic evidence of its presence.

Trematodes.—Flukes are found in man in the bisexual and hermaphrodite state. All of these parasites require an intermediate host, and all are flat and shaped like a leaf. Most have two suckers, with which they are attached to their host. Their alimentary system is branched.

Schistosoma haematobium.—The bloodfluke is found in North Africa and inhabits the veins, especially those near the bladder. The eggs have sharp points, and pierce the bladder, causing punctate haemorrhages which result in bleeding from the bladder into the urine. The ova, when they reach water, hatch out into embryos, especially sought after by a freshwater snail. Finally, the embryos, having developed a strong tail, leave the snail, penetrate the skin of a human being and thus reach the veins, where they mature. Mating takes place, the male, lighter in colour and slightly shorter, enfolding the black female in the gynaecophoric canal (Fig. 41) and taking her along with him until the smallest veins are reached. At this point the female goes on alone and deposits her eggs.

Fasciola hepatica.—Liverflukes also use the freshwater snail as an intermediate host. They affect sheep, causing liver-rot.

Insects

The part played by insects in the spread of disease is now re-cognized to be a very big one. Bacteria may be carried by the insect on its legs and proboscis, but sometimes the organism is carried about in its stomach and stored until an appropriate time arrives for the inoculation of a victim. Although the house-fly is not a blood sucker, it is capable of spreading disease from cesspool and garbage heap to larder and to living-room, and therefore it is as much a danger as the mosquito or the tsetse fly, which both spread dangerous diseases by sucking blood through a puncture in the skin of a human being. In Great Britain there are very few mosquitoes and no tsetse flies, since the climate, except in the south-west, is too cold. In certain of the Home Counties and near the streams, gnats and mosquitoes may be a nuisance by causing very irritating bites, which itch for several days afterwards, but there are only a few instances of fatal insect bites every summer, and we can say with certainty that the blood suckers are negligible. The fly, however, is a real menace to health, especially in a heat wave. The chief insects affecting health are mentioned below.

Cockroaches.—A plague of cockroaches is a serious thing in any household, because not only do these insects eat up large quantities of food, fabric, leather and other material of domestic value, but they have a habit of concealing themselves behind hot pipes and of getting well established in most inaccessible places. A cockroach may be quite an inch long. These insects usually come out at night and swarm over kitchens and larders. The method of killing them is by fumigation, but domestic minds are more primitive, and a mixture of flour and plaster of paris put out on the floor, with a handy saucer of water nearby to slake the thirst, is a barbaric ruse which is successful. Fermented and strong-smelling beer in a bowl, reached by a small inclined plane, also results in many casualties. D.D.T. powder may also be used.

Mosquitoes.—Two main varieties of mosquito are known, the *Culicini*, which are mostly harmless, and the *Anophelini*, which are the spreading agents of malaria and which are very rarely found in England. They are very like each other, being of most delicate construction with fine wings and very thin legs (Fig. 42). The female mosquito is the only danger to human beings since she is provided with a very sharp proboscis, capable of piercing deeply into the subcutaneous tissues when she searches for the blood which she requires while forming her eggs. The males live on the leaves of plants and on flowers. The female lays her eggs on a stretch of calm water, such as a stagnant pool or marsh; they may be found in groups. The larval stage is reached in 4 or 5 days, and the larvae are very active, moving about rapidly and eating hungrily; the insect may exist from a fortnight to several months in this stage, generally 14 days. The next stage is that of the pupa. This lasts less than a week. The pupa does not feed, but can breathe and move. Finally, the imago emerges and flies off to spend the rest of his short life, usually about 3 months. In suitable circumstances of climate the whole process from egg to imago takes 3 weeks (see Fig. 42). One type of culicine is the causative insect of yellow fever, about which so much research has been done. The anophelines have been identified in various parts of the country, but whether they inoculate us with the malaria parasite or no, we are safeguarded by the fact that in about 2 years the organism dies off in our blood. The climate of Great Britain is not kindly disposed towards malaria. Abroad, the disease is rampant in many places at which swamps exist or where improper drainage is the rule. Very satisfactory results have followed the drainage of waterlogged areas, and it is hoped to stamp out malaria altogether, but recurring epidemics have proved the need for much fresh research and new remedies. If a pool is sprayed with fine oil, the larvae may be suffocated. Various sprays in which pyrethrum, kerosene and other destructive drugs are employed have been used with success in houses, airplanes, camps and living quarters and offices. In malarial countries, no one would think of going to sleep without drawing round the mosquito net of fine gauze.

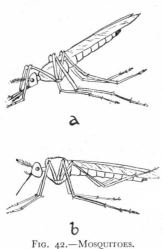

FIG. 42.—MOSQUITOES.

a, Anopheles, which carries malaria, with its typical tilted posture.

b, Culicida, does not convey malaria, and has horizontal posture.

The most serious aspect of malaria is its recurrences, which cause a high temperature for a certain number of days, corresponding to the changes going on, in the blood, of the malaria parasite. As each cycle is complete, the temperature rises and continues to do so every 3 or 4 days according to the type of parasite. In the more complicated varieties of malaria, it is essential that the undeveloped parasites should spend a period in the stomach of the mosquito. This is accomplished, and when ready the ripe parasite is brought back to the mouth of the mosquito and inoculated into the first victim bitten. Malaria is thus easily spread. A great amount of research has been done, and great progress achieved in the treatment of malaria, but it will be understood that discussion of this does not come within the province of hygiene.

The House Fly.—*Musca domestica* (the house fly) is of greatest importance because it is the most dangerous in the spread of disease. The structure of the house fly is shown in Fig. 43 and it will be seen that the feather-like feet and the long proboscis are ideal for the spreading of germs of disease.

Life History of the Common Fly.—Flies revel in dirt, and therefore their breeding place is the midden, the garbage heap and the dunghill. They appear to have an affinity for all forms of excreta, human included.

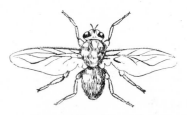

FIG. 43.—THE HOUSE FLY.
The fine hairs all over the body make germ transport easy.

The female deposits over 100 eggs in batches on moist filth, teeming with bacteria. The eggs can be recognized as white, sticky spindle shaped bodies occurring in clumps; 4 or 5 days after they are laid, the maggots are born. Within a week, during which they feed on the manure in which they lie, the latter are fully developed and they then go into the pupa stage, which lasts for another week. The fly crawls out, dries his wings and makes for the first larder. The rest of his life depends upon the hygienic education of his hosts. If he escapes the numerous devices to trap him, he may live just over a month. His best period is from July to September. In October the frost or a special fungus kills him off. Those who are destined to carry on the race do so in a pupa stage which resists the winter cold. It is thus almost impossible to stamp out the house fly, but it can be well controlled.

Dangers of Flies.—The fly is an ideal transport wagon for bacteria. His natural habitat is manure, and since no other matter is so suitable for germs, every time a fly alights it spreads a trail of microbes. But more than this happens. When a fly spends any time on a piece of meat or a bowl of milk it has a habit of bubbling its previously swallowed food through its mouth, therefore it leaves a filthy mess of microbes wherever it goes. In addition, it almost invariably defaecates and so leaves a further source of disease behind. In every way, then, flies are a menace to health. No matter how clean our houses may be, an invasion of flies soon transforms every part into a potential breeding ground for germs. The well known bluebottle fly is not so dangerous from a germ point of view as from the fact that it deposits its eggs on meat or even on an open sore, and maggots may hatch out in a few days. It has been proved that typhoid fever, paratyphoid fever, dysentery, summer diarrhoea of children and cholera can be spread by flies. They are always a danger to milk, which is an ideal medium for the breeding of microbes.

Fighting the Fly Menace.—There are three ways of getting rid of flies: 1. by preventing the breeding; 2. by killing the adult; 3. by protecting the food. It has already been mentioned that it is almost impossible to remove the fly from our midst. Numbers can be reduced, however, by keeping all dustbins covered, by covering up all excrement and by spraying manure heaps with oil or a disinfectant solution. Most of the advertised fly sprays are basically composed of formalin, paraffin or D.D.T. Burning of refuse (as described on pp. 46 and 47) is another method of prevention of breeding of flies. The fly itself may be trapped by simple devices such as the sticky papers universally sold, and made by smearing a mixture of castor oil and hot resin on sheets of glazed paper. Many fly papers are now impregnated with D.D.T., but it is essential that the fly, once it reaches the paper, should be held there. Various traps are also in use. Wire fly whisks mounted on long handles are sometimes employed when the flies are actively moving about. Finally, all foodstuffs should be kept in safes, refrigerators or larders, protected if necessary by fine muslin gauze. Milk should never be left uncovered. Most people find that a square of muslin weighted down by beads is satisfactory to put over the milk jug. Wire cages should always be placed over cold meats and anything of a perishable nature. The more larders and safes are scrubbed out the better. Condy's fluid is useful for floors and stone shelves; lysol is rather strong-smelling for the larder.

The Tsetse Fly.—This fly carries the trypanosome of sleeping sickness in the hot parts of Africa. Sleeping sickness is a tropical disease in which the victim is very drowsy and may be actually asleep or in a state of extreme torpor. This must not be confused with " sleepy sickness," or encephalitis lethargica, which is found, in Great Britain, and which is due to a microbe.

Methods of Disinfection

The routine adopted by the public health authorities to prevent the spread of infection is dealt with fully in Vol. III. Sect. 8 chap. 12. In the following pages, the principles of disinfection, the disinfectants used and the methods of using them are discussed.

Principles of Disinfection.—Assuming that the nurse is dealing with a disease treated at home, how is she to destroy the causative micro-organisms at every source? This question involves a knowledge of the chemicals used to kill microbes and of the physical processes which are adopted to render clothing and other things free of bacteria. A disinfectant is stronger than an antiseptic. The latter is represented by the weaker forms of antidote which merely retard the growth of germs; the former is also known as a *germicide* i.e. it results in the death of germs with which it has been in contact. Sterilization is a process of destroying all life. Before a nurse can be sure that her patient has ceased to be a source of danger to others she must make sure that the patient has ceased to harbour any germs, that the room and its furnishings are free of micro-organisms, that she herself and any person or persons who have been in contact with the patient are clear of infective material and that all clothing of the patient is similarly harmless to others. In most large towns and populous areas, the sanitary authority supervises the disinfection and no patient can be moved until a clearance certificate is granted. In certain cases, however, the nurse has to do a great deal in an ordinary routine way to prevent the spread of infection. The daily round is full of possibilities of transferring germs from one place to another, therefore the nurse must have a sound idea of the principles of disinfection. The great general stipulation is that the sickroom should be the limit of the infected area. Outside that, no microbe should pass. A moment's reflection will show that this covers the purification of the air, the cleansing of utensils, the toilet of the patient, the disinfection of clothing, the washing of clothing and the transport of food. Allowances must be made for the type of house; in some cases, the ideal is easy to reach; in others very great difficulties have to be overcome, and much depends upon the nurse's common sense.

Disinfectants.—First of all the common germicides must be enumerated. It must be remembered that although a thing has a strong scent it need not be disinfectant. We are too often put off by deodorants which create the strong antiseptic smell so powerfully impressive to the layman. Many of the strongest germicides have little or no odour at all, and some have to be coloured artificially so that they will be recognized. All disinfectants are specially tested against a known solution of carbolic acid (phenol). This is known as the Rideal-Walker test, and we refer to the strength of the germicide in terms of the Rideal-Walker coefficient. Disinfectants vary according to the strength of their solution and the time they are in contact with the microbe. They should not be too powerful and thus damage the skin or the article which they are disinfecting. It is obviously a mistake to use an acid which burns holes in clothing or a chemical which causes dermatitis.   Most of the best known germicides are members of the coal tar family, which includes phenol, cresol, carbolic acid, lysol and all the substances akin to it.   In addition to this, however, substances like formalin, chlorine, lime, potassium permanganate and perchloride of mercury all individually useful in certain cases, and the appropriate one must be selected when indicated by the case.   Disinfection by gases is brought about by using formaldehyde, chlorine or dioxide of sulphur.   Physical means of disinfection are those of incineration, boiling and steaming.

Phenol.—An old friend, phenol (carbolic acid) still remains in pristine favour.   Crude carbolic acid is complex, containing some cresol, which makes it more powerful.   The usual strength is 1 in 20, which kills bacteria in an hour, but does not injure textile fabrics or metals.   It is therefore recommended for faeces, urine, sputum, sheets, gowns and so on.

Cresol.—This substance, together with its emulsions—lysol, izal, cyllin and creolin, is very commonly used for drains and lavatories and for washing floors.   Most of these emulsions are stronger than carbolic acid, cheaper and not so dangerous. They form milky emulsions and become soapy in water.   They should be used in a strength of about one teaspoonful to the pint.

Formalin.—This disinfectant is made by adding 40 parts of formaldehyde to 60 of water.   It is generally employed in a spray and is used to treat large areas such as infected rooms.   It has rather an irritating odour, resulting from the fumes which rise easily from it.

Chlorine.—Chloride of lime, bleaching powder and similar substances act by liberating chlorine gas.   A 5 per cent solution destroys both bacteria and their spores in a few minutes.   It cannot be used for clothing or dyed fabrics because it bleaches them, but it is very useful for drains, traps and sinks.

Lime.—Ordinary slaked lime mixed with water forms whitewash, well known as an efficient disinfectant for walls and ceilings, especially in stables and cowsheds.   Milk of lime is a stronger solution useful for applying to dry closets and outside privies. The only disadvantage is its whiteness, which makes it visible, but it can be incorporated with distemper and is largely used in water paints.

Potassium permanganate.—Potassium permanganate is still used for disinfecting utensils, but it is not of much use for fabrics owing to the stains it leaves; it is a well known oxidizing agent.

Perchloride of mercury.—This substance, also known as corrosive sublimate, is used in the form of a clear solution which is usually tinted in order to save confusion with other solutions.   It is a very powerful poison, coagulating albumin rapidly and corroding metals.   In hospitals, it is commonly used in a strength of 1 in

1,000, which kills bacteria in half an hour; a solution double this strength will kill spores in an hour.

Fumigants.—In this group are included the gases mentioned above as disinfectants. These are employed when we want to destroy all the germs in a large room.

Formaldehyde gas.—Various lamps are used to produce formaldehyde gas; in the Paraform method the Alformant lamp is employed. In heating paraform, care must be taken that the room is sealed, since the fumes of formalin are very irritating. The advantages of formaldehyde are that it penetrates to every part of the room evenly, does not injure furniture or metal and kills microbes. Insects usually escape, however. It is customary to allow six hours for the gas to do its work properly. Occasionally formaldehyde is combined with potassium permanganate. In every 1,000 cubic feet of air space, we must allow at least 25 paraform tablets.

Chlorine gas.—If hydrochloric acid (spirit of salt) is added to bleaching powder, or sulphuric acid, common salt and manganese dioxide mixed together, chlorine gas is evolved. It was the first poison gas used in warfare. Owing to its weight, and to the cloud it forms with the vapour in the atmosphere, it should always be liberated from the top of a room. Cylinders of gas may also be used. Its disadvantage is that it is a very powerful bleaching agent.

Sulphur dioxide gas.—This gas, formerly thought to be of great disinfectant value, has been largely replaced by formalin. It is made by burning sulphur, in candle form, in a cast-iron pot, which resists the heat and which does not affect the sulphur. Sulphur is also used for disinfestation of vermin. Like chlorine, it can also be supplied in cylinders; it has a slight bleaching action.

Incineration.—The subject of incineration has been partly dealt with in the chapter on disposal of refuse. For soiled dressings, articles of clothing that can be destroyed and the general refuse of the sickroom, nothing is better than the domestic furnace.

Boiling.—Instruments and clothing of a certain type e.g. linen and cotton, can be dealt with by boiling, which kills all bacteria in a few minutes. Spores may resist for nearly an hour, however.

Steaming.—In large institutions, hospitals and infectious diseases centres, disinfection is done by steam. There are various ways of using steam, which is ideal for dealing with cotton or linen in quantity. Current steam, as used in the Thresh or Sack disinfector or Reck's stove, is steam constantly passed over material at atmospheric pressure, the articles being dried afterwards by hot air. In the pressure systems, in which steam at 250°–260° F. may be used, the pressure may be as much as 20 lb. The best known types of pressure steam disinfectors are the Autoclave and the Washington-Lyon apparatus. The former type is dealt with later; in the latter the entry to the machine is usually on one side of a wall and therefore in a separate chamber from the exit, which is on the other side of the wall. All materials are thus kept strictly free of reinfection once they are sterilized.

When the subject of infectious diseases is dealt with later, the whole routine of disinfection is described, but at this point a brief outline of the essentials of sickroom disinfection in a case of ordinary illness may be useful to the nurse.

Ordinary Disinfection in the Sickroom.—Regular dusting, together with bi-weekly scrubbing, will ensure that the first essential of cleanliness is provided for. In addition, the following precautions should be adopted.

Excrements.—Faeces and urine should be disinfected in order to protect the nurse and others. A 1 in 20 phenol solution may be used or cresol. A little should be left in the bedpan or urinal after it has been sterilized. After the excrement is passed, it may be necessary to add more carbolic and leave the utensil standing for 2 hours; quicklime may also be used. These things are important in places where there is no water carriage. In some cases faeces can be incinerated.

Nasal discharges.—Collect these in paper handkerchiefs or plain gauze and immediately burn in the fire.

Sputum.—Special cardboard cups are now made, but gauze can also be used. Both can be burned at once.

Fabrics.—These can be disinfected by soaking in 5 per cent phenol for twelve hours. Cotton and linen can then be boiled. Large textile articles can be taken to a steam disinfector.

Thermometer.—Always keep this in a little jar containing 1 in 20 phenol.

Hand lotions.—It is always advisable that the nurse should keep a lotion ready in a basin, so that she can disinfect her hands. Perchloride of mercury, 1 in 1,000, is recommended.

Air and light.—Keep all windows open in favourable weather, and do not allow the patient to lie in a semi-darkened room, unless it is desired to make him go to sleep.

Rubber gloves and overalls.—These should always be worn when doing dressings.

CHAPTER 7

HEATING

HEATING OF HOUSES.   COAL FIRES.   GAS FIRES.   ELEC-
TRIC HEATERS.   OIL STOVES.   COKE AND COAL STOVES.
HEATING OF HOSPITALS.   HOT WATER SYSTEMS.   ELECTRI-
CITY.   STEAM SYSTEMS.   HOT AIR SYSTEMS.   HOSPITAL
HEATING.   HOT WATER SUPPLIES.

THE rays of the sun supply a certain amount of direct heat to the earth, and the air temperature varies according to the situation of the district on the globe.   Another strong influence on climate is the direction of the wind.   We have already found that the temperature of the air, so far as Great Britain is concerned, is governed to a great extent by the Gulf Stream.

If people move about and are sufficiently clothed to maintain the temperature of the body at 98·4° F., there is no discomfort and no need is felt for artificial warmth.   In conditions of civilization, however, houses, although they are warmer than the outside air, are nevertheless incapable without artificial heating of maintenance at a high enough temperature to give us that feeling of comfort which we seek when we wear light clothes and lead a sedentary life.   Man has always been a fire worshipper and has learned of the peacefulness its warmth can bring to the human body.   He has therefore evolved systems of heating concurrently with his systems of housing and today our scientific methods of warming have been built up from the primitive open fire, which is the simplest form of extra heat supply, to the complex and carefully regulated systems of central heating.

Heating of Houses

In most houses of small to medium size, the heating is provided by open coal fires, gas fires, closed stoves or electric heaters. Sometimes oil is used, especially in country places.   While the temperature of a room may vary within wide limits, depending upon the time of the day, the thickness of the walls, the number of people in the room, the use to which the room is put (e.g. kitchens) and the habits of the occupants, it is generally agreed that the best temperature of a room is one between 60° and 65° F.

Humidity affects the comfort to a marked extent, as rooms that
are damp feel cold, thus weakening the occupant's resistance to
disease.   It has been proved that tuberculosis and rheumatism
are associated with dampness.   There are 3 ways of spreading
heat—by radiation, by convection and by conduction.   Radi-
ations may be either seen or unseen.   The cheering influence of
the sun and the joy at the prospect of a gleaming coal fire are
due to the visible rays which act on the skin and heat the blood
and the fat underneath the skin.   It must not be forgotten, however, that from both the fire and the sun, unseen (infra-red) rays
are constantly pouring out and warming the skin as well.   If we
have a good fire on in a room and the windows open, the temperature of the room can be kept at a normal level, because the
floor and the walls of the room are affected by the radiant heat
and constantly give off this heat to the cool air entering the room.
On the other hand, conduction of heat may occur by heating a
metal, one part of which is actually in contact with the flames
while the other takes up the heat by passing it on from particle
to particle.   A good example of this is provided if a steel poker
is put in the fire; even if the handle is far away from the flames,
it may be unbearably hot.   In kitchens, where iron furnaces for
heating water may be established, the heat is still present long
after the fire has gone out, and the whole area round the furnace
may remain appreciably warm all night.   This is the reason why
flies and animals congregate near furnaces although the fire
itself is out.   Convection heating is maintained by moving
particles of dust in the air, or by liquid particles in a boiling fluid
such as water.   Water which is hot always tends to rise to the
top of the container; this is the principle of the hot water systems
of houses.   Heated air also rises to the top of the room; this
allows the cold air to rush in, and thus a constant flow is assured.
These movements of the air and water are called convection
currents.   Artificial heating thus provides two things—extra
heat and efficient ventilation.   The term " airing " a house
which may have been standing empty for some time simply
means the drying of the walls and floors by radiation and the
setting up of convection currents which succeed in raising the
temperature of the whole house to normal levels.

Coal Fires.—Beginning with the old fashioned grate, which
burned a large quantity of coal and wood and which sent most
of its heat up the chimney, the coal fire has passed through many
changes.   It seems that we have now reached a stage at which
we can enjoy the sight of the flames and at the same time reap
the maximum benefit in heat.   Radiation is almost entirely the
method involved in coal fires, but the objects heated in the room
disperse their heat by convection, thus ventilation is helped, as
mentioned above.   The heat is quickly dispersed; thus, if we sit

close to a fire we may get our legs scorched whereas if we sit far
back we may not feel any heat at all. A coal fire must be carefully watched if it is to maintain the heat of the room at a certain
level. This is a very important point to be noted by nurses.
In the sickroom, the temperature must be kept up all night, when
the outer air is coldest, therefore a fire must be kept more active
than during the day. The advantage of a coal fire is that it

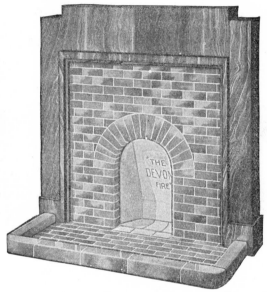

FIG. 44.—MODERN FIREPLACE IN WHICH ALL BARS AND
VENTILATING GRIDS ARE ABOLISHED.

Note that the fire burns in a well sunk below the level
of the kerb and that the back of the fireplace is inclined
forward, the whole arrangement giving the maximum heat
to the room.

(By courtesy of Messrs. Candy & Co. L:d. London.)

consumes all kinds of fuel—wood, peat, the special fuels made by
gas companies and coal itself. It can be allowed to burn slowly
by " banking " in the middle of the day, and when the temperature drops in the evening more solid fuel can be used. Hundreds
of types of " well " fires are on the market. The latest principle
to be adopted is that of combustion in a sunk brickwork " well,"
situated a few inches below the kerb, which is often raised. No
air inlet is necessary beyond the open fireplace, although some
fires have small metal shutters which regulate an air inlet. The

sides and back of the fire made of firebrick are set in " rifle-
back " slopes so that the flames strike them and are reflected
forwards.   There is no iron, either in the form of plates or bars.
By this method the minimum of heat goes up the chimney, the
maximum of heat is sent through the room and the combustion
is complete, with the minimum of waste.   While coal fires have
the communal disadvantage in that they pollute the air with

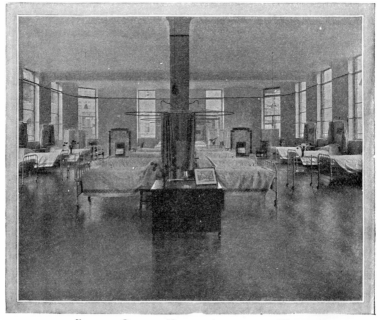

FIG. 45.—GAS AS A HEATING AGENT IN THE WARD
The cheerful effect of a gas fire is as important as its heating property.
(By courtesy of the British Commercial Gas Association, London.)

smoke, they seem destined, so far as Great Britain is concerned,
to be in vogue as the most homely ornament in the household for
many years.   The well fire is rapidly taking the place of the
antiquated bar fire with or without chimney-valves, metal
blowers and economizers set below the bars; it also prevents much
of the 75 per cent of loss of heat by flames and currents going up
the chimney (Fig. 44).

Gas Fires.—With the universal use of gas as an illuminant
came the inevitable heating devices.   Gradually gas has become
altered in composition to serve its purpose as a source of heat

rather than as a source of light; today gas fires are everywhere found. They are ideal for rooms which demand heat quickly, or heating for a short period only (such as bedrooms and dining-rooms). They have the advantage of being clean, efficient, economical and steady in their output, with exact regulation. Many varieties are produced, most of which depend upon the passage of a Bunsen flame through an openwork cylinder of specially treated fireclay, or through imitation coke or asbestos, which give the illusion of a coal fire. With a gas fire, the radiation is about 50 per cent and the conduction and convection supply 35 per cent, so that only 15 per cent is lost up the chimney. In using gas, therefore, there is much less of a loss than with coal; a minor disadvantage is that unless the chimneys are very efficient, the ventilation is poorer than that of a coal fire, and thus the room requires more efficient air supply. The air also tends to become too dry; for this reason it is customary to put a bowl of water in front of the fire. Gas may be slightly dearer than coal as a fuel factor, but its many advantages make it most popular, and it is ideal for the sickroom. All the modern gas fires and stoves are fitted with flues to lead the surplus fumes and air up the chimney (Fig. 46).

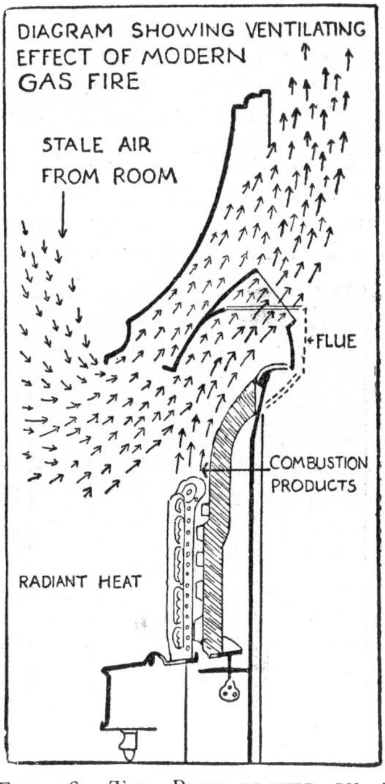

DIAGRAM SHOWING VENTILATING EFFECT OF MODERN GAS FIRE

STALE AIR FROM ROOM

FLUE

COMBUSTION PRODUCTS

RADIANT HEAT

Fig. 46.—The Part played by a Gas Fire in Heating and Ventilating a Room
(*By courtesy of the British Commercial Gas Association, London.*)

Electric Heaters.—The most cleanly method of heating is the electric radiator, and the time is at hand when the price can compete with coal or gas. There is no doubt that electricity is making great headway and it is more and more becoming established as the best form of heating for bedrooms. It gives out 100 per cent of its heat energy through its incandescent wires, divided up between radiation and convection as 3 : 1. It requires neither flue nor water and it can be regulated by switches. The only serious disadvantages are the sudden stoppages of supply of heat owing to fuses, general breakdowns and cuts made necessary by excessive load on the generating plant.

Oil Stoves.—In many places e.g. shops, offices, damp cellars and country houses, oil stoves are used. These are simply large lamps with proportionate container and wick, but instead of a glass globe, they have a cylinder of tin or other thin metal, with a shutter at the top. They act by convection, and are efficient, but their great disadvantage is their smell, which is distinctive and due to a substance called acrylic aldehyde. They also use up much of the oxygen. The Aladdin type of stove, however, represents a great advance in construction and general efficiency.

Coke and Coal Stoves.—In many cases, coke and coal are used for heating purposes in closed stoves. Both radiation and convection are in operation. Anthracite is a fuel commonly used for heating halls and passages because it is concentrated, clean, slow burning and regular in its output. Every anthracite stove is a danger when there is the slightest leak, and the carbon monoxide fumes have been known to poison people sleeping on the level of the chimney from which an anthracite stove was ventilated. The stoves are usually made of cast iron and are fitted with flue pipes leading to the outside air. They require to be attended to with care, and are found to be economical in use. The air near an anthracite stove is dry; the same applies to coke stoves.

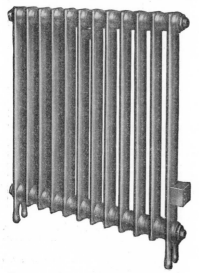

Fig. 47.—The Electrovex Hospital Radiator. This is heated by a system of electrical elements.

(By courtesy of Messrs. Benham & Sons, Ltd., London.)

Heating of Hospitals

In considering big heating schemes, it is convenient to take the example of modern hospital heating, which applies not only to other large buildings, but in part may be the same as that installed in dwelling houses big enough to require a central heating plant. Central heating is the term used to describe the warming of a large building by hot water or by steam. Hot air is sometimes used also.

Hot Water Systems.—The source of heat in this case is a coke boiler usually situated at the lowest part of the house or building, generally a basement. From this there runs a system of pipes to all parts of the building. In most cases the heat of each room is distributed by radiators, which are not radiators in the true sense of the word, since they act by the method of convection. Bright glossy green is the best colour, but many radiators are painted to conform to the colour scheme of the room or building, and thus lose a certain percentage of their efficiency as a sacrifice to art. The best place for a radiator is immediately under windows or in front of the incoming air shaft, in order to allow the air to be warmed. Heating by hot water has 3 systems available as described below.

1. *Low pressure system.*—In this the water is conducted in 3-inch cast iron pipes which run just above the skirting board of the room; the water is kept just below boiling point.

2. *High pressure system.*—The temperature of the water may be as much as 300° F. The pipes are less than an inch in diameter, and a considerable proportion is part of the furnace itself, in order to keep up the heat. It is akin to the locomotive boiler in many ways.

3. *The panel system.*—This is a newer method, adopted in some of the modern hospitals. Steel pipes conveying low pressure hot water end in panels made of asbestos and sawdust, which retain the maximum heat. In some cases metal plates 3 feet by 2 feet are fixed to the walls; behind them the pipes give out constantly a supply of heat which is radiated by these plates.

Gas radiators are sometimes used; in this system, the gas is lit below an ordinary water radiator. The disadvantage of steam or water radiators is that they often make a most disconcerting bubbling noise, which is annoying to patients.

Electricity.—There is a growing tendency to use electricity as a heating agent. The three illustrations (Figs. 47, 48 and 49) help to give an idea of the working of electrical heating systems. A power house generates the electric current, and from it cables carrying many wires pass on it making circuits in radiators, electric fires and other apparatus. Heating is by radiation, and unless care is taken in regulation of radiators (e.g. in a central heating system) the atmosphere tends to become overheated. Central heating by electricity is an ideal method, as it saves labour, does not produce harmful products and is easily controlled.

Steam Systems.—Many American houses are heated by steam, and the temperature of the room on the average is rather higher than 65°. In hotels which cater for American visitors, the central heating is often unbearable to English people.   The system is much the same as the water system, except that steam is passed through, and as it condenses water is formed which must be conducted back to the boiler.   Great care must be taken to have all joints firmly united.

Hot Air Systems.—Forced ventilation in cinemas, theatres, public buildings and schools may be combined with a hot air system.   The incoming air is warmed and delivered to the various rooms as previously described.   The heating occurs by convection in the air and is rarely efficient in very cold weather, when it has to be amplified.

Hospital Heating.—Various methods of heating are in force. Some modern hospitals have the radiating plate method; the older ones are supplied by low pressure systems.   The aim in all wards should be to prevent cold draughts, to avoid moisture, and to allow the floor of the ward to be well warmed, while the air circulating at the level of the patient lying in bed should be slightly cooler and in gentle motion.

Hot Water Supplies

One of the essentials in modern house construction is the provision of constant hot water.   In many cases, large blocks of houses are provided with a communal hot water supply.   In ordinary dwelling houses, however, the old system of putting a copper boiler at the back of the fireplace has been replaced by up to date apparatus which depends upon the heating by coke of a water jacket which surrounds a central furnace.   Many excellent varieties may be inspected at home exhibitions and building exhibitions.   Nurses are often faced with the problems of hot water supply, and an understanding of the general principles may be helpful.

There are two essentials in a successful hot water supply: 1. a reliable and satisfactory apparatus; 2. a common sense direction of it.

The action is very simple and depends upon the fact that hot water always rises to the top of a container.   The water to be heated is supplied to the water jacket direct from the hot water tank.   The jacket is therefore never empty.   The hot water tank is generally placed below the level of the cold water cistern, and supplies the bathroom and other rooms on the ground and first floors.   As the water heats in the water jacket, it rises to the intermediate tank and collects on the top, the cold water circulating until the whole tank is full of hot water.   Special safety valves are provided to prevent pipes bursting as a result of excessive pressure.   Once the tank is full of boiling water it is a simple

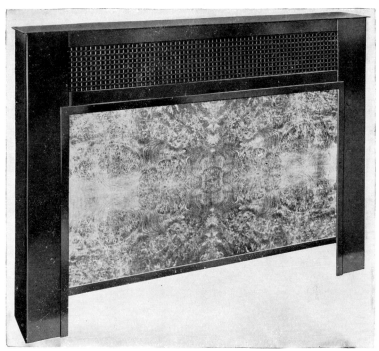

FIG. 48.—PANEL METHOD OF CENTRAL HEATING BY ELECTRICITY.
(*By courtesy of Messrs. Benham & Sons, Ltd., London.*)

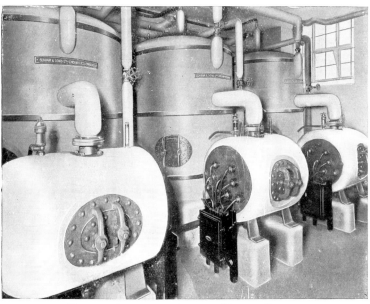

FIG. 49.—ELECTRICAL CENTRAL HEATING PLANT.
(*By courtesy of Messrs. Benham & Sons, Ltd., London.*)

matter to keep up the supply. The great thing to remember is that water should not be drawn until the intermediate tank is completely hot. This can easily be tested by the hand. When a bath is run, fresh water immediately runs into the bottom of the tank and circulation is again begun until once more the tank is hot. Constant hot water is assured if the furnace is kept going well as long as there is a demand for hot water. Once the demand has passed, the fire can be damped down, like an ordinary furnace. The normal amounts used in the household, sickroom, washbasins and so on, can easily be maintained if the tank has time to make good its heat loss, in some cases only a matter of 10 minutes. In this way the water is kept steadily at a very high temperature. Pipes from the top of the intermediate tank supply all the hot pipes of the house. The cold water enters at the base of the

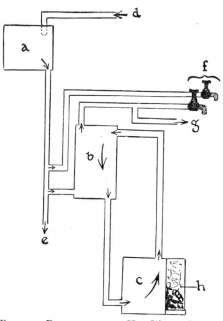

FIG. 50.—DIAGRAM OF THE HOT WATER SYSTEM OF A HOUSE.

a, Storage tank, supplied by pipe from main (*d*). The course of the water is indicated by arrows. Various pipes are led off to supply cold water taps (e.g. *e* and *f*). One pipe goes to the intermediate tank *b*, supplying it with cold water. The water from *b* passes to a boiler (*c*) placed in relation to a fire (*h*). As the water in *c* heats, it rises to the top of the tank *b*, and can be used at *f* and *g*, which are bathroom and lavatory hot water taps.

tank. These tanks and their pipes may be of lead, copper or special iron structure. They rarely go wrong. When difficulties arise in heating systems, it is usually the stoker who is wrong. The furnaces themselves are very useful in burning up all the refuse of the house; thus the maximum economy of fuel is assured (Fig. 50).

CHAPTER 8

LIGHTING

NATURAL LIGHTING. SUNLIGHT. INSOLATION. ANALY-
SIS OF LIGHT. NATURAL LIGHTING OF HOUSES. WINDOW
SPACE. ARTIFICIAL LIGHTING. CANDLES. OIL LAMPS.
COAL GAS. ACETYLENE. ELECTRICITY. LIGHTING AND
EYESIGHT. THE IDEAL ARTIFICIAL LIGHTING. HOSPITAL
LIGHTING.

Of recent years the subject of lighting, both from the artificial
and from the natural point of view, has become much more
important than formerly. The health of a community is
definitely influenced by the amount of clear sunlight available,
and now it is understood that much of the ill health found in
slum areas is due to smoke, fog, dust or small window space
which interrupt the passage of the sun's rays. Improved methods
of artificial lighting have also brought with them devices for
provision of artificial rays analogous to those emanating from
the sun. The craze for sunbathing and for outdoor life has as
its stimulus the desire to expose as much of the body to the
valuable ultra-violet and infra-red rays of the sun, normally
shut out by ordinary glass.

Natural Lighting

Sunlight.—There is nothing which can surpass the natural
rays of the sun, both from an illuminant and from a health point
of view. A few hours of good daylight are better than many
hours of even superlative electric lighting. Sunlight has an incalculable moral effect on the individual, amply proved by con-
trasting the temperament of those who live in warm, sunny
climates with those who inhabit countries in which rain and cloud
are common. We ourselves know that on a bright day in June
our spirits are the opposite of those on a dismal, dark day of
November. The energy derived from the sun is enormous, and
although it is certain that the sun is gradually losing its power,
it will be millions of years before there is any appreciable effect;
as far as we are concerned, therefore, it need not cause any
apprehension.

Insolation.—This is a term which is used to define the amount of radiation from the sun on a given area of the earth. Several factors influence insolation. For instance, the length of time that the sun's rays are fixed on the ground is not entirely responsible for the effect of sunlight. The amount of sunlight depends upon the season, which in turn depends upon the way the earth is tilted towards the sun in its orbit. Distance from the sun also varies, and can be appreciated. In January we are nearer to the sun than in July, and this affects to a certain extent the extremes of climate. At any time, it must be remembered, the sun is over 90,000,000 miles away. Another point is that the angle of the sun's rays as they strike the ground have an effect on the radiation; comparison of the overhead vertical rays of the tropics with the slanting rays of the cooler regions is ample proof of the difference in radiation. The atmosphere takes up a certain amount of energy from the sun's rays so that if a beam has longer to travel, it will have less power of insolation.

Analysis of Light.—All light has a certain index of strength called the candle power, and sources of light are estimated according to this convention. Lighting is gauged in units, known as unit foot-candles. The foot-candle may be defined as the light received on a surface, every point of which is one foot in length from a point source of light of one candle power. The strength of the sun is impossible to assess with any certainty. Scientists have now decided and proved that the spectrum (which is a band of colours passing by gradual stages from red, through orange, yellow, green, blue to violet, and formed when light is passed through a prism) does not show all the rays constituting the so-called pure white light. Indeed, two of the most important rays are invisible: one belongs to one end of the scale (the infra-red group); the other is found at the other end of the spectrum (the ultra-violet group). These two sets of rays—the infra-red and the ultra-violet—are of incalculable benefit to health and probably constitute the strongest part of the sun's rays, which, although they may contain light, heat and other types of ray, depend upon the two above mentioned for their great hygienic effect on the individual and their detrimental effect on bacteria.

When we observe the sun tanned nudist or the bronzed skin of a person fresh from the open air life of the camp or seaside, we see particularly the effect of the ultra-violet rays. The coloration is a response of the pigment of the skin to protect the human being against too much of the sun; it is in fact a demonstration that the body has accommodated itself to the solar radiation. These rays may be trying to the eyes, especially when there is much white about as in chalky districts, or in white-washed rooms or in working with anything having a high gloss. The eyes always require to be protected against ultra-violet rays, hence the universal use of goggles with tinted glass. The sun may also cause nervous irritability as in sunstroke. Generally, however, a simple subterfuge can be adopted to overcome the harmful effects of sun and to reap the maximum harvest of the beneficial rays. Heliotherapy has become an important method of treatment during the past few years, and every nurse should

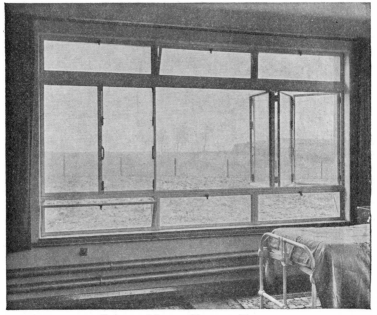

FIG. 51.—MODERN HOSPITAL WINDOWS.

These should be regarded as consisting of three parts. The upper and lower panes are worked on the hopper principle, and can be used to ventilate the room when the weather is bad. Normally the middle leaves can be folded outwards by sliding them in a series of swivel wheels. Thus the maximum direct sunlight and fresh air are admitted to the ward or sickroom, and there is an unobstructed view.

(By courtesy of Crittall Manufacturing Co., Ltd., Braintree.)

understand how much benefit can be obtained from the sun. It is certain that we do not take the full advantage of the health giving rays which cost nothing and are always offered us. Those who seek perfect sun conditions may go to the mountains, where, say, in Switzerland, the average sunlight is about twice as much as that of the big towns. In addition to this, there are more ultra-violet rays in the mountain areas, especially when there is a clear blue sky. For further information see Vol. III, Sect. 7 chapt. 9.

Natural Lighting of Houses.—If we could ensure that every house was taking full advantage of the sun, we should be far on the way to better health. Modern ideas of building concur in recommending as much space as possible for windows, and a glance at present day architecture in all parts of the world will show that schools, factories and dwelling houses have great areas of glass. Ordinary lead glass does not allow the passage of either infra-red or ultra-violet rays, but nowadays special glass (e.g. Vita Glass, Holviglass) acts like quartz in allowing these beneficial rays to pass through. Many buildings are furnished in this fashion and it is claimed that the general health of the inhabitants is improved thereby, so that the minor ailments are prevented; work is more efficient and energy is increased.

Window Space.—While the aim of the older architects was apparently to shut out as much light as possible, the newer school, prompted by hygienic advice, allow at least one-tenth of the floor space, and often twice as much as this. Indeed the window is one of the most important considerations in any room (Fig. 51). If the sun is shining directly, the opening can be freed of its glass screen by the use of casement windows, which are more easily operated than sash windows and do not have the disadvantage that the latter have in leaving at the best one-half of the window space covered with glass, a great drawback in hot weather. We have long since passed the stage of worrying over the fading of curtains and fabrics by sun, realizing that it is better to take the colour out of our furnishings than to live behind the funereal venetian blind. The position of the window is important; the higher up the window extends towards the ceiling, the better for the supply of light. In some hospitals the whole side of a ward may be constructed of glass, fitted in folding doors or sliding windows. In schools, the light should come from the left side, as this ensures the best condition for reading and writing. All possible measures to increase the supply of daylight by fixing up reflectors outside windows and by painting the ends of buildings white are indicated in congested areas, because daylight is always better than artificial light, no matter how good the illumination of a lamp may be. This has been amply proved by research workers. (See also p. 19, Fig. 3, and p. 12, Fig. 6.)

Artificial Lighting

Before going on to the subject of artificial light in its proper sense, we must refer to the production of artificial sunlight. This can be accomplished in several ways by electricity. Lamps may be used of a special construction, with filament and filling of a type which results in rays containing both ultra-violet and infra-red rays, and a carbon arc lamp is also in common use.

The best apparatus is, however, the mercury vapour lamp. The employment of these lamps is undoubtedly of great value in cases of rickets, debility and other troubles due to poor hygienic conditions, but in no circumstances should they be used by others than experts, either doctors with special knowledge or medical electricians who have obtained approved certificates. More harm than good may be done by the promiscuous use of the ultra-violet and infra-red rays. (See Vol. III, Sect. 7 chapt. 9.

Artificial lighting can be provided for by combustible oils or gases, or by electricity. Each method is dealt with in turn below.

Candles.—The paraffin wax candle, although both its wick and its fats are carefully purified, is a primitive form of lighting, only used in emergencies and for decorative effects. The disadvantage, as in all other combustion methods, is the amount of carbonic acid gas generated. This may amount to as much as that produced by 5 people, so that the atmosphere is soon vitiated. In addition to this, candles are dirty, because they never use up the oil completely, thus much soot and smoke goes into the room, especially if there is the slightest draught. The unpleasant smell and the extra heat also cause discomfort to the occupants of the room.

Oil Lamps.—In many country places, oil lamps, chiefly operated by kerosene, are still in active use. The principle is the burning of a wick kept saturated by dipping into a metal or stout glass container. Glass globes tightly fixed round the wick increase the illuminating effect, and often burnished metal reflectors are added. Here and there we find the incandescent principle applied to oil lamps, but with the advance of electricity we can assume that the day of the oil lamp is ending. It has a certain soothing and warming effect, especially in winter time, but in addition to all the disadvantages possessed by the candle, the oil lamp is unsatisfactory because it is dangerous unless the wick is carefully fitted into a keeper which is screwed into the oil container, and the latter must be heavy, free from leakage and safe from accidents by explosion or sudden fire.

Coal Gas.—For a time coal gas was the universal illuminant, but gradually its value has diminished and now we consider coal gas chiefly as a source of heat. To begin with, coal gas was used in the simple butterfly burner, which gave a characteristic flame. The Welsbach incandescent burner took its place, however. This consists of a central Bunsen burner, sending up a fine jet of gas, which is made incandescent by a surrounding network of fine asbestos gauze containing a certain substance—sulphate of zirconium. In addition to improved lighting, the incandescent burner uses less oxygen, gives off less CO_2 and is more economical than the ordinary burner. In all coal gas lighting the danger of carbon monoxide poisoning is a great disadvantage, especially when tubes and burners are old and unreliable.

Acetylene.—For a long time, acetylene gas was used on motor cars, and it is still employed as an illuminant in country halls and churches. In warfare it may be used to light operating tents and other parts of field hospitals, and has been of great service. It is best made in large metal drums by adding a steady but small amount of water to calcium carbide. It gives a splendid white light but it is very explosive and has a smell which is easily recognized. Some bicycle lamps burn acetylene, which is manufactured on a small scale in containers carried on the bicycle.

Electricity.—There is no comparison between the value of electricity and all the other methods of lighting. Electricity is apparently in its infancy, and there is no saying what results may be obtained by its development. Already the United Kingdom is prepared for universal supply through a grid system, and in time there will not be a single hamlet without its complete facilities for electric light. Electric light depends upon the heating to a white heat of a fine filament at the end of a circuit, and for this purpose, glass bulbs, free of air, or containing a special gas (e.g. argon, an inert gas) are used. They vary in candle power, and are graded in units known as watts. Every lamp is marked with the voltage of the supply, 100, 200, 230, or whatever it may be, and the strength of the lamp in watts, e.g. 25, 40, 60, 75, 100 and so on. All nurses should understand about these things, as it is unsafe to fit the wrong type of lamp to a terminal, while the best results are obtained only when the appropriate lamps are used. In most cases, tungsten is the substance used in the filament lamp, the gas in the bulb being non-combustible, acting really as a " cushion " to prevent the filament from breaking up. When it is realized that only 5 per cent of the electricity is transformed into light, it will be quite evident that electric bulbs heat the air, but they have certain advantages over the other forms of lighting in that they do not use up oxygen, and do not give off any CO_2. Probably the greatest attribute of electric lighting is its cleanliness. It is also an advantage to have light under such easy control, although the fuse system and the occasional generating station breakdowns are the causes of temporary lack of supply.

In the carbon arc lamp, used for searchlights, stage effects, film work and street lighting, the source of light is a white-hot flame which passes as an electric arc across the points of two carefully adjusted carbon pencils. The carbon arc lamp is powerful, but it is spluttering and messy, and the source of light " jumps " considerably. Development in electrical methods of lighting is going on rapidly, especially in the provision by special lamps of daylight effects and with shadows reduced to the minimum.

Lighting and Eyesight.—With ever increasing electrical power, the question of eyestrain becomes more and more important; inadequate lighting causes eyestrain, and this should be carefully avoided. The subject of glare, especially on roads used by cars, in factories and in schools, is occupying the minds of ophthalmic specialists. In schools, a good deal of research has been done on the colouring for walls, red, stone colour and a certain tone of yellow being found most suitable, but the greatest factor is the absence of high degree of reflection, so that occasional strong beams do not strike the delicate retina. The ideal light for school children is one which is just above their heads, and the lamps should be enclosed in white opaque globes which cast an even amount of light all round, avoiding sharp shadows (Fig. 52). The same problems affect the industrial worker, some trades being worse than others. In many cases, strong lights are a danger to the eyes, e.g. in glass blowing and welding. In any circumstances which involve the sudden glare of a strong beam, coloured goggles should be worn, the glass being tinted blue, green, brown or red, depending upon the occupation. The constant change of light from weak to strong and vice versa is very tiring to the iris, and leads to eyestrain.

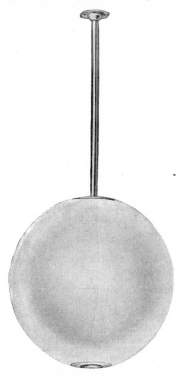

FIG. 52.—A COMBINED FORM OF ELECTRIC LAMP SPECIALLY USED IN MODERN HOSPITALS.

Inside the large globe is a 150 watt lamp which is used when full illumination is required; during the night a small 25 watt lamp shown at the bottom of the globe may be used.

(*By courtesy of the British Electrical Development Association, Inc., London.*)

The Ideal Artificial Lighting.—Already it has been proved that the bare electric bulb is trying to the eyes, and tinted or frosted glass bulbs are commonly used. The frosted glass diffuses the light in a softening way; the colours are soothing and result in

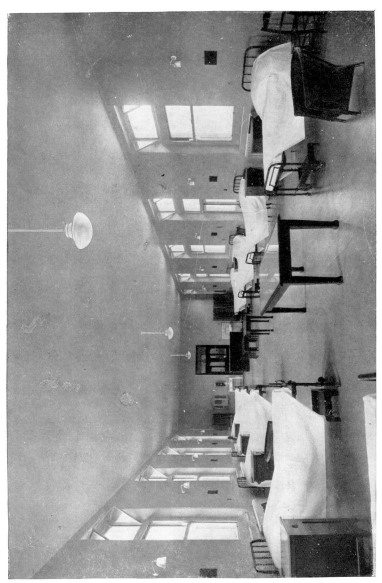

FIG. 53.—MODERN LIGHTING. A WARD OF AN ENGLISH ISOLATION HOSPITAL.

(*By courtesy of the General Electric Co., Ltd., and the British Electrical Development Association, Inc., London.*)

a certain type of " atmosphere " important to domestic perfection. But the greatest advance in lighting recently has been the adoption of concealed lighting, which is light indirectly supplied by causing the lamps to shine from cornices and picture rails on to the roof. The softness of this diffusion produces the most harmonious and nerve soothing effect, and when combined with a system of opaque glass fittings, results in perfect lighting, causing the least strain to the eyes and not forming any shadows.

Hospital Lighting.—As far as general lighting is concerned, hospitals are best dealt with by indirect lighting. The special lighting of theatres and similar offices is referred to later on (Vol. III, Sect. 6 chapt 8). The individual patient, lying in bed, needs something just above his head; the modern wall lamps, enclosed in opaque white glass, are very satisfactory. If a bedside lamp is used, it should be provided with an ample, green lined screen, and should not cause a glare on the patient's face. The use of special dimming bulbs for hospitals is to be recommended; otherwise, nurses must make provision for the safe covering up of lights which may have to be left on while the patient is asleep (Figs. 52 and 53).

CHAPTER 9

FOOD AND NUTRITION

CHEMICAL CONSTITUENTS OF FOOD. PROTEINS. CARBO-
HYDRATES. FATS. VITAMINS. MINERALS. WATER.
SPECIAL ARTICLES OF FOOD. MILK. CHEESE. BUTTER.
MARGARINE. EGGS. MEAT. TABLE OF FOODS IN ORDER
OF DIGESTIBILITY. VEGETABLES. FRUIT. NUTS. CEREALS.
ALCOHOL. BEVERAGES. CONDIMENTS. READY RECKONER
FOR DIET, BY CALORIES. PROPRIETARY PREPARATIONS:
VALUE AND DANGERS.

THE art of nutrition is the application of our knowledge of various food factors needed by the body for normal function.

Good nutrition is an essential factor in the maintenance of good health for all age groups and for the social and economic life of a community. The importance of this was recognized by the British Government when establishing a Ministry of Food to plan and carry out a nutritional policy which proved to be a valuable contribution towards maintaining the health and morale of a large number of people during the strain of a world war.

The successful treatment of sick people is largely based upon good nutrition; the object of this chapter is to give a basic knowledge of food and dietary principles needed in the education of the modern nurse.

Children and adolescents require a full share of the protective foods. Old people require easily assimilable foods; there is no scientific evidence to prove that their nutritional requirements are less than those of the younger age groups.

Chemical Constituents of Food

Food is derived from animal, vegetable and mineral sources and is classified into the following groups: proteins, carbohydrates, fats, vitamins, minerals and water. These have all been referred to already so far as their physiology is concerned (see Vol. I, pp. 210–226) but a fuller study must be made now.

Proteins.—These are to be found in every cell, the chemical

124

structure being peculiar to the particular type of cell. The protein of egg albumin is different chemically from nucleoprotein of glandular tissue.

Proteins are composed of chemical compounds called amino acids, these being building stones of which there are many kinds; they all contain oxygen, hydrogen, carbon and nitrogen, and some contain sulphur and phosphorus. Nutritionists divide amino acids into two groups: essential and non-essential. Essential amino acids must be taken in the diet as they cannot be formed in the body; non-essential amino acids can be synthesized or built up in the body from other amino acids.

Biological value.—Proteins have a biological value, which is a measure of the extent to which any protein can supply the nutrient requirements of the body. The terms, first class protein and second class protein, are still used, but a better and more accurate definition is that in which the terms complete and incomplete, protein are used; the former contains all the essential amino acids whereas the latter lack some essential amino acids. Protein of good biological value comes from animal sources: meat, game, poultry, fish, milk, cheese and eggs. Protein of lesser biological value is to be found in peas, beans, lentils, nuts, cereals and vegetables; the value of these proteins is supplemented when they are eaten with animal protein, hence the need to mix the proteins in a diet.

Uses of protein.—Protein is used by the body for growth, repair of tissue, energy, reproduction and lactation. Protein hydrolysates are polypeptide and amino acid products obtained from the hydrolysis or digestion of animal protein with acid or trypsin. Owing to their unpalatable properties oral administration should be judicious and only given in certain conditions. All proteins have the same calorie value, one gramme being equal to 4 calories.

Carbohydrates.—Carbohydrates are compounds composed of carbon, hydrogen and oxygen, the latter in the same ratio as is present in water.

Carbohydrate is present in vegetables and fruits in the form of starch and sugar, in milk as lactose, in liver and shell fish as glycogen. Cellulose is a form of carbohydrate forming the skeletal structure of plants; it is not digested in the human alimentary tract but forms bulk in the intestines. Herbivorous animals can with bacterial aid obtain a good deal of nutriment from plant cellulose. Sugar is pure carbohydrate which is quickly absorbed by the body as a source of heat and energy. There are many different kinds of sugar and some have a sweeter taste than others, but weight for weight the calorie or energy value of each is the same.

Sugars.—Cane and beet sugar are of the same chemical structure; sugar is extracted and manufactured into cubes or granulated crystals, or pulverized into castor and icing sugar.   Brown demerara is a less refined form of sugar.

Lactose is present in all types of mammalian milk; it is the least sweet of the sugars.   Maltose or malt sugar is formed by enzyme activity upon starch; dextri-maltose is an intermediate product of maltose and dextrin often used in infant feeding.   Glucose or dextrose is present in plants, fruits and honey; it is also the physiological sugar of the blood; the liver stores glucose as glycogen; it is released into the circulation again as glucose. Fructose is one of the sugars of fruit and honey and is considered to have the sweetest taste of all sugars.

Starch.—This is the main constituent of breakfast cereals, grains and their flours, potatoes, arrowroot, macaroni, tapioca, rice, semolina and the pulses.   To test the presence of starch in food drop some iodine on to a portion; its presence is indicated by the appearance of a blue-black colour.   It may be necessary to dissolve some foods in water before testing.

Saccharin.—Although saccharin has a sweet taste, it is not a sugar and has not any food value.   It is a white crystalline product of coal tar and can be used as a sweetening agent by persons suffering from diabetes and in any condition in which sugar is contra-indicated.

The calorie value of all carbohydrates is 4 to one gramme.

Fats.—Fats and oils for human nutrition are obtained from animal and vegetable sources, their chemical constituents being the same as the carbohydrates viz. carbon, hydrogen and oxygen in a different and more complex ratio.   Fat can be stored in the body as a reserve food of high concentration; the oxidation of one gramme of fat provides 9 calories.   Olive oil and lard have no fat soluble vitamin content; fish liver oil is a rich source of vitamins of this type.   The food sources of animal fat and oil are cream, butter, suet, dripping, lard and fish.   The food sources of vegetable fat and oil are fruit and leaves and seeds of plants. Examples are olive and cotton seed oil, linseed oil, and nut oils from which margarine is manufactured.   The nutritive value of fat and oil is in proportion to the vitamin content.

Vitamins.—The vitamins are chemical substances present in small amounts in certain foods; they are important for normal growth and good health.   The two main groups consist respectively of water soluble and fat soluble vitamins; many vitamins act as catalysts in the process of metabolism; they are capable of bringing about or accelerating chemical processes in the body without losing their identity.   When vitamins were first discovered their composition was unknown and they were named after the letters of the alphabet.   With the development of our knowledge they are now often called by their correct chemical names.

Water soluble vitamins.—A number of vitamins are soluble in water, hence the use of this term.

Vitamin C (ascorbic acid) is a simple derivative of the hexose sugars and can be prepared from glucose. It is not very stable but much can be done to prevent loss in the preparation and cooking of vegetables. Locked up in the active cells is a plant enzyme, ascorbic acid oxidase; this is liberated when the plant is damaged or wilted and activates the oxidation of ascorbic acid. Vegetables should be prepared immediately before cooking; they should not be shredded too finely and the smallest amount of boiling water should be used for cooking, thus reducing appreciably the loss of vitamin C; the oxidase is destroyed by heat.

Ascorbic acid is not stored in the body apart from the tissue cells; when the tissues are completely saturated any excess is excreted in the urine, therefore it is necessary to maintain a daily intake from dietary sources. A deficiency of ascorbic acid in the body is associated with infantile and adult scurvy, a condition in which there is marked fragility of the capillary walls. Bleeding occurs in the gums, under the skin and in many other organs of the body; large painful swellings occur over the bones due to subperiosteal bleeding. Ascorbic acid is a contributory factor in the healing of wounds and bone injuries and in raising the resistance to infection.

The chief dietary sources of ascorbic acid are green leaf vegetables and fresh fruits. Green leaf vegetables are only good sources when they are fresh. Oranges, lemons, grape fruit, black currants, strawberries and tomatoes are very good sources.

Root vegetables and tubers can be reliable dietary sources, although the amount present is small. Fruit and vegetables canned quickly after harvesting retain most of their vitamin C content; dried fruits and vegetables are poor sources of this vitamin. Cow's milk supplies insufficient amounts; the amount in human milk varies with the amount taken in the mother's diet.

Vitamin P, also known as hesperidin, is closely allied to vitamin C in therapeutic properties; it is a factor associated with the treatment of vascular purpura. Vitamin P is present in paprika and in all sources of vitamin C.

So far as vitamin B is concerned, B_1 (aneurin in Great Britain; thiamin in America) and B_2 complex are the most important ones in human nutrition. The first to be discovered was vitamin B_1 and the remainder were grouped together as B_2 complex. Of this complex the most important are riboflavin, nicotinic acid, pyridoxin, pantothenic acid, choline and folic acid.

Aneurin is an important factor in carbohydrate metabolism; during this process an intermedial breakdown product called pyruvic acid is produced. Aneurin by its catalytic action aids in the complete conversion of pyruvic acid into carbon dioxide and water. A test for aneurin deficiency is the estimation of pyruvic acid in the blood. The best food sources of this vitamin are yeast, liver, bacon, ham, egg yolk, nuts, peas, beans and whole-meal bread. Deficiency of aneurin in the diet will give rise to loss of appetite, constipation and peripheral neuritis; when the deficiency persists beriberi occurs, this being followed by de-generation of the central nervous system, enlargement of the heart and oedema beginning in the legs and becoming general-ized.

The substance riboflavin is obtained in the form of orange crystals—the name gives the clue to its composition (ribose—a sugar, and flavin—a yellow fluorescent pigment). Food sources are milk, yeast, liver, meat, eggs, cheese and green vegetables. A deficiency of riboflavin in the body gives rise to lesions of a particular type affecting the epithelium: sores and cracks appear on the lips and at the corners of the mouth and the skin covering the vestibule of the nostrils is dry and scales away. The papillae of the tongue are flat instead of raised and the tongue has a smooth discoloured surface. This condition is known as cheilosis.

Nicotinic acid, although in some respects related to the nico-tine of tobacco, is not the same as and does not contain the toxic properties of nicotine. Nicotinic acid deficiency is responsible for the development of pellagra, a disease with characteristic symptoms in which scaly, dark red lesions appear on the upper surface of the arms, hands, feet, legs and face, in fact the areas exposed to the light of the sun. As the disease progresses there is marked degeneration of the nervous system followed by dementia. Pellagra is seldom seen in Great Britain but it is a serious nutritional problem in some countries in which the chief articles of diet consist of maize, white flour and sugar to the exclusion of other foods. Nicotinic acid is present in meat, fish, liver, eggs, yeast and green vegetables.

Pyridoxin is concerned with the metabolism of fat and protein. The food sources are egg yolk, liver, yeast and wholemeal bread.

Pantothenic acid: little is known about the influence of this substance in human nutrition; it prevents dermatitis in chickens. The food sources are wheat germ, liver and yeast.

Choline is a lipotropic factor i.e. it has an affinity for fats and oils and is thus a factor preventing the formation of fat in the liver. A deficiency of choline from the diet allows the liver to synthesize more fat than is needed from carbohydrates; this fat accumulates in the liver causing fatty infiltration of the hepatic cells. The food sources are eggs, meat and cereals.

Folic acid occurs as a bright yellow pigment in grass, asparagus and green leaves and is also found in liver and yeast.   Folic acid is used in the treatment of pernicious (macrocytic) anaemia.

Fat soluble vitamins.—These are essentially the vitamins in foods of a fatty nature: the livers of cod and halibut, and of the sheep and ox are the richest sources; other food sources are cream, butter, egg yolk, cheese and fish (tinned or fresh).

Vitamin A.   The precursor of this vitamin is carotene, a yellow pigment present in carrots, tomatoes, fruits and green plants.   The body is capable of converting carotene into vitamin A; fish obtain carotene by feeding on green sea plants, which they can convert into vitamin A and store in their livers.   In human nutrition vitamin A is a factor required for normal growth and development, for the integrity of the epithelium and for the prevention of night blindness.   A deficiency test for vitamin A is the dark adaptation test of the human eye.   Present in the retina is a photochemical pigment known as visual purple; this pigment is bleached by light and formed again in the dark when vitamin A is present.   In the absence of vitamin A the regenerating process takes very much longer and the individual suffers from night blindness.   In gross deficiency of vitamin A keratinization of the cornea develops, and if this is not treated xerophthalmia occurs, a condition of permanent damage and blindness.   Good food sources of vitamin A are cod and halibut liver oil, liver, butter, eggs and cream.   It is stored in the human liver.

Vitamin D is well known as the antirachitic or rickets protector vitamin.   It can be stored by the body in the liver and skin. Vitamin D is present as a natural vitamin in the liver oil and bodies of fat fish, sardines, herrings and salmon, also in egg yolk and butter; it is now introduced into margarine (vitaminized margarine).

Vitamin D_2, or calciferol, is obtained by irradiation with ultra-violet light of a substance present in food and known as ergosterol. Milk can be irradiated with ultra-violet light with a subsequent increase of its vitamin D_2 content.   Sunlight can also increase the natural Vitamin D_2 content of the body by its action upon a substance in the skin called dehydrocholesterol (vitamin D_3); the vitamin is then absorbed by the blood.

Vitamin D is necessary for the proper development of bone structure because it maintains a supply of calcium and phosphorus in the blood serum which is used in the formation of bone cells.   This in turn affects the absorption of calcium from the intestine.   Deficiency leads to failure of normal bone development which in infants is called rickets and in adolescents and adults osteoporosis; a more severe type is osteomalacia.   The dietary intake of vitamin D is of the utmost importance.   It should be the responsibility of all who are in charge of infants and young children to give a daily protective dose of vitamin D in one of the preparations available. Expectant and nursing mothers should also be supplied with information regarding the importance of a daily optimum dose of the vitamin.

Vitamin E is also called tocopherol. There is still a good deal unknown about the activity of this vitamin in relationship to human nutrition. It is a factor associated with the fertility of some animals and it also exhibits oxidation reduction properties. Food sources of vitamin E are green leaf vegetables, wheat germ oil, wholemeal flour and egg yolk.

Vitamin K is necessary for the maintenance of an adequate amount of prothrombin in the blood. Prothrombin is formed in the liver and for the proper absorption of vitamin K, bile salts are necessary. If there is a deficiency of prothrombin in the blood caused by biliary obstruction, vitamin K must be injected in conjunction with bile salts. Vitamin K is of no value in the treatment of bleeding associated with haemophilia. The food sources are green leaf and root vegetables, fruit, egg yolk, liver and tomatoes.

Minerals.—Mineral salts are very important constituents of food, without which human life as we know it would entirely cease. Minerals have many different functions to perform; the normal irritability of living tissues depends upon the presence of mineral salts in the fluid that bathes them. There is a certain concentration of mineral salts in the blood and it is vitally essential that this level should be kept constant. The structure of bone and teeth depends entirely upon minerals absorbed from food. In addition there are certain minerals in the blood known as trace elements which are important for certain metabolic processes. It is important to maintain an optimum dietary intake of minerals to make good the loss in excretion which is essential in the metabolic breaking down and building up processes of the body.

Calcium.—Calcium, with phosphorus, is the chief constituent of bones and teeth; increased amounts of calcium should be given in the diets of infants, children, pregnant and nursing mothers. Calcium is an essential factor in the clotting of blood and for the normal excitability of nerve and muscle fibres. A low blood calcium is associated with tetany.

Food sources of calcium are milk, cheese, eggs, the pulses and green leaf vegetables. Water in some districts has a high calcium carbonate content; this could be regarded as a dietary source. Calcium carbonate is also added to National flour to replace calcium rendered unavailable in wholemeal bread because of the formation of insoluble calcium as a result of the action of phytin.

Phosphorus.—Phosphorus is an integral part of all cells, animal

and vegetable. It is distributed in a very wide range of foods
—milk, cheese, meat, fish, egg yolk, liver, cereals, fruits and
vegetables. It is an essential mineral of all body fluids and a
component of the cells of the central nervous system as well as
glandular organs and their secretions.

Iron.—The amount of iron required by the body is small. Iron
is needed for haemoglobin, which has the property of carrying
oxygen in the blood. A deficiency of iron in the diet gives rise
to nutritional anaemia; the oxygen carried is lessened, and this
causes breathlessness. Food sources of iron are corned beef,
liver, kidney, meat, eggs, oatmeal, green leaf vegetables, cocoa,
black treacle, dried fruits and National flour. A certain amount
of iron is absorbed by food from iron kitchen utensils, such as
mincers and unlined iron cooking pans. Milk is a poor source
of iron and if for any reason milk is to be the staple diet, iron salts
should be added.

Copper.—Copper is necessary for the proper utilization of iron;
this was discovered in the treatment of animals suffering from
nutritional anaemia. When iron alone was given the anaemia
persisted, but when green leaves were added to the diet the
condition improved; the curative property in the green leaves
was inorganic copper. The best food sources of copper are the
iron-containing foods.

Iodine.—This is a component of thyroxine, the active principle
of the thyroid gland. Unless the dietary intake of iodine is
sufficient the thyroid gland becomes enlarged, and goitre develops. Dietary sources of iodine are milk, fish, green leaf vegetables and fruit. Iodine is particularly rich in foods grown near
the sea; in the goitre districts, the food does not contain sufficient
amounts of iodine for human requirements. Iodized salt should
be included in the diets of people living in these areas.

Sodium Chloride.—This is common salt and is usually taken in
the diet in almost all foods; it is also added as a condiment.
Sodium salts are present in all body fluids in physiological proportions; they have many functions of vital importance to perform. The secretion of hydrochloric acid in the gastric juice is
influenced by sodium chloride whereas sodium bicarbonate acts
as a buffer in the blood against excess of acid products of metabolism. Sodium chloride contributes to the osmotic pressure of
body fluids. In certain conditions in which the sodium chloride
loss is excessive (such as Addison's disease), and among people
who work hard in a hot atmosphere, there is a fall in blood volume
with dehydration; these people complain of fatigue, cramp,
muscular weakness and lack of power to concentrate mentally.
The condition responds to a sufficient intake of salt; the salt
should be added to beverages and drinking water.

Potassium.—This salt is present in all articles of diet; it acts as a buffering agent and regulates the osmotic pressure of body fluid. It is one of the essentials in contraction of cardiac muscle.

Magnesium.—Magnesium is associated with calcium in the formation of bones and teeth; it also plays a part in enzyme activity. Food sources include green vegetables, fruits, meat, fish and cereals.

Water.—This is of the utmost importance in nutrition; it constitutes more than half of the total weight of the body. Water is a solvent for all nutrients and a carrier of these elements in the systemic circulation. Water is excreted from the body in urine, faeces, perspiration, vapour from the lungs and by vomiting. Deficiency of water leads to a rise in the osmotic pressure of the plasma protein, dehydration and finally death. It is imperative that unconscious and semiconscious patients should be supplied with sufficient water to prevent dehydration. Dietary sources of water are drinking water, beverages, soups, gravies, the water in solid foods and water from oxidation of foods. In the normal metabolism of the body the water intake should balance the water output.

Water Requirement.—It is estimated that infants require daily $2\frac{1}{2}$–3 ounces of fluid per pound body weight. The amount of fluid required by the average adult varies with the temperature of his environment. In a country of variable temperatures 3–4 pints of fluid (including the water content of solid food) is sufficient, but in tropical countries the fluid requirement may be 4 times this amount. In disease the fluid requirements vary; they may be within normal limits or they may increase.

Special Articles of Food

The protective foods are those foods which contain substances essential for the prevention of deficiency diseases. The main examples are given below.

Milk.—Milk is a valuable food from birth to old age. It can be incorporated into diets in many attractive ways to humour the most capricious appetite. It is discussed in the following chapter (p. 141).

Cheese.—Cheese is made from whole or skimmed milk; the caseinogen is precipitated by clotting with rennet or with a weak acid such as vinegar. The whey is extracted by pressure, the degree of pressure determining the consistency of the cheese i.e. whether it is a hard or soft variety. The harder the cheese the less whey it contains and the higher the nutrient value for weight. The precipitated clot is allowed to ripen under conditions peculiar to the type of cheese required. As an article of diet cheese is excellent; it provides in a concentrated form protein, fat, minerals and vitamins.   Cheese is a very nutritious and digestible food for children and sick persons; it can be grated and made into sandwiches or sprinkled in soups or over vegetables.

Butter.—Butter is formed by the agitation of cream in a churn.   The fat globules adhere to each other until a solid mass is produced.   The fluid left in the churn is buttermilk.   Butter is always a good source of vitamin A but a good source of vitamin D only in the summer months or when the cow has had additional vitamin D in her diet.

Margarine.—This substance is manufactured from unsaturated fats, whale oil and vegetable oils; the unsaturated carbon atoms are saturated by hydrogen.   This process produces a fat of butter-like consistency.   Vitamins A and D are added. The caloric or energy value is the same as that of butter.

Eggs.—Eggs are good sources of protein, fat, calcium, phosphorus, iron and vitamins A and D and B_1.   The colour of the shell has a surface value only; a brown shell is no indication of the interior quality of the egg.   It is now known that cooked eggs are better utilized by the body than raw eggs.   Lightly boiled or poached eggs are digested in less time than hard boiled or fried eggs.

Preservation of Eggs.—The end point of all forms of egg preservation is to prevent evaporation of water and carbon dioxide through the porous egg shell.   This may be achieved by the use of sodium silicate or water glass, or by encasing the shell in a coating of fat, or by painting the shell with a special type of preserving varnish.   Another method of egg preservation is by drying.   The yolk and white are pulped together; the liquid is then forced through fine jets into a chamber, through which warm air circulates.   The water content of the eggs is quickly evaporated and the dried egg is deposited as a powder on the floor of the chamber.   The temperature is carefully controlled to prevent scorching of the egg.

Meat.—Meat includes the flesh and offal of all animals, poultry and game.   Meat contains protein of a high biological value, fat, mineral salts, riboflavin and nicotinic acid.   The flavour of meat is due to the presence of extractives.   The water content varies with the age of the animal; the younger the meat the higher is the water content; leg of mutton is 45 per cent water; veal is 75 per cent water.   The tenderness of meat is dependent upon the length of the bundles of muscle fibres; the shortest fibres are the muscles used the least—the sirloin, loin and middle ribs.   The most tender meat is breast of chicken. Tougher joints are the muscles which have been well exercised e.g. the leg, shin, neck and flank.

Pork.—Pork should not be given to young children and persons suffering from gastric lesions, owing to its indigestible properties. Because of the large amount of fat interspersed between the muscle fibres, the gastric juices require much longer to gain access to digest the fibres of pork, and the process of digestion is therefore slowed down.

Corned Beef.—This is a valuable addition to the diet; it is also a good source of iron and has the advantage of being cooked ready for eating.

Liver.—Liver should whenever possible be given to children and adolescents. It is easily digested and is a valuable source of iron, vitamins A and B_1, also riboflavin and nicotinic acid.

Sweetbread.—The term, sweetbread, is applied to the thymus gland of the lamb and calf and the pancreas of the sheep and ox; all are rich in phosphorus and nucleoprotein and are easily digested.

Bacon and Ham.—These are examples of cured pork; during the curing and smoking process the flesh is partially cooked. Both are easily digested by young children and invalids; they should not, however, be given to patients suffering from acute gastric conditions for whom a bland diet is required.

Tripe.—Tripe is the lining of the stomach of the ox, cleaned and boiled. It contains a large amount of collagen which, when cooked, is converted into gelatin. As it is lacking in extractives tripe lacks flavour, but this can be added during the cooking by the vegetables used.

Fish.—The nutritive value of fish depends upon the type of fish to some extent. Fat fish, in which the fat is distributed throughout the body of the fish (herring, turbot, mackerel and salmon) yield a higher calorie value weight for weight than the white fish (cod, plaice and fresh haddock) in which the fat is stored in the liver. Fat fish is also a rich source of the fat soluble vitamins A and D. Fish as an article of diet supplies protein equal to the protein of meat, also phosphorus and other minerals. Sea fish is also a good source of iodine in the diet. Fish has a higher water content than meat: one and a half ounces of white fish or one and a quarter ounces of fat fish is equal in calorie value to one ounce of meat.

Tinned fish—sardines, herrings, pilchards and salmon—are of a high nutritive value and a good source of calcium, iron and the fat soluble vitamins.

Shell Fish.—These fall into two groups—mollusc and crustacean. The former include oysters, clams, scallops and mussels; the latter have crust like shells and are represented by lobsters, crabs, shrimps and prawns. All are of a high nutritive value and some are more easily digested than others. The crustacean group have denser and more fibrous tissue than those of the mollusc group.

TABLE OF FOODS ARRANGED ACCORDING TO THEIR COMPARATIVE DIGESTIBILITY

(With acknowledgments to Gilman Thomson and James Burnet)

1. *Easily Digested:* Oysters, soft-boiled eggs, sweetbreads, boiled white fish.

2. *Light Diet:* Boiled chicken, lean roast beef, lean steak, scrambled eggs, tripe.

3. *Ordinary Diet:* Roast mutton, fried bacon, roast chicken, liver, roast lamb, mutton cutlets.

4. *Heavy Diet:* Veal, ham, rabbit, salmon, herring, pork.

COMPOSITION AND CALORIE VALUE OF CERTAIN MEATS (AFTER PAVY)

	Lean Beef.	Fat Beef.	Lean Mutton.	Fat Mutton.	Veal.	Bacon.	Chicken.
Protein per cent	19·3	14·8	18·3	12·4	16·5	9·8	26·5
Fat per cent .	3·6	29·8	4·9	31·1	15·8	48·9	10·0
Salts per cent .	5·1	4·4	4·8	3·5	4·7	2·3	3·8
Water per cent	72·0	51·0	72·0	53·0	63·0	39·0	59·7
Calories per oz.	35	100	36	95	63	145	60

Vegetables.—Vegetables should occupy an important place in the dietary of all age groups. How important this is in the nutrition of the nation is shown by the policy of the Ministry of Food in bringing to the notice of the general public the necessity of growing more vegetables in gardens and allotments, and having grown the vegetables to know how to utilize them to the best advantage.

Vegetables may be divided into the following groups: 1. green leaf vegetables and salads; 2. roots and tubers (carrots, swedes, turnips, parsnips, potatoes, artichokes); 3. legumes or pulses (peas, beans, lentils); 4. gourds (cucumbers, marrows, pumpkins); 5. bulbs (leeks, onions, shallots, garlic, chives); 6. stems (celery, asparagus, mushrooms).

Nutritional Value of Vegetables.—Green leaf vegetables and salads are good sources of vitamin C, carotene, riboflavin, nicotinic acid and folic acid, also calcium and iron. As their calorie value is low they can form bulk in reducing diets.

Salad vegetables such as watercress, mustard and cress, radishes and raw, shredded tender cabbage or brussel sprouts should be introduced into the daily menu as often as possible.

Potatoes are a good source of carbohydrate and minerals. In

the winter months, when other vegetables are in short supply, they are a staple source of vitamin C.

Carrots, swedes, turnips and parsnips contain carbohydrate and variable amounts of vitamin C, carotene, calcium and iron.

Beetroot is a very useful vegetable for use in certain diets, as its carbohydrate is in the form of sugar. The red pigment in beetroot is very soluble in water and is intensified by acid; the addition of vinegar to beetroot for salads produces a brighter colour effect. Another interesting point is that the red pigment is excreted in the urine when large amounts are ingested.

Peas, beans and lentils provide protein which is not of such a high biological value as that of meat; this can be balanced by the addition of a complete protein such as bacon to beans, cheese to lentils and so on. All the pulses are good sources of iron, calcium, aneurin and pyridoxin.

Cucumbers, marrows and pumpkins all contain minerals; their water content is approximately 96 per cent; their calorie value is therefore low. Their value in the diet is more in the nature of an accompaniment to foods of a higher nutritive value.

Leeks, onions, shallots and similar bulbs are also rich in cellulose and should therefore be used with discretion in the diets of young children and sick persons.

Celery and asparagus are both good sources of inorganic minerals; owing to their low carbohydrate value and the ease with which they can be incorporated into reducing diets they have a satiety value.

Dried and canned vegetables.—The nutritive value is the same as when fresh. Modern methods of drying vegetables involves preliminary scalding; this preserves the colour, flavour and smell. By the addition of water the vegetables revert to their original form.

Dehydrated potatoes and carrots require to be soaked in hot water for two hours; ordinary cooking should then be done.

Mashed potato powder is dehydrated cooked potato; when reconstituted with water it is used in the same way as mashed potato.

Fruit.—Fruit is included in the protective foods because of its valuable vitamin C content. Blackcurrants contribute the highest amount of vitamin C; strawberries, oranges and grapefruit come next in order; gooseberries, raspberries, blackberries and tomatoes have lesser amounts. Apples, with the exception of Bramley seedlings, are a poor source of vitamin C.

Bananas are high in calorie value; they contain a large amount of starch which is changed into maltose as the fruit ripens. The natural sugars of fruit—fructose and glucose—are also present. This is the reason why ripe bananas are well tolerated by children suffering from coeliac disease.

The peel of the citrus fruits—oranges, lemons and grapefruit— contains large amounts of vitamin C and should be used for flavouring or, dried and grated, should be added to puddings.

The acid of fruit is oxidized in the body to carbon dioxide and water leaving an alkaline base residue. Fruits may be given generously to patients in whom an alkaline base is desirable.

Dried fruits, such as prunes, dates, figs, raisins and apricots, have a concentrated nutritive value; some are good sources of iron and calcium.

Nuts.—These contain fat and protein in a concentrated form and they can be used in the diet in a variety of ways.

Nut products such as canned nut meat, nut sandwich spreads, nut soups and peanut butter are all valuable articles of food. The chestnut has a high carbohydrate content and in some countries provides part of the staple diet of the peasants. Groundnuts are largely used for the extraction of oil for use in the manufacture of margarine and cooking fat.

Cereals.—Farinaceous or flour-producing foods are classed as cereals. Cereals include oats, wheat, barley, rye, maize and rice. Cereal products are manufactured from these and some of these include cornflakes, macaroni, noodles and vermicelli, all of which are made from wheat or wheat flour. Semolina contains more protein as it is from the aleurone or protein layer of wheat grain. Cornflour is almost all starch prepared by the refining of maize. Oatmeal contains more protein, fat, calcium and iron than any other cereal product.

Soya bean flour is a very valuable cereal; it has a very low carbohydrate content which is present in the form of dextrin; the fat and protein content is also high. A milk of high nutritive value is made from soya bean flour and is used extensively in some countries.

Alcohol.—Alcohol has a high energy value; it is quickly absorbed into the blood stream and its value in an emergency is well known. Alcohol also has its dangers; under its influence the central nervous system is depressed, resulting in dullness of accuracy and of good judgment. Alcohol is present in varying amounts in beers, wines, spirits or liqueurs; it may be 5 per cent as in beer or 35 per cent as in whisky.

Wines are made from fermented fruit juices, usually grapes; they may have an alcohol content of 20 per cent.

Medicated wines, of which there are some now on the home market, are usually port, sherry or burgundy to which meat extracts and proteolytic preparations such as peptones and polypeptides have been added. Their calorie value is parallel with that of other wines.

Beverages.—These serve a useful purpose in nutrition; they can be a means of introducing in solution all the food factors; they also possess stimulating properties.

Tea.—Tea consists of the leaves and buds of the tea shrub which have gone through a process of fermentation and dehydration. Tea contains a stimulant—caffeine, and also an astringent—tannic acid. Green tea is also obtained from the shrub; the leaves and buds only are dehydrated in this case; this type of tea contains the same percentage of caffeine and tannic acid as other tea. The food value of tea depends upon the amount of milk and sugar added.

Coffee.—Coffee is the bean of a small shrub; the characteristic flavour and aroma are developed by the technique employed in roasting the beans. The stimulating property is due to the presence of caffeine, and its nutritive value is parallel with the amount of cream and sugar added.

Cocoa.—This is obtained from the ripe seeds of the cocoa bean. Cocoa contains valuable nutrients. One ounce of cocoa powder yields 128 calories and also 4 milligrammes of iron. The carbohydrate is present in the form of starch which is insoluble; when making the beverage the best results are obtained by thoroughly cooking the cocoa with water before adding milk and sugar.

Condiments.—Condiments take their place in nutrition as flavouring agents and stimulants to appetite. Appetite may exist without actual hunger; herbs and condiments may be used as a means to promote appetite for food which in itself may be far from appetizing. It is on record that the victorious seamen of Nelson's fleet were deterred from mutiny only by the arrival of pickles, without which they were unable to consume their rations of salt pork, weevil-infested biscuits and mouldy cheese.

Pepper.—This is a product of the fruit from a creeping vine—Piper nigrum; white pepper is obtained from the ripe fruit and black pepper from the ground unripe fruit. Paprika is made from the ground ripe fruit of capsicum. Cayenne, or red pepper, is from the ground pods of capsicum.

Mustard.—This is derived from the powdered seeds of the mustard plant. English table mustard is made by blending ground mustard seed with turmeric and wheat flour to absorb the volatile oils and retard fermentation.

Vinegar.—Vinegar can be made from barley, molasses, wine and juice of fruits. Malt vinegar is a product of yeast-fermented barley; acetic acid gives the piquant flavour which is the characteristic property of all vinegars.

Salt.—The physiological value of sodium chloride has already been mentioned. The value of salt as a condiment has been universally appreciated down the ages, and much has been written in favour of it as a flavouring agent. The addition of salt to sweet dishes, cakes, sweetmeats and coffee enhances the

READY RECKONER FOR DIET, BY CALORIES; UNIT, ONE OUNCE

CALORIES

Over 250.	200–250.	150–200.	125–150.	100–125.	75–100.	50–75.	Less than 50.
Dripping (262)	Butter (225)	Chocolate (178)	Cheese (130)	Oatmeal (120)	Jam (98)	Brown bread (72)	Half-egg (38)
Lard (250)	Margarine (223)	Bacon (165)		Thick cream (120)	Currants (96)	Lean meat (65)	Liver (37)
				Pork (118)	Marmalade (96)	Salmon (65)	Lean mutton (36)
				Dried peas (114)	Raisins (96)	Chicken (60)	Rabbit (35)
				Sugar (114)	Fat mutton (95)	Sardines (59)	Green peas (32)
				Dried beans (112)	Honey (95)	Herrings (57)	Potatoes (30)
				Dried lentils (110)	White bread (90)		Plums (23)
				Ham (104)	Syrup (67)		Milk (20)
				Macaroni (104)			Bananas (19)
				Flour (103)			Tripe (17)
				Sago (103)			Apples (14)
				Tapioca (103)			Beetroot (12)
				Rice (102)			Carrots (10)
				Fat beef (101)			Oranges (10)
							Greens (8)
							Turnips (8)
							Onions (7)

The figures after each article indicate the average number of calories. Most vegetables and fruits not mentioned above have a calorie value of from 5–10.

flavour.   Salt is also a valuable property in food preservation.

Proprietary Preparations : Value and Dangers

Owing to the shortage of protein in Western Europe, the bulk of proprietary foods on the home market have as their base one or sometimes more of the cereals, wheat, oats and barley, to which other ingredients are added.   Their particular identity is associated with the technique employed in the preparation. They may be processed or partially cooked, or they may contain a diastase to predigest the starch.   No proprietary food should be prescribed in infant feeding without a basic knowledge of its ingredients and calorie value.

The dietary value of proprietary foods depends to some degree upon the requirements of the individual and the indications present for incorporating any particular one into the diet.   Meat extracts are valuable as flavouring agents; they cannot be regarded as having a very high nutritive value.   Tinned meats and fish are a valuable addition to the protein ration and should be made use of whenever possible.

Tinned milk is obtained as dry milk powder and as unsweetened evaporated milk or as sweetened condensed milk.   All tinned milk contains valuable nutrients which can be used in infant feeding, and should be given in the correct proportions with added vitamins.

CHAPTER 10

MILK

COMPOSITION OF MILK. SOURCES OF CONTAMINATION.
DIRT IN MILK. ADULTERATION OF MILK. STORAGE
AND PRESERVATION OF MILK. NORMAL TREATMENT
OF ORDINARY MILK. DISEASES ASSOCIATED WITH MILK.
DESIGNATED MILKS. HEAT STERILIZATION. TUBERCULIN-
TESTED MILK. ACCREDITED MILK. PASTEURIZATION OF
MILK. OTHER METHODS OF TREATING MILK.

From every point of view, there is probably no more important food than milk. We frequently speak of it as a perfect food, since it contains the 6 constituents of food necessary for life. Milk is part of the dietary of almost every man, woman and child in Great Britain, being almost as essential as water. Furthermore, the production of milk on the large scale necessary is an undertaking demanding the application of every modern and scientific device to maintain its standard of purity, and the laws controlling its preservation, storage and sale are far reaching and exacting. Knowing how easy it is for cow's milk to act as the vehicle in the spread of infectious diseases, particularly tuberculosis, we need not be surprised that supervision of this food is carried out from the time the cow is milked until the bottle of milk is deposited at the door. Of recent years, not only the distribution but also the quality of milk has been carefully controlled, and the time seems to have come when we can regard the supply as the best obtainable in present circumstances. There is no doubt that the solution of the milk problem is the solution to many other dependent problems affecting the general health of the community.

The fundamental constituents and the general properties of milk have already been mentioned (Vol. I, pp. 214 and 215), and later on (Vol. III, Sect. 7 chapt. 7) the food value of milk is discussed from the dietetic point of view. In this chapter we must confine our studies to the purely hygienic side of milk, dealing chiefly with the publc health aspect.

Composition of Milk

The constituents of milk are caseinogen, lactalbumin, a trace of lactoglobulin, which are first class proteins; fats; lactose (sugar of milk), a disaccharide; and the various salts already mentioned.   If milk is to be termed " good milk," its fat content should be 3·5 per cent and above.   The fat of cow's milk is all-important.   It consists chiefly of butyrin, from which butter is derived.   This fat rises to the top of the milk when the latter is allowed to stand for a few hours and is known as cream.   The quality of milk is often determined by its fat content, and naturally this depends upon the type of cow, the method of feeding and the possible dilution of the milk by the retailer.   There is also a seasonal and diurnal variation in the quality of milk; in the last quarter of the year milk is richer in fats than at any other period and it is well-known to dairymen that a cow gives her " fattest " milk in the evening.   Jersey cows are closely followed by Ayrshire cows in showing the highest percentage of fat in their milk.   Three gallons of milk a day per cow is a good yield in a dairy; the average is about 15 pints.   Milk is soured after a certain time by the formation of lactic acid.   Initially cow's milk is neutral, but it turns acid owing to the splitting up of lactose by bacteria into lactic acid and this change has usually occurred before the milk is delivered.   The process of splitting up goes on steadily until ultimately the milk may be turned sour. Since cow's milk is used extensively for the feeding of children, its vitamin content is important.   Vitamins A, B_1, B_2, C, D and E may all be found in cow's milk.   When grass is plentiful vitamin A, containing carotene, is abundant, but this vitamin is almost absent in the winter months.   Pasture fed animals give milk with a higher vitamin A, C and D content than those which are stall fed. Vitamins B and C are variable.   The practice of giving children orange juice or substitutes with their feeds ensures that plenty of vitamin C is provided.   Calcium is one of the main properties of milk, and in combination with phosphorus, calcium phosphate is formed which is chiefly concerned with the structure of teeth and bones.   Absorption of calcium phosphate is complete only if vitamin D is present.   Calcium salts are believed to play a special part in muscle contraction, and are essential for blood clotting outside the blood vessels.   Iron is weakly represented; its deficiency is made good by the iron of the water.

Sources of Contamination

Before dealing with the subject of impure milk, we must understand what is meant by the term " clean milk."   The law insists on certain standards of fats and non-fatty solids, but it also makes regulations for the cleanliness of milk.

Clean Milk.—It is impossible to maintain a normal milk distribution without allowing for the presence of some bacteria.

A dirty milk contains millions of bacteria but a clean milk has very few; this is the simple method of designating the cleanliness of milk. When we consider the conditions of great difficulty under which the dairyman has to work, it is surprising how clean milk may be rendered; the two chief methods are by killing off the bacteria and by taking measures to keep the milk free from contamination during its journey to the consumer. If any milk is found to contain more than ·0001 per cent of dirt it is unfit for human consumption.

Dirt in Milk.—Dirt can get into milk in various ways.

1. *In the Dairy.*—The difficulties of milking a cow in the old fashioned cowshed are self evident. Even with all the modern improvements, there is still a possibility of soiling the milk when it is passing from the udder to the pail. Manure is the main source of contamination, and it is made more dangerous on account of the fact that it dissolves in part in milk. Millions of bacteria may thus find their way into the milk at the start and by multiplication add to the uncleanliness of the already soiled milk. It must never be forgotten that milk is an ideal medium for the breeding of microbes. Every modern dairy farmer knows that in addition to the cow herself, there are many sources of uncleanliness. The hands and the clothes of the milker, the milk pails and cans, the house fly and many other factors must be the subject of careful study. Apart from the tubercle bacillus the chief bacteria found are the bacillus coli, the streptococcus and the bacillus of lactic acid.

2. *In Transit.*—While the law is very strict in controlling the cleanliness of milk at all stages of its journey to the table, potential sources of dirt may become operative. Thus there may be contamination while the milk stands in a dairy, and cream which is skimmed off from wide basins may contain numerous bacteria, since they rise to the surface. Again the milk cans may be tampered with on carts, on the railways or at the distributing centres. The retailer may be responsible for tainted milk by careless methods of handling. Lastly the consumer himself may allow the milk to become infected in his household by leaving it exposed to flies and dust or by letting it come in contact with dirty utensils. It is therefore clear that the problem of clean milk is a serious and difficult one, and is not to be wondered at that it has been made a national one.

Adulteration of Milk

For over 40 years the regulations controlling the standard of milk have given the following 3 essentials.

1. That if the milk fat is less than 3 per cent it is presumed

that some of the original fat has been extracted or that water
has been added.

2. That if milk contains less than 8·5 per cent of non-fatty
solids it is similarly under suspicion.

3. That separated, or skimmed, milk must contain more than
8·7 per cent of total solids.

Under the Food and Drugs (Adulteration) Act of 1928, milk
must be " of the nature, substance and quality demanded by the
purchaser," and it must be free of any injurious mixture.   Milk
therefore includes its full cream, and it is an offence to take away
any of its normal constituents.   The time has come when the
village pump is no longer a substitute for the recalcitrant cow.
It is indeed a smart dairyman who succeeds in eluding the law
for any time on the matter of milk adulteration.   Milk is a food
which must be kept as near as possible to the condition found
when the milk is at its exodus from the udder; even the addition
of any preservative is now illegal.   These restrictions are not
harsh; investigations prove that the standards of milk are not too
high; indeed many types contain a much higher percentage of
fats and non-fatty solids than is required by law.

Storage and Preservation of Milk

Under this heading we study the methods in use to ensure the
safety of milk until it reaches the consumer, and we also deal with
the grading of milk, a classification of great importance.   On
examination milk may appear clean, but it may not be safe to
drink.

Normal Treatment of Ordinary Milk.—The regulations
insist on certain precautions regarding the cows, the cowsheds,
the milkers, the dairy premises, the containers and the transport
of milk.   In the Acts and Orders pertaining to the milk trade,
registration of dairymen, management and handling of cows,
prevention of disease and its spread and clear directions as to
the disposal of milk are provided for.   All cows must be prevented from infection of any kind.   As a result, the modern
dairy farmer must carry out a scrupulous toilet of his cows prior
to milking.   This should include daily grooming, especially of
the long hairs near the udders, washing the udders thoroughly,
and rinsing with water to which a weak disinfectant has been
added.   Suspicion that he is a carrier of infection may fall on
an attendant, and if indeed the latter is proved to be a carrier
immediate exclusion from milking is necessary.   A medical
examination, with a satisfactory report, is essential before the
attendant can resume work.   The farmer's premises must be
hygienic, and he must be prepared for casual visitations from
the sanitary inspector and the veterinary surgeon; his milkers

must wear clean aprons and caps, must sterilize the hands and keep them dry when milking; the milk pails should be covered or have a very narrow inlet, preferably at the side. Immediately the milking is over, the milk must be cooled to about 50° F. or not more than 5° above the temperature of the water used in

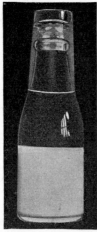

Fig. 54.—How to keep a half filled milk bottle free from contamination by means of a tumbler.

(*By courtesy of the National Milk Publicity Council.*)

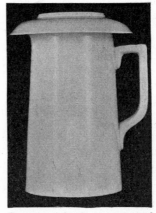

Fig. 55.—A hygienic method of keeping a milk jug free from flies and other forms of pollution.

(*By courtesy of the National Milk Publicity Council.*)

cooling it. This is of vital importance in limiting the multiplication of germs. After the milk is cooled, it can be stored in proper receptacles, and all the utensils must be sterilized by boiling or by steam under pressure. Space does not allow a consideration of the numerous refinements of milk treatment and storage carried out by the large dairy companies, who, in dealing with great volumes of milk, arrange for its perfect preservation. Nor can we deal with the special types of mechanical milkers and other cowshed refinements which make the modern dairy entirely different from its predecessors. The illustrations show how far reaching is the advance in modern hygiene. In the delivery of milk to the consumer, undoubtedly the introduction of the glass bottle with patent sterilized cap is a wonderful improvement on the old milk can.

The nurse should make the storage of her patients' milk a special duty. Caps should be kept clean and replaced immediately any milk has been taken out of the bottle. All milk left in jugs and open bowls should be covered with fine gauze weighted down with beads, so that flies are kept out. The importance of boiling all utensils is paramount. When possible milk should be kept in a refrigerator. All these precautions must be adopted for the prevention of the various infections of milk which are described below.

Diseases Associated with Milk.—Undoubtedly modern science has succeeded in stamping out many of the diseases spread by milk, but tuberculosis is still the chief danger, and this despite elaborate precautions. The bacillus found in the cow (the bovine type) is not the same as that active in phthisis in adult man, but children who suffer from bone and abdominal tuberculosis are found to harbour the bovine bacillus in 60 per cent of cases. Now, milk is universally drunk by children, and the question of tuberculosis is therefore a most vital one for the race. Children from birth, if bottle fed, to 15 years of age, consume more milk than adults do and it is in this age group that non-pulmonary tuberculosis is most fatal. Statistics tell their own tale. It has to be admitted that over 25 per cent of all dairy cows suffer from tuberculosis in some form. About 2 per cent have tuberculous udders and thus the T.B. are transferred to the milk direct. But in the majority of cases, milk containing T.B. is not infected from the udder, and we have to face the fact that at least 10 per cent of the milk sold in London contains the tubercle bacillus. The percentage varies in different towns, but the menace has not passed off. It is an offence to sell tuberculous milk.

Other diseases known to be spread by milk are typhoid fever, paratyphoid fever, cholera, diphtheria, scarlet fever, dysentery, summer diarrhoea of children, foot and mouth disease and septic sore throat; the last is a type of tonsillitis which is caused by the streptococcus and which may be passed to the milk from an inflamed udder. Malta fever is a peculiar infection common formerly in soldiers stationed in **Malta**, and traced to goats' milk.

Designated Milks.—Milks are classified according to their purity or to their special treatment. Professor J. R. Currie and Dr. A. G. Mearns of Glasgow give the following classification of designated milks in England and Wales:

1. Tuberculin-tested milk;
2. Accredited milk;
3. Pasteurized milk.

Thus 3 grades or designations are now recognized, but as tuberculin-tested milk is delivered raw, it must be labelled " tuberculin-tested (certified)." This milk is bottled at the farm and heat has not been applied to it. If protected against tuberculosis and other milk borne diseases by pasteurization, then all bottles are labelled "tuberculin-tested milk (pasteurized)," after being firmly sealed.

There are 4 designations of milk in Scotland as follows:

    1. Certified;
    2. Tuberculin-tested;
    3. Standard;
    4. Pasteurized.

No dairyman is allowed to have a special licence for the production of these milks unless he can at least come within 50 per cent of the ideal in method and equipment.

Heat Sterilization.—It must be kept constantly in mind that much of the artificial treatment of milk is due to the desire on the part of the dairy farmer to retain the sweetness of the milk for as long a period as possible. Formerly antiseptics such as boracic acid and formalin were allowed, but now there are not any preservatives in use. Boiling, or sterilization, for 5 minutes, kills all the microbes, but it makes a big change in the essential constituents of the milk, turning the calcium and magnesium salts out as precipitations, altering the vitamins, especially vitamin A and vitamin C, and coagulating the lactalbumin so that it forms a thick skin, containing some of the fat, on the surface of the milk. There is a distinct change of taste and generally speaking the milk is less palatable and less digestible. Nevertheless it must be realized that often there is no alternative to boiling. Pasteurization is the best method of heat treatment. This is discussed below.

1. *Tuberculin-tested Milk.*—If bottled at the farm, this grade of milk is labelled *Tuberculin-tested Milk (Certified)*. If bottled at the dairy it is labelled *Tuberculin-tested Milk*. If pasteurized, it contains fewer bacteria, and it is labelled *Tuberculin-tested Milk (Pasteurized)*.

All animals concerned in this category must be examined at least twice a year by a veterinary surgeon; similarly the tuberculin test must be carried out at the same interval. The most careful precautions are taken to exclude tuberculous cows from the herd, which should be kept by itself, with a register of each cow. The milk is collected, and after cooling, put into sterilized bottles on the premises. Bottles are specially sealed with airtight caps, fully describing the origin and nature of the milk. Any heat process is forbidden, and milk should be cooled immediately to 50° F. or lower. Further, the milk must satisfy various tests for purity and cream content: 30,000 bacteria per cubic centimetre is the limit of contamination, while no colon bacillus must be demonstrated in ·1 cubic centimetre.

2. *Accredited Milk.*—The cows are not submitted to a tuberculin test, but are examined every 3 months by a veterinary surgeon. All doubtful cows must be removed or isolated. Other rules

concerning the herd are similar to those laid down for tuber-culin-tested milk. Bottling and labelling requirements are also similar, but farm bottled milk must be labelled *Accredited Milk Farm Bottled*. If sent to a dairy, the label reads *Accredited Milk* only. No heat should be applied, unless for pasteurization pur-poses. The bacterial tests are not so strict; the limit for bacteria

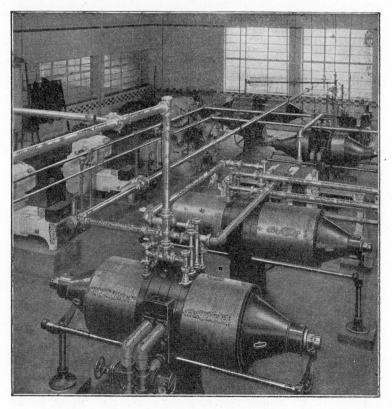

FIG. 56.—MILK PASTEURIZING PLANT.
(By courtesy of United Dairies, Ltd., London.)

is 200,000 per c.cm.; no colon bacillus must be found in ·01 cubic centimetre.

3. *Pasteurization of Milk.*—This is a common and accepted pro-cess, and is much cheaper than the first 2 methods of obtaining a pure milk, since it eliminates many veterinary and transport charges. There are no regulations regarding the cows. Bottles and containers are used only for pasteurized milk. If milk is

pasteurized, the label must be distinctly printed *Pasteurized Milk.*

In pasteurization of milk, the principle is the raising of milk to a certain temperature at which the germs are destroyed, but none of the other changes associated with boiling occur. There are two methods, the flash method and the holder method. In the former, the milk is passed through an apparatus which provides for the sudden and momentary exposure of the milk to a temperature of about 165° F. Rapid cooling is arranged for. This method is not popular, as it is supposed to be uncertain in its action. The system used by most of the big dairy companies is the holder method, which keeps the milk at a temperature of between 145° F. and 150° F. for half an hour, then immediately

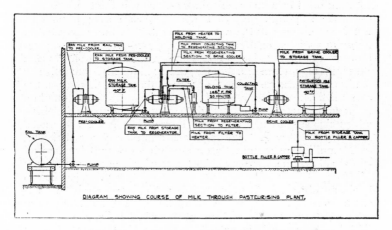

FIG. 57.—HOLDER METHOD OF MILK PASTEURIZATION.
(*By courtesy of United Dairies, Ltd., London.*)

cools it down to 40° F. In ordinary pasteurized milk, a count of less than 100,000 bacteria per cubic centimetre (c.cm.) is stipulated. There is no doubt that the holder method is a great benefit to the human race. We can be certain that there is little or no alteration in the constituents, except that the bacteria are reduced by about 95 per cent and vitamin C is destroyed. The only doubtful germ is the T.B., and research is still proceeding on its characteristics. In large centres requiring huge daily amounts of milk, pasteurization must be regarded as of superlative benefit in the restriction of disease.

Other Methods of Treating Milk.—Drying milk reduces it to a fine powder, containing all the necessary constituents unchanged in value. The method used is that of passing the milk through very hot roller machines, which quickly drive off the water. Seven parts of water must be added to one part of powder before use. Desiccated milk forms the basis of many proprietary infant foods. Evaporated milk is milk reduced 50 per cent by heating. Homogenized milk is supplied commonly in London; it represents an attempt to retain the fat in small globules through the body of the milk. Milk may be skimmed by hand or by a centrifugal machine; in the latter case it is also called separated milk, and is, if sweetened, unfit for infant feeding. Condensed milk is evaporated milk to which sugar has been added.

CHAPTER 11

PREPARATION AND SERVING OF FOOD

METHODS OF COOKING. BOILING. BAKING. BRAISING.
STEWING. STEAMING. FRYING. GRILLING OR BROILING.
MAKING OF SOUP. PRACTICAL SICKROOM COOKERY.
RECIPES FOR SICKROOM COOKERY. BEEF TEA. JELLIES.
JUNKET. WHEY. PEPTONIZED MILK. CITRATED MILK.
LACTIC ACID MILK. HYDROCHLORIC ACID MILK. GRUEL.
ARROWROOT. ALBUMEN WATER. BARLEY WATER. EGG
DISHES. BEVERAGES FOR INVALIDS.

It is important in the application of dietary principles for nurses
to have a basic knowledge of the general principles of cooking
and of the changes which take place in some foods during the
process of cooking. In addition to physical changes which occur
during the cooking of food, the destruction of bacteria responsible
for souring and putrefaction takes place. There is also the
psychological element associated with well cooked appetizing
food.

Cooking increases the digestibility of some vegetables and
cereals by softening the cellulose envelope surrounding the
starch cells; the cells absorb water, increase in size and rupture.
The result is that either a gelatinous or a flour like condition is
produced which is parallel with the amount of water absorbed
by the starch cells. The short crisp texture of biscuits is a condition obtained by absorption by the ruptured starch granules of
fat and sugar.

The palatability of meat is increased and its mastication is
made easier by cooking. Physical changes occur, the protein is
coagulated and the collagen or gristle is converted into gelatine;
water is also evaporated during roasting. As a result a certain
amount of shrinkage takes place. It is now established that
undercooked meat is more easily digested than well cooked meat;
the amount of heat required for the easy digestion of meat should
not be sufficient to change the colour of the haemoglobin from
red to brown.

Methods of Cooking

Boiling.—In this method food is submerged in cold or boiling

151

water and the water is kept boiling until cooking is completed. This is the general principle adopted in cooking meat, vegetables and specially prepared pudding mixtures. It is not a practical method for cooking fish owing to the great loss of minerals and of flavouring which takes place. Meat may either be placed in cold water and brought to boiling point or plunged into boiling water. The loss of soluble properties in the meat is the same for either method employed.

Baking.—Baking is a process of cooking by the circulation of hot air around the food inside a gas or electric oven. Meat should stand on a rack placed inside the baking tin to allow the heated air to circulate freely under the meat. As meat is a slow conductor of heat, 45 minutes per pound at an oven temperature of 300° F. is required for thin small pieces of meat; for solid joints of meat 25 minutes per pound is sufficient at the same oven temperature. The surface of the meat should be basted with hot fat every 15 minutes to prevent undue hardening and loss of moisture. Meat should never be punctured by piercing with a sharp instrument during the process of cooking.

Braising.—This is a combination of dry and moist cooking, it is a suitable method to employ for cooking game and small joints. An oven casserole with a well fitting lid is a suitable receptacle in which to cook the food. The surplus fat is trimmed off the meat, which is then lightly fried on both sides and the prepared vegetables are sliced and browned in the frying pan; they are then placed in the casserole to form a foundation or bed for the meat. The meat is then placed on the vegetables and sufficient stock is added to surround the vegetables without covering the meat. The casserole is put into a moderately hot oven and the meat is allowed to cook in the savoury vapour of the vegetables. One hour should be the time allowed for cooking a small bird, rabbit or small piece of meat.

Stewing.—Stewing is an economical method of cooking the cheaper joints such as shin of beef and scrag end of mutton or breast of mutton; any vegetables in season may be added for flavouring. All surplus fat should be removed from the meat, and sufficient stock added to cover the meat and vegetables. The correct heat required for stewing is 180° F. A stew should never boil. Stewing is a process of long, slow cooking.

Steaming.—This is a cooking process in which heated vapour is employed. It is very suitable for cooking puddings when a light spongy mixture is desired, but it is not an economical one to employ in the cooking of meat because many of the soluble nutrients escape into the water contained in the steamer. The modern high pressure steamers are excellent as the temperature can be raised much above boiling point and food cooked very quickly with correspondingly less loss of soluble nutrients.

Frying.—Frying is the cooking of food in heated oil or fat. Careful attention is necessary to obtain good results. The fat should reach a temperature of 360° F., which is indicated by the appearance of blue smoke rising from the surface. Deep fat frying is an economical method used in large scale frying; less fat is absorbed by the food, and the fat can be used many times for the same purpose. Shallow frying is the term applied when sufficient fat only is allowed to prevent the food adhering to the bottom of the pan. It is a suitable method for bacon, sausage, small fillets of steak and cutlets. Fried food is appetizing and popular, and quite suitable for many patients. It is estimated that the vitamin C loss in chip potatoes is 20 per cent less than when potatoes are boiled. A certain amount of fat is absorbed by food during the process of frying, a point to be remembered when a reducing diet is prescribed.

Grilling or Broiling.—These terms are used to describe cooking by direct heat from a bright glowing fire, or under the deflector of a gas or electric grill. It is a very suitable method for the quick cooking of rashers of bacon, fillet of steak, chops and kidneys. The surface of the food should be brushed with fat to prevent excessive scorching and the heat should be maintained until the food is cooked throughout. A properly cooked grilled steak or chop should be of a deep brown colour on both sides, with a puffy raised centre; the meat should be elastic to the touch.

Making of Soup.—The basis of soup is stock, which may be obtained from meat, fish or vegetable sources. The stock is the vehicle for both soluble and insoluble nutrients.

Soups are grouped into 2 classes, thin or thick. Broths and *consommés* (or clear soups) are in the former class; and *potages* in the latter class. The dietetic value of soup will largely depend upon the ingredients used for making the soup. Hot soup is valuable as a stimulant when given to persons suffering from exposure to cold. The following is the correct proportion of ingredients for 1 pint of soup: ½ lb. meat, ½ lb. vegetables, 2 oz. soaked peas, beans or lentils. The following additions may be made before a soup is served; egg yolks, milk, cream or wine.

A well prepared soup should have a good flavour from the blending of meat, vegetables and condiments. It should be free from grease; this may be achieved by careful skimming throughout the process of making the soup. The texture should be smooth and free from lumps and the colour should be suitable so that the soup is in all respects appetizing.

Practical Sickroom Cookery.—When preparing meals for sick persons, any of the above methods may be employed to suit the individual patient's requirements. Whenever possible the best ingredients obtainable should be used for the preparation of all sickroom dishes.

Serving of Meals

The following observations may help in the serving of the meals.

1. Meals should be served punctually. This is especially important when the meal is for a gastric or diabetic patient.

2. Serve small quantities at first on plates or dishes of the correct size. Second helpings may be given when asked for. When this principle is adopted there is less plate wastage.

3. Whenever possible, serve the food from individual portion dishes. This is more attractive than a helping from one large dish.

4. Every effort should be made to provide the patient with hot food on a hot plate; alternatively when a cold dish or jelly is to be served it should remain in the refrigerator until required for the patient.

5. Care should be taken in garnishing the food; a coloured tray cloth and elegant china add to the general appearance of the meal as a whole. Many patients dislike changes from food to which they are accustomed. This is a most important point missed often by doctors and nurses. New flavours and new kinds of food should be introduced into the diet gradually, together with some other food with which such patients are familiar.

Recipes for Sickroom Cookery

Beef Tea.—The value of this preparation lies more in the stimulant rather than the nutritive properties. It is known that meat protein is coagulated at 160° F., therefore to obtain the maximum amount of protein in solution the heat employed during the preparation should be gradually increased and should not exceed 180° F. If coagulation of the meat protein is allowed to occur a mass of cooked meat will remain in the bottom of the cooking vessel, and there will be a corresponding loss in the amount of soluble protein present in the beef tea. The most suitable meats to use for beef tea are rump steak, fillet of steak or topside, which are juicy and easily disintegrated. Shin of beef is not suitable owing to the toughness of its texture.

Method for Ordinary Beef Tea.—1 lb. beef steak to 1 pint cold water, salt to taste. Remove the skin, gristle and fat from the meat; cut the meat into thin strips in the direction of the muscle fibres. It is then scraped and placed in an earthenware jar containing 1 pint of cold water and salt and allowed to stand for 30 minutes; during this time the meat is pressed against the sides of the jar to assist the disintegration of the meat. The jar is covered with greased paper and placed in an oven at a temperature of 180° F. for 3 hours; at the end of this time the beef tea should be strained through muslin or a large mesh strainer. The fat should be skimmed from the surface and any fat remaining after skimming should be removed by absorbing it with kitchen paper from the surface. The finished beef tea should have the appearance of a light brown smooth liquid; marmite may be added to supply vitamin B and salt.

Raw Beef Tea.—The ingredients are the same as for ordinary beef tea. The meat is also prepared in the same manner, cold water and salt being added and the meat and water allowed to stand for 1 hour during which time the meat is frequently pressed or pounded against the sides of the jar in order to extract all the soluble properties. It is then strained and served in a coloured glass.

Chicken Broth.—Ingredients: the carcase, legs and wings of a chicken, 1½ pints water or stock, 2 carrots, 3 cloves, 6 peppercorns, 1 onion, 1 teaspoonful chopped parsley. Salt to taste.

Method: chop the carcase into pieces and cut the meat from the legs and wings; place all the ingredients into a saucepan with the stock or water and simmer gently for 3 hours, then strain. Cereal pearl barley or rice may be added to the above ingredients. The breast of chicken may be minced and served as a separate dish or made into a fricassee.

Jellies.—These are classified as clear (or transparent) and opaque. Transparent jellies are solutions of gelatine in water; fruit juices, wine and brandy may be added. They should just be sufficiently stiff to support their own weight when turned out of the mould. Opaque jellies are solutions of gelatine in milk, egg or port wine. The dietetic value of jelly is to refresh and stimulate; although the nutritive value is low, jelly has a very definite place in the diet of the sick person.

Gelatine is prepared from animal tissues including the skin, bones, ligaments and tendons; it goes through various processes of refining before it is finally produced as commercial gelatine. Gelatine should never be boiled or overheated; when this occurs the gelatine becomes sticky and unusable. The best results are obtained by placing it in a cool solution and gradually increasing the heat to 160° F.

Isinglass is a refined form of gelatine prepared from the

swimming bladder of the sturgeon; it is tasteless and has a higher setting property than gelatine.

Agar-agar is prepared from seaweed; it is valuable for vegetarian cookery.

Calves' Foot Jelly.—This jelly is set by the gelatine extracted from calves' feet by prolonged boiling. Ingredients: 2 calves' feet, 5 pints water. To make the stock for the jelly, wash and scrape the feet and cut them up into pieces; remove the marrow and fat and wash in warm water. Blanch the feet by placing them in a pan of cold water and bring to boiling point. Pour away the water and rinse the feet. Put the feet into an enamel pan, cover with 5 pints cold water, bring slowly to boiling point and simmer for 5–6 hours until the water is reduced to half its volume. Strain through muslin or a fine mesh sieve and leave until cold.

Clear Calves' Foot Jelly.—Ingredients: the rind and juice of 2 lemons, 4 oz. sugar, 2 oz. sherry, 4 cloves, stock, 1½ pints from the calves' foot jelly described above, the whites and shells of 2 eggs. Method: remove any fat present on the surface of the jellied stock and wipe it over with a clean damp cloth. Place all the ingredients in a deep enamel lined pan, wash the lemons and peel off the rind thinly, wash the egg shells and crush them; these act as a filter when the jelly is strained. Add the 2 egg whites and whisk into the other ingredients over a moderate heat. Care should be taken to keep all the ingredients at a temperature of 160° F.; if the temperature is allowed to rise beyond this the egg albumen will coagulate and the jelly will not be so clear. Cease whisking and allow the jelly to reach boiling point. Strain the jelly through a flannel jelly bag.

Egg Jelly.—Ingredients: 1 pint liquid to include the juice of 2 lemons and water. The rind and juice of 2 lemons, 4 oz. sugar, 2 eggs and ½ oz. gelatine. Method: place the gelatine in a saucepan and add the sugar, lemon rind and 1 pint of water and lemon juice. Stir over moderate heat until the gelatine is in solution. Whisk the eggs and add them to the mixture; strain and pour into wet moulds.

Milk Jelly.—Ingredients: ½ pint milk, ¼ oz. gelatine, the thin rind of a lemon and 1 oz. sugar. Method: dissolve the gelatine in the milk and add the sugar, then the thinly pared lemon rind. Strain the jelly and pour into wet moulds and allow to set.

Junket.—Ingredients: 1 pint unboiled milk, 1 teaspoonful castor sugar, 2 teaspoonfuls essence of rennet, flavouring, nutmeg. Method: warm the milk to blood heat, pour into a glass bowl, add the sugar and rennet, stir lightly. Leave the mixture undisturbed in a warm place until set. Grate a little nutmeg over the surface.

Whey.—This is prepared by adding 2 teaspoonfuls essence of rennet to 1 pint unboiled milk at 100° F. A clot will form; this is broken up with a fork or knife and strained through muslin. If the whey is required for use in infant feeding it should be boiled before using.

Sherry Whey.—Add 2 oz. cooking sherry to 1 pint of unboiled milk at 160° F.; this will curdle the milk; strain through muslin and the whey is ready to use.

Peptonized Milk.—Peptonizing milk is a process of pre-digesting the protein of cow's milk by active pancreatin. One pint of milk is warmed to 100° F. and the active enzyme added, the whole being kept in a water bath at 100° F. for 20 minutes and then brought to boiling point to destroy the enzyme. If the milk is allowed to peptonize for longer a bitter flavour develops. There are several preparations of pancreatin obtainable; they all possess the same properties of the active pancreatic enzymes and directions for use will be found with each preparation.

Citrated Milk.—This is made by adding sodium citrate (1–2 grains) to a feed of whole cow's milk; if quantity of the feed is over 7 oz., another grain of sodium citrate should be added. Sodium citrate is an alkali; its addition to cow's milk breaks up the casein into a flocculent formation and it is more easily digested by some infants or by patients with gastric ulcer.

Lactic Acid Milk.—To 1 pint of cooled boiled milk add, drop by drop, 40 drops of lactic acid (BP), stirring all the time; the milk is then ready for use. If the milk is warmed above 98° F. it will curdle. Another method employed in the feeding of infants is to add the lactic acid to the feed in the feeding bottle, allowing 2 drops of lactic acid to each ounce of milk.

Hydrochloric Acid Milk.—This is used in some types of infantile eczema. Boil 1 pint of milk and cool; remove the surface skin of lactalbumen, make up the infant's feeds to the prescribed amount and put into feeding bottles. Before the infant is fed, warm the feed to 90° F. and add 2 drops of dilute hydrochloric acid to each ounce of cow's milk in a feed.

Gruel.—Ingredients: ½ ounce, or one dessertspoonful of groats or fine oatmeal to 7 oz. of milk; sugar and salt to taste. Method: mix the dry ingredients into a paste with a little cold boiled water, boil the milk and stir into the mixed paste. Return the mixture to the saucepan and cook for 5 minutes.

Arrowroot.—Allow 1 dessertspoonful of arrowroot to ½ pint milk. Mix the arrowroot into a paste with cold water, add ½ pint boiling milk stirring constantly, return to saucepan and cook for 5 minutes. Add salt and sugar to taste.

Albumen Water.—The white of an egg is placed in a bowl and divided by cutting through with a knife or scissors; add 5 oz. cold boiled water.   Albumen water may be used as a demulcent in some cases of acid swallowing; it is of little dietetic value, since raw egg albumen is not properly absorbed in the gastro-intestinal tract.

Barley Water.—Ingredients: 2 oz. pearl barley, 1 pint boiling water, the rind and juice of ½ lemon, sugar to taste.   Method: blanch the barley by placing it in a saucepan of cold water and bringing it to the boil, strain away the water and put the barley into a jug.   Add the pint of boiling water, sugar, lemon rind and strained juice.   Cover the jug and allow to cool, then strain; the barley water is then ready for use.

Egg Dishes.—Eggs can be cooked in many ways.   A few of the principal methods are described below.

Baked Custard.—Ingredients: 1 egg, ½ pint milk, ½ oz. castor sugar, 6 drops vanilla flavouring (or grated nutmeg).   Method: warm the milk, whisk the egg and sugar together, add the vanilla essence and strain into a greased pie dish.   Place the pie dish in a larger tin and surround it with water.   Bake in a moderate oven for 30 minutes.

Cup Custard.—Ingredients: 1 egg, ½ pint milk, ½ oz. castor sugar, 6 drops vanilla essence.   Method: beat the egg with some of the milk, heat the remainder of the milk and add to the beaten egg.   Strain the egg and milk mixture into a double saucepan and cook over a moderate heat until the custard thickens and coats the back of the spoon; stir continually and do not allow the custard to boil.   Add the vanilla essence and the sugar.   Cool and serve in custard glasses.

Egg Flip.—Ingredients: 1 egg, 1 tablespoonful brandy or sherry, ½ teaspoonful sugar, 5 oz. milk.   Method: separate the white from the yolk, warm the milk and whisk it with the egg yolk; add the wine and sugar.   Whisk the white until slightly frothy and fold it into the yolk and milk mixture.   Serve in a glass.

Poached Egg.—Ingredients: 1 round buttered toast, 1 egg, salt.   Method: butter the toast and place in a hot oven.   Half fill a small frying pan with water, add salt and bring to simmering point.   Break the egg into a cup and slide it gently into the water at side of pan.   Cook for 3 minutes and the egg white will be set.   An egg poacher may be used instead of a frying pan.

Buttered or Scrambled Egg.—Ingredients: 1 round buttered toast, 1 egg, 1 tablespoonful milk, ¼ oz. butter, pepper and salt, ½ teaspoonful chopped parsley.   Method: melt the butter in a small saucepan, beat the egg, add the milk and seasoning.   Add the egg to the butter in the saucepan and stir briskly over the heat until a creamy texture is obtained. Pile on to the hot buttered toast and garnish with the chopped parsley.

Savoury Omelette.—Ingredients: 2 eggs, $\frac{1}{2}$ oz. butter, $\frac{1}{2}$ teaspoonful chopped parsley, pepper and salt. Method: first clean the pan thoroughly with salt to obtain a smooth surface. Heat the butter in the pan and beat the egg with the parsley and seasoning. When the butter is hot, pour in the mixture and stir until the texture is creamy. Smooth the top and fold the omelette quickly. Brown lightly. Turn out on to a hot dish and serve.

Beverages for Invalids.—From the large selection available, 5 of the best known invalid beverages have been chosen and are described below.

Appleade.—Ingredients: 1 large ripe apple, 1 dessertspoonful castor sugar, 1 pint boiling water, 1 tablespoonful lemon juice. Method: wash the apple and cut it into thin slices; sprinkle the sugar over the apple and place all into a jug. Add 1 pint of boiling water, cover the jug with a close fitting lid and allow the contents to cool. Strain and add the lemon juice.

Lemonade.—Ingredients: 1 lemon, 1 tablespoonful sugar, $\frac{1}{2}$ pint boiling water. Method: peel the rind from the lemon thinly, extract the juice from the lemon. Place the rind, juice and sugar into a jug and add the boiling water. Cover closely and allow to cool. Strain and serve. Ice may be added.

Cocoa.—Ingredients: allow 1 teaspoonful cocoa and 5 oz. milk per person. Method: place the cocoa in a small basin, boil the milk, mix the cocoa to a paste with hot water, add to boiling milk and cook for three minutes. When this method is used the cocoa will be in solution and will not be deposited at the bottom of the cup. The flavour is also fully developed.

Coffee.—Ingredients: 2 oz. of coffee to each pint of boiling water. Heat the coffee jug and put in the coffee, pour on the boiling water and let the whole stand in a warm place for 5 or 6 minutes, then strain. Serve equal quantities of coffee and boiling milk.

Blackcurrant Tea.—1 tablespoonful blackcurrant jam to 7 oz. boiling water. Place the jam in a jug, pour boiling water over the jam and press jam to sides of the jug to extract the juice and sugar from the fruit. Strain and serve in a glass.

CHAPTER 12

HYGIENE OF THE WARD AND SICKROOM

WARD HYGIENE. SICKROOM HYGIENE. CHOICE OF A SICK-
ROOM. CLEANING OF THE ROOM. HEATING. VENTILATION.
DISINFECTION. HYGIENE OF AGE. MIDDLE AGE. OLD AGE.

THE application of the principles discussed in the foregoing
chapters constitutes the practical hygiene of the ward or of the
sickroom. In most cases, hospitals have by alteration or modern
building conformed to the latest ideas about hygiene and the
carrying out of the health-bringing rules is a matter of ordinary
routine. In private houses, however, the nurse will have to use
her common sense, and apply her special knowledge to the
conditions as she may find them. It is a sign of good training
when a nurse, faced with big odds in the sickroom, does not
grumble at her difficulties and sigh for the amenities of her old
wards, but strives with all her ingenuity to make the place as
perfect as possible within the limits of her power.

Ward Hygiene.—A few words will suffice for this part of
the subject. All wards are heated, ventilated and lighted by
systems approved by architects and engineers after consultation
with the medical authorities, and the nurse's duty is to see that
the standards are maintained. She should make herself acquainted
with the methods of airing, the workings of the heating pipes
including the adjustment of the valves, the sanitary arrangements
connected with the ward, the lighting fuses, the plugs available
for extra lighting, x-ray, and heating, the storage of food and the
routine of cleaning. All these things help to keep the machine
going and the parts well oiled.

Sickroom Hygiene.—It is when the nurse goes out to a
private case that all her hygienic education is of full value. For
instance she may find that she has to nurse an old farmer, lying
in an upstairs room, with poor lighting, primitive heating and
very primitive sanitary provision. Or she may go to a very
well appointed town flat and find that the room is overcrowded
with too many adjuncts to comfort and luxury, which may
hamper the patient's progress. In both cases she has to use all
her powers of construction and her executive ability.

160

Choice of a Sickroom.—The best room in a house is a first floor room near the bathroom and lavatory. This is handy and comparatively quiet, and away from the traffic of the ground floor. The outlook should be to the south, west, or south-west, so that the cold winds are avoided. The patient can thus enjoy the afternoon sun and he is not disturbed by the glare of the morning sun shining through his window too early. If there is a back stair nearby to the kitchen it is a very great benefit, as food does not become easily cooled and the nurse may manage to go occasionally to the kitchen to do a little special cookery for her patient. The more light in the room the better. If a door is opposite a window, provision must be made to prevent unduly severe draughts from passing through the room. A room with a door opposite the fireplace is better avoided. While everything should be done to encourage an atmosphere of hygienic perfection, the temperament of the patient must be studied. It is all very well to strip off curtains and pull down pictures, and make life impossible for even the most resistant microbe, but the moral effect on the patient of good pictures, bright fabrics and cheerful surroundings is better than the best antiseptic aura. In most cases the nurse will find that the artistry of her furnishings is as effective as the strength of her disinfectant in the progress of her patient. While there is no need to retain dust-harbouring ornaments, useless books, uncomfortable cushions and other furnishings, it is just as unnecessary to replace them by medicine bottles, phials and instruments that constantly remind the patient that he is ill. Such apparent trivialities as flowers, fruit, the bedside table (a very important outlook for the patient) and the drawing of the curtains may have far-reaching effects on the speedy recovery of the person confined to bed. The more a nurse uses her imagination and the more she sees life through the eyes of her patient, the better will she be able to minister to his needs, and make a success of her treatment.

Cleaning of the Room.—This has already been referred to (pp. 25 and 26). On no account should dust be raised. Rather than upset the nerves of the patient by carpet sweepers and vacuum cleaners, it is better to remove rugs and mats and clean them elsewhere. The woodwork, windows and furniture can be wiped daily with a damp cloth containing 5 per cent phenol or lysol.

Heating.—A temperature between 60° and 70° F. is satisfactory and usually easy to maintain. An old person requires more heat than a young person. Premature infants require an atmosphere of 70° F. and above. A coal fire ventilates the room, but is difficult to keep at a regular output; gas fires can easily be regulated and they are clean, but they are not so cheering to the patient. A bowl of water should be kept in front of gas fires. Nurses on night duty should carefully stoke up the fire during the night, using gloves to lift the coals as noiselessly as possible on to the fire. Electricity should be utilized to the full when available (see Fig. 59). If patients are sitting up in bed,

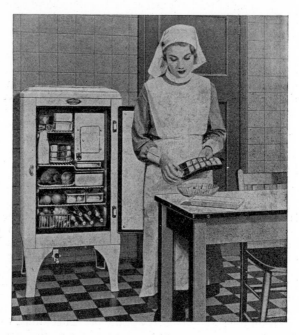

Fig. 58.—A constant supply of ice can be maintained by the modern motorless refrigerator, which, in addition to ensuring the perfect preservation of foodstuffs, functions as an all weather larder at constant low temperature.

(By courtesy of Electrolux, Ltd. London.)

even when the room is above 60°, a shawl or bed jacket should be worn.

Ventilation.—Various devices can be used to keep the room well aired. As long as there is no draught the windows can be opened at the top and at the bottom. The nurse is referred to Chapter 2 for guidance as to regulation of ventilation. During the night, the bottom sash may be lowered. In cold weather, the windows may be shut and the door opened. A screen is always of great use in protecting the patient against draughts.

Disinfection.—The nurse should see to the cleansing of all

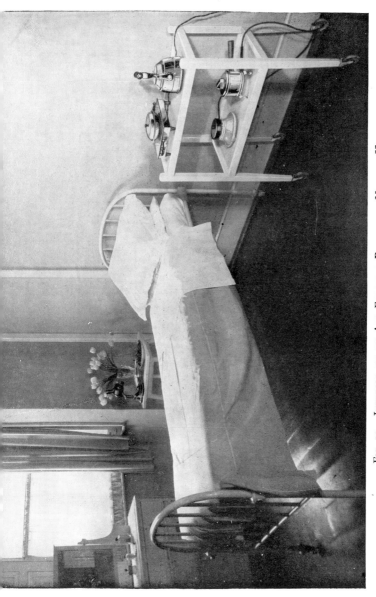

FIG. 59.—INTERIOR OF AN ALL ELECTRIC ROOM IN A NURSING HOME.

Showing how electricity can be used in nursing. On the table at the right hand side of the bed is a Bandolero fan. The trolley on the left hand side contains, on the top shelf, a 150-watt copper warming plate and a 650-watt Magnet kettle of nickel plate. Below is a small boiling plate and a 300-watt saucepan, useful for heating milk and other fluids.

(*By courtesy of the British Electrical Development Association, Inc., London, and the Scottish Nursing Home, Maida Vale.*)

sanitary utensils; excretions should be removed, disinfected and disposed of, as soon as they are passed. Feeding cups, plates, cups, knives and forks should all be kept for the patient's own use, preferably in a handy cupboard not far from the sickroom. They should be sterilized in boiling water after each meal. Food should be carefully selected, cooked and served, and the utmost care should be taken that no harmful microbes are present. The danger of flies has already been stressed. The kitchen and larder should be periodically cleared out and the walls, window sills and shelves sprayed with D.D.T. solution. Great care must be taken to see that none of the solution falls on food. While spraying is in progress, all naked lights must be extinguished. A good refrigerator is a great asset (Fig. 58).

Hygiene of Age.—The hygiene of the infant, of the growing child and of the pregnant woman are discussed elsewhere, but brief reference must be made to the differences which are met with in the prime of life, in middle age and in old age. With regard to the first, accidents, pneumonia, acute appendicitis and other casualties of the " twenties " and " thirties " are usually overcome without incident.

Middle Age.—After the age of 40, a man begins to feel that Nature leaves him less scope than before. Constipation, increasing weight and inability to take active exercise may make a man less fit, and when he is ill he requires more attention and a longer time to recover. After the age of 50 the rise of blood pressure, the hardening of the arteries and the wear and tear of the system make diseases like cancer and kidney trouble more prevalent. Once the body gets into a low condition of health it does not readily recover, so the nurse has much more to do than with a younger person. This applies to the mental as well as to the physical aspect of the case.

Old Age.—Senility is not much different from infancy. The patient may be quite helpless, and the nurse may require all her mental and physical strength to stand the strain of the heavy work involved. All the tissues are shrunken, the muscles are wasted and the organs are worn out. The individual is more easily affected by the changes of temperature, light and food. Sleep is an essential, and must be encouraged by hypnotics if prescribed. The limbs are cold owing to sluggish circulation, and bed stockings may be necessary. Constipation should be carefully avoided.

SECTION IV

BACTERIOLOGY AND CLINICAL PATHOLOGY

CHAPTER 1

BACTERIA

MAIN DIVISIONS. DESCRIPTION. SIZE. LIFE HISTORY OF
BACTERIA. REPRODUCTION. COMPOSITION. ESSENTIAL
FACTORS IN BACTERIAL GROWTH. FOOD. MEDIUM. MOIST-
URE. ATMOSPHERIC CONDITIONS. TEMPERATURE. LIGHT.
SPECIAL PROPERTIES OF BACTERIA. SPORULATION.
MOTILITY. FERMENTATION. PUTREFACTION. CHROMO-
GENESIS. DISTRIBUTION OF BACTERIA AND RELATION TO
DISEASE. AIR. WATER. SOIL. MILK. CONTAMINATION
OF FOOD. DECOMPOSITION OF FOOD. BOTULISM. CAR-
RIERS. FOMITES. TRANSMISSION OF DISEASE BY INSECTS.
INFECTION.

THE science of bacteriology embraces the study of minute vegetable organisms known as bacteria, each of which consists of one
cell only; the bacterium perpetuates itself by a process of fission.

Main Divisions.—Bacteria may be considered under the following headings.

1. Those which are pathogenic (disease producing) to
man;

2. Non-pathogenic organisms or commensals; these occur
on the skin or in certain parts of the body e.g. the mouth,
throat and intestines, without exerting any harmful effects
on man or animals i.e. they are saprophytic in action.

It must always be remembered however that under certain
conditions commensals may become pathogenic, especially if
they find their way into organs of which they are not normal
inhabitants; for example, the *bacillus coli communis* is normally
found in the intestines, but if it makes its way into the urinary
tract it may cause serious infection of the tissues concerned. In
such circumstances the bacteria concerned are classed as potential pathogens. Under normal conditions these non-pathogenic
organisms, which are constantly found in the air, in water and
in foodstuffs, are protective in action; some are of commercial
value in the preparation of foodstuffs, wines and chemicals.

Description.—Each bacterium is a complete and independent unit of life, consisting of protoplasm enclosed in a cell wall through which it is able to absorb food and water and to excrete waste products. Bacteria are devoid of chlorophyll and have no well defined nucleus.

Size.—The unit of measurement adopted is the *Micron* which is equal to 0·001 millimetre or approximately $\frac{1}{25000}$ inch, and is represented by the Greek letter μ.

Life History of Bacteria

Reproduction.—Organisms usually multiply by a process of transverse fission, the cell elongating and becoming constricted in the centre and finally dividing to form two distinct organisms. Should conditions for multiplication prove to be favourable, it may progress with great rapidity; one organism can become a grandfather in less than an hour.

Composition.—The protoplasm of the organism contains protein substances similar to those found in animal and plant tissue; some of these are abundantly supplied with fats and mineral salts ; water is also a substantial constituent (about 80 per cent).

Essential Factors in Bacterial Growth

Food.—Bacteria require organic material i.e. proteins, carbohydrates and mineral salts, all of which must be in a soluble form for absorption.

Medium.—Most bacteria prefer a slightly alkaline medium, since acidity inhibits growth.

Moisture.—The majority of bacteria are composed mainly of water, which is essential to growth; water also acts as a vehicle by which the soluble foodstuffs are able to diffuse through the cell wall of the organism.

Atmospheric Conditions.—Some bacteria grow only in the presence of free oxygen and are then classed as obligatory aerobes e.g. the tubercle bacillus. Others cannot exist in the presence of oxygen and are known as obligatory anaerobes e.g. the bacillus of tetanus. A third group is indifferent to atmospheric conditions and its members flourish equally well whether oxygen is present or not; such organisms are described as facultative anaerobes, and it is in this category that the majority of pathogens may be enlisted.

Temperature.—The temperature at which pathogenic bacteria grow most satisfactorily is that of the human body—98·4° F. Low temperatures tend to inhibit the growth of the organism whereas high temperatures destroy it. Spores are much more resistant to heat than the organisms which do not form spores. Moist heat is more destructive than dry heat.

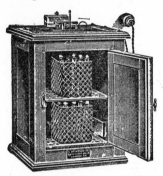

Fig. 60.—Incubator for Bacterial Cultivation at 37°C. (98·4° F.).

(By courtesy of Messrs. Hearson & Co. Ltd., London.)

Light.—Sunlight and, to a lesser degree, the electric arc, are very injurious to certain kinds of bacteria, a reaction being set up by the ultra-violet rays. Accordingly water and milk can be sterilized without the occurrence of an appreciable rise of temperature by exposure to the ultra-violet rays given out by a quartz mercury lamp.

Special Properties of Bacteria

Sporulation.—Certain types of bacteria possess the property of forming spores e.g. bacilli, and occasionally spirilla. When sporulation is about to take place, a granule appears in the protoplasm, slowly enlarging to form a highly refractile round or ovoid body enclosed in a tough membrane.

Spores exhibit very great resistance to heat, desiccation and chemical agents. Bacteria are thus able to preserve their species in most disadvantageous circumstances and as soon as conditions are favourable again, the capsule or membrane ruptures and the organism resumes its bacillary form.

Spores are named according to their position in the cell as follows.

Equatorial spores, the spore being in the centre of the cell;

Terminal spores, the spore occurring at either end of the cell;

Sub-terminal spores, the spore visible between the centre and the end of the cell.

Motility.—Most bacteria, particularly bacilli and spirilla, are capable of motion; they possess delicate elongations of their protoplasm, known as flagella, by which they are able to move about in the fluid medium in which they grow. These processes vary in number from a single one attached to one extremity of the bacillus to as many as 20 or more which are attached to all parts of the organism.

Fermentation.—The power of hydrolysis of carbohydrates is possessed by certain bacteria. Most bacilli and many cocci are capable of fermenting substances made up of carbon, hydrogen and oxygen and reducing them to organic acids, alcohols and simple gases (such as carbonic acid gas), a property very useful in the identification of an organism. Bacteria are used commercially in the manufacture of alcohol and vinegar from carbohydrates.

Putrefaction.—Nitrogenous substances such as proteins (including animal and plant proteins) are decomposed by bacteria; the insoluble albumins are first converted into albumoses and peptones and finally completely digested to the state known as putrefaction. Indole is one of the final products of protein decomposition and is a great aid in bacterial diagnosis.

Chromogenesis.—Chromogenesis, or the production of pigment, is an important characteristic possessed by certain organisms and is useful in identification. Sometimes a definite coloration is imparted to tissue fluids and pus when a chromogenic organism is the infecting agent.

Distribution of Bacteria and Relation to Disease

Organisms are found everywhere—in the air and the soil; in food and in water; in dust from houses, streets and roads; on and in the human body.

Air.—The number of bacteria found varies considerably, but they rely largely upon the amount of organic matter present in the air. On mountain tops there are comparatively few germs, but in the air of towns, in crowded rooms, in theatres and in picture houses they are ubiquitous, because of the amount of organic matter present and the number of objects which may give rise to them. Some of these organisms are pathogenic and are exhaled from the air passages of infected persons who are harbouring them—for example the diphtheria bacillus which may be present in their throats.

Water.—The distribution of bacteria is variable, but surface water may come in contact with excretal infection from leaking drain pipes and thus cause disease. Typhoid fever, cholera, paratyphoid fever and dysentery are the principal water borne diseases, although poliomyelitis, sore throat, conjunctivitis, suppurative otitis media and frontal sinus suppuration may be traced in certain circumstances to visits to swimming baths used by infected persons.

Most bacteria tend to settle to the bottom of a bulk of water and this process of sedimentation is an important factor in the self-purification of water. Storage is a very important method of purification of water on a large scale.

Deep wells.—Deep well water, because of its passage through the earth, must be subjected to a process of natural filtration and therefore should be free from pathogenic organisms unless contaminated from some outside source, such as seepage from farm effluent into the well.

Tap water.—Tap water, on account of its constant movement and chemical purification, should be pure, although when it is allowed to stand for a lengthy period in the pipes, it is liable to contamination, hence the necessity for running off for some time water left in the cistern all night before it is collected for drinking purposes.

Distilled water.—Distilled water is only reliably pure if it has been recently treated and carefully bottled.

Soil.—Earth may be generally considered fairly free from bacteria in the deeper layers. On the surface it may be contaminated by organisms such as the tetanus bacillus and its spores, or the anthrax bacillus and its spores.

The Tetanus bacillus.—The tetanus bacillus is found very frequently in cow and horse dung, more rarely in human faeces. It is constantly present in newly manured land and may set up the disease, tetanus, by entering a scratch, an abrasion or superficial cut or a wound caused by a rusty nail or broken glass.

The Anthrax bacillus.—This organism affects cattle, sheep, pigs, horses and goats; the animals with anthrax die with infected blood around the nostrils and anus; thus the spores are left on the field and infect the soil.

Milk.—Milk is one of the foods most easily contaminated; this may be due to direct infection from the cow.

Tuberculosis.—Cattle are susceptible to tuberculosis and in the case of the cow the tubercle bacillus reaches the milk. The term, bovine tuberculosis, is used, this including any of the following tubercular conditions: tuberculous adenitis, tuberculous peritonitis, tuberculous meningitis and certain infections of the bones and joints occurring in children fed on cow's milk.

Streptococcal infections.—Cows suffering from mastitis, which is a haemolytic infection of the udder, may cause epidemics of tonsillitis among milk drinkers; moreover the milker handling the cow or milk can infect the milk in this way, causing outbreaks of scarlet fever and other debilitating streptococcal infections.

Typhoid and paratyphoid fever.—Usually a carrier is the cause of infection of this type; the person handling the milk or milking the cow may spread the disease; further, the use of infected water for washing the utensils, or dilution of milk with infected water, may cause pollution.

Diphtheria.—The cow's udder may become infected with the bacillus of diphtheria with formation of ulcers, which may be a cause of infection of milk. As diphtheria is one of the carrier infections, the organisms from nasal and faucial infection may gain access to milk when an infected person deals with it in any way.

Abortus fever.—This infection of the cow gives rise to abortion, the causative organism being the *Brucella abortus.* In human beings who consume milk thus infected, a malady known as undulant fever may be set up.

Contamination of Food.—The organisms of typhoid fever, dysentery, and in tropical countries, cholera, may infect food from several sources. Such organisms may be transmitted by sewage-contaminated water, infecting oysters and other shell fish in the sea and watercress in streams. In this connexion the danger of inefficiently cleansed salads must be kept in mind. Carriers or persons with unwashed hands who have attended patients with these diseases, and who have then prepared the food, must also be under suspicion.

Decomposition of Food.—Gaertner's bacillus is often the cause of epidemics of meat poisoning and has been traced in meat from pigs, cattle, horses and fish. The eating of tinned meats or fish pastes insufficiently sterilized, in which anaerobic organisms have been allowed to flourish and produce toxins, gives rise to symptoms of sudden and acute poisoning. The infected meat is usually normal in appearance, taste and smell, and may be eaten without causing suspicion. These epidemics are sometimes traced to infected sausages, brawn and meat pies.

Botulism.—Botulism is an intoxication caused by the *bacillus botulinus*, a spore-forming organism which attacks the nervous system, giving rise to thirst, nausea, double vision and many other symptoms and signs. The organism may be found in tinned meats, including meat paste, and fish paste when these have been insufficiently sterilized; the spores are thus left unaffected so that they flourish and produce toxins.

Carriers.—The human carrier may be

1. a person suffering from a mild form of a recognized attack of a disease;

2. a person who has apparently quite recovered;

3. a person who is not suffering and never has suffered, but who merely acts as an intermediary or carrier of infection; here organisms may be found in the mucous membranes of the nose and throat.

Fomites.—Infection may be transmitted by fomites—articles which have been used by a patient with an infectious disease or which have come in contact with the patient (handkerchiefs, towels, dressings, bedpans, sputum mugs, toys, books, drinking utensils). Another method of infection by fomites is that in which disease is caused by children sucking toys, pencils and so on, which have been in contact with other infected children.

Transmission of Disease by Insects.—This can be effected into two ways: 1. biologically, when the pathogenic organism is actually taken into the body of the insect by sucking blood from an infected person; 2. directly, when insects convey organisms on their mouths, feet and other parts to human beings, but do not actually bite. In biological infection the organism undergoes a stage of development in the body of the insect. This is well illustrated in the condition of malaria.

Mosquitoes. — The Anopheles mosquitoes — the carriers of malaria—are two-winged insects which act as intermediate hosts for a parasite and convey the organism from man to man. The female mosquito, which alone sucks the blood from the infected person, itself becomes infected; once inside the mosquito, the malarial parasite undergoes a sexual cycle and it is then ready to be injected into the next unfortunate person. The mosquito may bite when in search for more blood, and it is in this new blood that the parasite undergoes asexual reproduction.

Stegomyia fasciata (Aëdes Aegypti) a species of black and silver mosquito is a carrier of yellow fever, a disease due to a filterable virus; it does not convey the infection until about 12 days have elapsed after it has bitten the infected person. During this period the mosquito cultivates the virus in its body cavity.

Ticks.—Particularly in the warmer climates, blood sucking parasites are proved to be responsible for the conveyance of a number of diseases among both man and animals e.g. African relapsing fever or African tick fever, which infects sheep, horses, dogs, fowls and cattle as well as man.

Fleas.—The flea which commonly attacks man is *pulex irritans*; the latter is not definitely credited with the spread of disease, although the rat flea (*xenopsylla cheopis*) has been proved to be the carrier of the germ of bubonic plague to man. The flea sucks the blood from an infected animal, which contains large numbers of the bacillus; these multiply in the stomach and proventriculus of the flea, which on the death of the animal deserts it for a human host, regurgitating the organisms when it bites the new victim.

Tsetse fly.—The tsetse fly (*glossina palpalis*), found only in Africa, is closely associated with the spread of sleeping sickness, acting as a mechanical carrier; it feeds on an infected being and carries the trypanosome in its alimentary canal until it bites a healthy person and thus causes infection.

Lice.—The body louse (*pediculus corporis*) is regarded as a carrier of typhus, relapsing fever and trench fever. Typhus is predisposed to by overcrowding, poverty and generally bad hygienic conditions, being spread by lice. The virus is a filter-passing organism the *rickettsia prowazeki*, only found in the intestines of lice which have fed on typhus patients.

The house fly.—Of the non-biting species of insects, the *musca domestica*, or common house fly, is foremost as a carrier of disease, and so emphatically is it credited with being one of the chief carriers of typhoid fever that it has been suggested that it should be given the title of typhoid fly, in preference to the usual one of house fly. Its presence indicates filth. Flies revel in filth, and therefore their breeding places will be in the midden, the garbage heap and the dunghill; the fly is born in filth, it lives in filth, feeds on filth and carries filth on its wings and feet, leaving organisms of disease on any food on which it may alight. As it is incapable of breaking up solid food when it comes in contact with it, it is obliged to empty the contents of its stomach (human liquid faeces) in order to soften the food, at the same time leaving numerous pathogenic organisms on the food, ready for man to consume.

The diseases commonly carried by flies include typhoid fever, cholera, epidemic diarrhoea, dysentery, diphtheria, poliomyelitis and ophthalmia.

Infection.—When bacteria gain entrance to the tissues, they grow in them, injuring them and producing symptoms of malaise; when this occurs, the changes are known as infection.

Portals of entry.—There are certain routes by which bacteria gain access to the body and the pathway chosen by an organism is important in determining the nature of the infection, because each type of disease organism selects its own particular route.

The routes most generally chosen are as follows.

1. Through the skin by means of inoculation, any small cut, abrasion or prick; even a thin and delicate membrane—such as the conjunctiva covering the eye—can serve as a portal of entry for pathogenic organisms. Bubonic plague, tetanus and syphilis are examples of inoculation by the skin.

2. Through the respiratory tract, by means of inhalation of certain pathogenic organisms exhaled by infected persons from the respiratory passages during talking, coughing or breathing. The temperature of the atmosphere varies between 50° and 80° F., and many exhaled organisms soon die under such conditions, therefore infection of this type depends upon proximity and immediate inhalation of harmful germs. Whooping cough and influenza are both contracted by this method. The tubercle bacillus is a well known exception as it can withstand both cold and dryness for considerable periods.

3. By the mouth and gastro-intestinal tract. The organism may be swallowed in food or water, causing diseases of the alimentary tract, such as typhoid fever, paratyphoid fever, dysentery, cholera and summer diarrhoea and food poisoning.

STAINING AND CULTIVATION OF BACTERIA

As already mentioned, bacteria are invisible to the naked eye. In order to identify them, magnification is made by means of the microscope, but it is essential first to stain the organisms with dyes of various types. Bacteria may be also cultivated, so that in the mass they form colonies of certain construction and character according to the organism present.

Staining of Bacteria

The use of aniline dyes in staining bacteria has been in practice for a period of over 60 years, and is one of the most useful, quick and satisfactory methods. These dyes were introduced about 1880 by 3 early and famous bacteriologists—Koch, Weigert and Ehrlich. Reaction to certain stains aids differentiation microscopically of one organism from others.

Stains.—Although there is a large variety of dyes in both colour and type, only a few are employed in the laboratory; of these the best known are fuchsine, methylene blue, methyl violet, gentian violet and Bismarck brown. Research has shown that the staining power of the dyes is considerably increased by the addition of a certain class of mordant which has the power of adhesion both to the bacterium and to the dye. The most commonly used mordants are alum, phenol, aniline oil and tannin.

The stains in actual use are prepared from stock solutions of the dyes, owing to the fact that the staining capacity of most of them does not last long when made up with water; these stock solutions are prepared by adding the dye to alcohol until the alcohol is saturated and cannot take in any further dye without precipitation. The greater number of stains used in the laboratory are made up as a dilute alcoholic solution or as a solution of a basic dye that is partly alcoholic and partly aqueous, with the addition of a mordant; methylene blue is an exception to the rule and does not deteriorate in an aqueous solution. All saturated solutions should be stored in the dark in coloured glass stoppered bottles.

Methods.—In preparation for staining, the coverslip or slide should be thoroughly free from grease and dirt; this may be achieved by boiling for 10 minutes and keeping the slides stored in methylated spirit.

Smear preparations of pus, sputum, urine or broth cultures are made by spreading a thin film of the material evenly on the slide with a sterile platinum needle. The smear is allowed to dry. It is then warmed by passing the slide over the flame of a Bunsen burner, a process known as " fixing." The smear should never be exposed to direct heat on account of the danger of scorching. When the slide is quite dry, the dry film is covered with Loeffler's methylene blue and left for 2 minutes. The stain is then poured off by putting the slide under a gentle stream of water from the tap, until the water is clear of the blue dye; the slide then is blotted between filter paper and allowed to dry. A small drop of Canada balsam is placed in the centre of the slide and a cover-glass put on if the film is to be mounted; it may be examined unmounted by using an oil immersion lens, in which case a small drop of cedar wood oil is placed on the film. Single colour stains are often used for a quick diagnosis of the morphology of the organism.

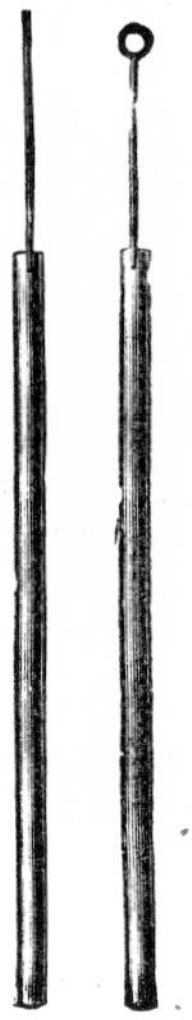

A   B

FIG. 61.—(A) PLATINUM NEEDLE, (B), PLATINUM LOOP.

(*By courtesy of Messrs. Baird & Tatlock, Ltd., London.*)

Gram Stain.—One of the most generally used stains employed for classifying bacteria was devised by a scientist named Gram (1884); it was known as a differential stain because it differentiated bacteria into two main groups referred to as Gram negative and Gram positive respectively.

The film is prepared in the usual way and then covered with a solution of gentian violet in which it is allowed to remain for 30 seconds; it is then washed off with a gentle stream of water.

Lugol's iodine is then applied for one minute and then dried off with filter paper. The slide is washed for 10-20 seconds in absolute alcohol. A counter stain, carbol fuchsin, is then used for 15-30 seconds. In this method of staining if the purple coloration be retained after washing with alcohol, the organism is termed Gram positive, and if decolorized after this process Gram negative.

Ziehl-Neelsen Method.—This staining method is invaluable in the diagnosis of tuberculosis and is used for staining smears of sputum and other materials suspected of containing the tubercle bacillus (T.B.). Especially in the case of sputum stained by this method, the organisms are clearly shown as bright red rods— the only red objects visible in the smear—lying in the blue field.

Method of staining.—Spread a thin film of the material for examination on a slide and fix in the usual way, especially using any small thick purulent particles present; pour hot carbol fuchsin on to the slide and leave the material exposed to the stain for 5 minutes, keeping the stain hot all the time; rinse with water and decolorize by dipping in 25 per cent sulphuric acid. The red colour of the stain changes to a yellowish brown. After the slide has been immersed in the acid for one minute wash with water; the red colouring re-appears and this process should be repeated until the colour becomes a pale pink. Wash well again in water, counterstain for 2 minutes with Loeffler's methylene blue and finally wash and dry.

Stains Used for Diphtheria Bacillus.—The diphtheria organism is Gram positive, and as confirmatory stains, Pugh's or Neisser's stains can be used.

Pugh's stain.—Stain the film for 3 minutes with toluidine blue, wash and dry; this stain shows the diphtheria bacillus as light blue in colour and the granules as a reddish purple.

Neisser's stain.—In this method the film is flooded with Neisser's mixed A and B stains for 15 seconds, then washed in distilled water; it is counterstained with chrysoidin, washed in water, and blotted dry. The films will show the bacilli stained brown by the chrysoidin, and the granules blue-black in colour.

Acid-fast Bacteria.—A large number of important bacteria, notably those which are encased in a fatty or lipoidal envelope, are distinguished from other varieties by the fact that they are stained with great difficulty, but when once exposed to carbol fuchsin, a bright red and powerful stain, they resist decoloriza- tion by acids, and it is for this reason they are said to take an acid-fast stain. They do not give up the stain, even when the slide is immersed in alcohol, as in the case of many bacteria, and can only be decolorized by means of a solution of 25 per cent sulphuric acid, as described above.

Some of the principal acid-fast organisms, in addition to the tubercle bacillus, are the bacillus of leprosy, the non-pathogenic smegma bacillus and the butter bacillus, found in specimens of butter and milk.

Cultivation of Bacteria

A culture medium has often been described as the soil in which organisms are planted for the purposes of laboratory study, and if any material is to be used as a culture medium, it must meet certain fundamental needs.

Culture Media: Essentials.—These are summarized below.

1. The medium must contain certain food elements. All bacteria need protein in some form in conjunction with carbohydrates, the ordinary mineral salts (such as sodium chloride and phosphates) and water.

2. The medium must be of correct chemical reaction. Most organisms are very sensitive to acidity and develop most satisfactorily in a medium which has a neutral or slightly alkaline reaction.

3. The medium must be sterile. Very few kinds of media, when made, are free from bacteria, hence the need for their sterilization before use; further, the medium must be kept sterile until the organisms for investigation are planted in it.

Uses of Media.—Culture media are primarily used to support growth, but certain types serve other purposes. Some serve the purpose of demonstrating the physiological activities of the organisms, such as the power to ferment sugars, others are prepared in order to differentiate one kind of bacterium from another or to encourage the growth of a particular kind so as to help in the identification of the species. The basis of the medium in everyday use in the laboratory is a watery extract of meat, which should roughly correspond in composition and reaction to the body fluids.

The stock media commonly used consist of either a fluid known as *bouillon* (more generally named broth) or a solid medium of agar or gelatin. These solid media have actually a broth basis and the agar and gelatin have been added merely for purposes of solidification.

Nutrient Broth.—Prepare lean meat or ox heart by freeing it of any fat; mince very finely and add one litre of distilled water to a pound of the flesh; leave the mixture in the refrigerator for 24 hours. At the end of this period strain through muslin, finally expressing any fluid left in the meat by means of a meat press. The fluid should be bright red in colour on account of the retention of haemoglobin. Any trace of fat which may have accumulated on the surface of the fluid must be separated by skimming with filter paper. The fluid should then be boiled for 15 minutes, a process which makes it turn into a dark brown turbid liquid; it is then filtered and made up to its original volume by the addition of distilled water; the fluid becomes bright yellow; it is now ready for the addition of peptone to the amount of 2 per cent, a replacement made necessary because of the fact that in the process of heating the protein is removed by coagulation. Sodium chloride content is increased by the addition of 1 per cent common salt.

Standardization.—It will be found that the reaction of the fluid is too acid for growth of the majority of bacteria; therefore it should be neutralized by the addition of an alkali (sodium hydroxide); it is steamed to precipitate phosphates, filtered through coarse filter paper and the reaction readjusted; then the fluid is bottled and finally sterilized in an autoclave. Nutrient broth is a suitable fluid culture medium for organisms such as those belonging to the coliform group.

Digest Media.—To the ordinary media, digested protein is added in the form of a peptone, but in the preparation of digest media, meat which is digested by the action of trypsin is used, and the products of this digestion are made the basis of the medium. Preparations of this type of medium are used in culturing the diphtheria bacillus.

Solid Media.—Agar-agar, a constituent of Japanese seaweed, is used in the form of a powder and added to ordinary broth until there is a proportion of agar amounting to 2 per cent. The mixture is heated in a Koch's steam sterilizer for 1 hour, cooled, cleared with the white of an egg and then filtered through Chardin filter paper. The filtrate is placed in an autoclave for half an hour and then put up into test tubes or bottles. This medium is much in use in bacteriological laboratories.

Some organisms will not grow on ordinary agar medium unless the latter is enriched by the addition of certain uncoagulated body fluids. Examples are given below.

Blood Agar.—Sterile blood is added to the agar just before it begins to solidify; the tube into which this medium is put is then rolled in the hands in order to mix the contents and the mixture is allowed to cool and solidify in a sloped position.

Serum Agar.—Sterile horse serum is added to cooled melted agar. It is a valuable medium used in the growing of streptococci, pneumococci, meningococci and gonococci.

Boiled Blood (Chocolate) Agar.—This medium is made by adding 10 per cent of defibrinated blood to melted agar and boiling slowly for a few minutes; the blood is coagulated, changing in colour to a dark brown (chocolate colour). This medium is useful especially in the cultivation of *B. influenzae, B. pertussis* and *streptococcus viridans.*

Glucose Agar.—This is prepared by the addition of glucose, 1 per cent, to ordinary nutrient agar, and is used in the cultivation of yeasts and moulds.

Sabouraud's Medium.—This is prepared by the addition of 4 per cent maltose to ordinary agar, and is a successful medium for the cultivation of fungi such as the organisms of ringworm and favus. This medium, after inoculation, should be kept at the ordinary temperature of the laboratory for about 10 days, the period during which the organisms incubate.

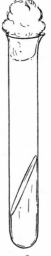

Fig. 62.—
Blood Agar
Slope in Test
Tube.

Gelatin Media.—Gelatin is an animal protein which is usually derived from tissues such as bone cartilage; in the animal tissues it exists as an albuminoid collagen and is extracted by a process of hydrolysis. Gelatin medium consists of single strength broth, to which is added 10–15 per cent of pure gelatin. It sets at 24° C., and does not allow incubation at body temperature; frequently a cold incubator at 22° C. is used, or cultures are incubated in the laboratory at room temperature. This medium requires very careful handling in its preparation; if it is heated too much it will not set; if it is insufficiently heated it goes bad because of lack of adequate sterilization, and because of the presence of germs. Gelatin produces a very acid reaction in a medium, and it is found necessary to add an alkali and to restandardize before use.

Selective Media.—Media of this type contain substances which assist the growth of the bacterium required to be cultivated and which at the same time restrain the growth of other organisms present in the culture, especially when the organisms for investigation are present in small numbers.

MacConkey's Bile Salt Agar.—This medium is used for organisms which cannot be distinguished by their microscopical appearance or their method of growth on ordinary agar, but by the appearance of their colonies on special media. It is especially used to distinguish the bacillus coli from organisms of the typhoid and dysenteric groups. Its use depends partly on sugar reactions and partly because it contains bile salts which have the required effect of inhibiting the growth of organisms which do not belong to the group under investigation.

The medium contains sodium taurocholate (bile salts), peptone, lactose and tap water and is coloured with neutral red. If a solid medium is wanted, agar is added.

The bacillus coli ferments the lactose and produces a red colony; the typhoid bacillus and other organisms of the typhoid group have no effect on lactose and produce colourless colonies.

Desoxycholate Agar.—This is a medium now used even more generally for the isolation of the dysentery, paratyphoid and salmonella groups of organisms.

Dorset's Egg Medium.—This medium is made from fresh eggs beaten up and mixed with distilled water and strained through muslin in order to remove any air bubbles; the mixture is then run into test tubes and solidified in the sloped position: it is used for cultivating tubercle bacilli. A modified form of this medium known as Lowenstein-Jensen's medium is used for the growth of both human and bovine tubercle bacilli.

Loeffler's Blood Serum.—This consists of sterile serum from the blood of an ox, sheep or horse, added to glucose broth, and slowly coagulated by heat. It is used in the cultivation of the diphtheria bacillus.

Bordet-Gengou Medium.—This medium is made of nutrient agar added to a certain amount of freshly made potato extract; it is useful in cultivating *B. pertussis*, the causative organism of whooping cough.

Methods of Cultivating Anaerobes.—Anaerobes, as previously mentioned, are organisms which are unable to grow in the presence of oxygen, although such organisms require oxygen for their metabolism, which they obtain by breaking down the constituents of the medium instead of getting it direct from the air.

Only the simpler methods are described here.

1. *Stab culture.*—The medium is boiled in a test tube in order to release free oxygen and is then cooled. A sterile platinum needle is inoculated with the material for culture and plunged straight down into the medium. After the stab is made the upper portion

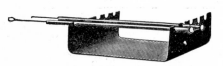

FIG. 63.—PLATINUM NEEDLE AND LOOP ON REST.
(*By courtesy of Messrs. Baird & Tatlock, Ltd., London.*)

of the medium is gently warmed to seal off the needle-track.

2. *Shake cultures.*—A tube of medium is boiled and allowed to cool to 45° C.; the material for culture is then added in semi-liquid or liquid form by means of a Pasteur pipette. The tube is well rotated between the hands in order to mix the contents, and the material is allowed to set in the upright position; the tube should be sealed with liquid paraffin.

Extraction of Oxygen from a Medium.—Buchner's tube is an apparatus used for media contained in a test tube. It consists of a tube of wide bore, the lower end of which is blown out to form a bulbous part; above the bulb is a constriction on which the test tube containing the medium rests. Pyrogallic acid crystals are placed in the bottom of the Buchner's tube and then sodium hydroxide is run down the side of the tube. Sodium pyrogallol is produced which rapidly absorbs any oxygen. The medium and culture are quickly added and the tube is immediately sealed with a rubber bung, which should be coated with vaseline.

McIntosh and Filde's Method.—This method depends on the principle of combustion of hydrogen and oxygen in the presence of palladium which acts as a catalyst. The apparatus consists of an aluminium jar approximately 8 in. in height, and 6 in. in diameter, provided with a metal lid, which can be clamped down in order to make an airtight joint. The lid contains 2 valves, one by which hydrogen can be introduced and one which acts as an exit for air; it is also provided with a porcelain spool covered with palladinized asbestos surrounded by a coil of resistance wire; the ends of the wire are connected to the terminals on the top of the lid. When the apparatus is used, the inoculated tubes or plates are introduced into the jar, the lid is replaced immediately and screwed down, the joint being made completely airtight with tallow; then both valves are adjusted and hydrogen is allowed to stream in for 2–3 minutes; the valves are shut off and the palladinized asbestos is heated by passing an electric current through the coil. After an interval of a few minutes a little more hydrogen is introduced in order to replace that lost by combustion; the valves are then closed and the jar is placed in the incubator.

Animal Inoculation.—This method, used in the cultivation of bacteria, takes advantage of the susceptibility of certain animals to certain bacteria, and may be required 1. to intensify the virulence of an organism, which has become attenuated through culture on media; the infective agent may be injected alone or with another pathogenic organism or with a toxin, in order to lower the animal's resistance; 2. to enable an organism to be identified or to determine its virulence; 3. as a means of obtaining a pure culture.

The animals employed for this purpose are the guineapig, rabbit, white mouse and white rat. These animals may be injected subcutaneously or intraperitoneally. The white mouse is very susceptible to pneumococcal infection and sputum in this infection is generally laden with a variety of organisms. When a specimen of sputum from a positive case is used in inoculating the mouse, the animal dies of pneumococcal septicaemia and a culture is made from a drop of blood from the heart; this culture yields a pure growth of the pneumococcus.

The tubercle bacillus is obtained in a pure culture from the sputum by inoculating some of the specimen into a guineapig.

The rabbit, owing to the fact that it is prone to mange, snuffles and so on, is kept more for experimental work than for diagnostic purposes, especially in the production of immune sera, used for routine laboratory diagnosis.

CHAPTER 3

CLASSIFICATION OF BACTERIA

VARIOUS methods have been used in the past in the classification
of bacteria, but now these have been superseded by the classification of the Committee of the Society of American Bacteriologists
of 1920, in which morphology, staining, reactions and physiological characteristics are taken into consideration. This classification, in a modified form, has been adopted in Great Britain,
although many of the old names such as cocci and bacilli are still
in use, and for the sake of familiarity and convenience are, in
fact, used in this work.

Varieties of Bacteria.—The main types of true bacteria have
been referred to on pp. 164–165. At this stage, however, we
may expand our classification considerably. Bacteria comprise
the types given below.

1. Cocci: spherical in shape; e.g. streptococci.

2. Bacilli: straight rod-shaped organisms; e.g. *bacillus
typhosus.*

3. Vibrios: curved or comma shaped rods; e.g. *vibrio
cholerae.*

4. Spirilla: long filamentous types of bacteria; e.g.
spirillum minus.

5. Viruses : ultra-microscopic bacteria, which cannot be
seen even with the highest magnification of the ordinary
microscope, but which are visible when ultramicroscopical
methods are used.

6. Spirochaetes : organisms which have spiral filaments,
which are so thin that they can only be seen by means of a
special method of microscopical examination known as
dark ground illumination.

7. Yeasts and moulds; these organisms are classed as
" fungi " and are more highly organised than are bacteria.

Cocci.—The word, coccus, is of Greek derivation and means
" a berry "; the cocci are classified morphologically as follows.

1. Micrococci ; cocci in which special grouping of cells
is absent.

2. Diplococci; cocci appear in pairs and are seen usually with the adjacent sides of the organisms in close contact.

3. Staphylococci; the cocci are arranged in clusters like bunches of grapes.

4. Streptococci; the cocci are arranged in chains.

5. Sarcinae; cocci arranged in regular packets of 8, or multiples of 8.

Pyogenic cocci are associated with pus formation and are found in various acute inflammatory and suppurative conditions and for descriptive purposes are classified Gram positive cocci and Gram negative cocci.

Description of Organisms.—Bacteria are subdivided into main divisions and subdivisions. In the following pages the characteristics of each organism are set down in tabular form, the principal headings being those of group, organism, morphology, cultural characters, resistance, habitat, pathogenesis and chemotherapy. It is hoped that these tables will serve the purpose for which they were devised viz. speedy reference and concise summary.

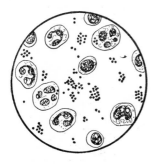

FIG 64.—STAPHYLOCOCCI.

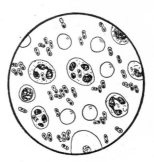

FIG. 65.—PNEUMOCOCCI.

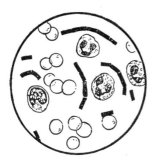

FIG. 66.—ANTHRAX BACILLI IN
BLOOD FILM.

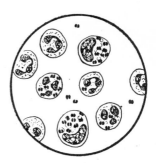

FIG. 67.—GONOCOCCI LYING IN
PAIRS MOSTLY WITHIN THE
LEUCOCYTES.

BACTERIOLOGICAL TABLES

Group	Organism	Morphology	Cultural Characters	Resistance	Habitat	Pathogenesis	Chemotherapy
Gram Positive Cocci.	Staphylococcus pyogenes aureus.	Spherical in shape, and arranged in grape-like clusters; is non-motile, does not form spores. Size 0·8-0·9µ in diameter.	Aerobe and facultative anaerobe. Grows well at room temperature and at blood heat. Virulence of cultures persists for many months. Broth—a general turbidity forms within 18 hours. Gelatine—liquefies readily. Agar and blood serum—a thick streak is seen at first pale yellow, and then golden yellow.	Exposure to moist heat for one hour required to kill some strains. Killed by exposure to 2 per cent phenol for 15 minutes.	The surface of the body normally. Found in dust, earth and water; its presence in these is probably accidental.	Found in ulcerative endocarditis, furunculosis, osteomyelitis empyema, boils, carbuncles, abscesses, in the blood in septicaemia.	Sensitive to sulphathiazole and penicillin.
Do.	Staphylococcus albus.	Similar in growth to S. aureus but is unpigmented and white in colour.	Whitish growth on agar. With gelatine —slow liquefaction. In broth, a greyish white turbidity is produced.	Similar to S. aureus.	Commonly present on the skin, in the mouth and throat.	Present in the pus of boils, stitch abscesses, carbuncles, septic discharges, in chronic prostatitis and infection of the kidney due to calculi.	Same as S. aureus.
Do.	Staphylococcus citreus.	Non-pathogenic saprophyte.	Bright lemon colour on solid medium.	—	—	—	—

Group	Organism	Morphology	Cultural Characters	Resistance	Habitat	Pathogenesis	Chemotherapy
Gram Positive Cocci.	Micrococcus tetragenus.	Spherical or ovoid cells arranged in fours with a capsule.	Slowly develops on gelatine as a thick white growth and ferments glucose with the formation of acid.	—	Skin.	Found in phthisical cavities, sometimes in pus of acute and chronic abscesses, though it is usually a saprophyte.	—
Do.	Sarcinae.	Spherical cocci, slightly larger than staphylococci; arranged in cubes of eight, forming small blocks.	Grow well on agar and produce a deep yellow pigment in broth; fluffy deposits at the bottom of the culture; slow liquefaction of gelatine.	—	Air, water, dust.	May be found in sputum, normally non-pathogenic.	—
Do.	Pneumococcus (Diplococcus pneumoniae)	Occurs typically in pairs of ovoid or lanceolated and encapsulated cocci, with rounded ends together. Size 1μ in its long diameter.	Addition of blood or agar is necessary to ensure growth. On agar, growth consists of small transparent dew-drop-like colonies which tend to remain discrete. On broth, the growth shows at first a uniform turbidity, but later a granular deposit is visible in the tube. Gelatine is not liquefied.	—	—	Important human pathogen causing lobar pneumonia, empyema, pericarditis, otitis media, sinusitis, meningitis, suppurative arthritis, peritonitis.	Dramatically successful with the use of sulphonamides, especially sulphapyridine, and of penicillin.

BACTERIOLOGICAL TABLES

Group	Organism	Morphology	Cultural Characters	Resistance	Habitat	Pathogenesis	Chemotherapy
Gram Positive Cocci.	*Streptococcus haemolyticus.*	Chain-like formation containing 10 or more spherical cocci measuring 0·5 to 0·75µ in diameter; the organism is non-mobile.	Aerobic and facultatively anaerobic. On agar, the colonies are small, discrete and transparent. Gelatine—no liquefaction occurs. Broth—some turbidity is visible with granular deposits. The most important character of this organism is its power of lysing red blood cells, which can be seen in cultures made on blood agar.	Killed in 30 minutes at about 55° C.; destroyed by prolonged application of disinfectants.	—	Causative organism of scarlet fever, tonsillitis, puerperal fever, erysipelas, cellulitis, septicaemia and numerous suppurative conditions.	Sensitive to sulphonamides and to penicillin, which have now replaced antitoxins in the treatment of streptococcal infections.
Do.	*Streptococcus viridans.*	Similar in morphology to streptococci of the haemolytic group; its virulence is low. Arranged in chains which are short in formation.	Similar to haemolytic streptococci, but no true haemolytic reaction occurs on blood agar.	Killed by heating at 60° C. for 30 minutes.	Many strains probably non-pathogenic and the organism is often found in the human mouth and throat, gum margins and teeth, frequently in the faeces.	When associated with disease, it may be found in the blood in subacute and chronic endocarditis.	Some strains are insensitive to penicillin.

BACTERIOLOGICAL TABLES

Group	Organism	Morphology	Cultural Characters	Resistance	Habitat	Pathogenesis	Chemotherapy
Gram Positive Cocci.	Streptococcus faecalis.	Chains of cocci, of short length and generally arranged in pairs or singly.	Grows well on ordinary media, showing separate transparent colonies on agar slightly larger than those of the haemolytic group. Similar growth in broth and gelatine.	Resistant to heat at 60° C. for 30 minutes.	Normal commensal of the faeces.	When certain strains are pathogenic, they are usually of low virulence, and are known to cause urinary infections and ulcerative endocarditis.	Results of penicillin treatment still under investigation, but until now has proved to be insensitive though the organism is sensitive to sulphathiazole.
Gram Negative Cocci. (The Neisseria are gram negative cocci and are usually arranged in pairs.)	Gonococcus or Neisseria gonorrhoeae.	A diplococcus, each measuring about 0·7 by 0·5μ, and shaped rather like a coffee bean and grouped in pairs: the flattened sides of the two organisms are adjacent; aerobic.	Grows easily on serum, or blood agar, enriched with hydrocele fluid. The colonies are semi-transparent discs about the size of a pin head. Broth—gives slight turbidity; Gelatine—no action; Glucose—on this it has a fermentative reaction but none on maltose, lactose or saccharose.	Sensitive to heat (killed in 10 minutes at 60° C.), to antiseptics and to sunlight.	In the male—mucosa of the urethra. In the female—cervix, urethra, glands of Bartholin, vulva, vagina and uterine tubes.	Suppurative inflammation with a purulent discharge.	Sensitive to sulphonamides and to penicillin; the efficacy of the latter treatment has been established without doubt.

BACTERIOLOGICAL TABLES

Group	Organism	Morphology	Cultural Characters	Resistance	Habitat	Pathogenesis	Chemotherapy
Gram Negative Cocci	Meningococcus or Neisseria meningitidis.	Diplococcus with opposed surfaces flattened; very susceptible to cold, and infected swabs and other material intended for culture must be kept at body heat.	Does not grow on ordinary agar, broth or gelatine. On blood agar, the colonies appear as small transparent greyish discs. The meningococcus ferments maltose and glucose with the production of acid, and fails to ferment sucrose.	Killed by moist heat at 55° C. in 5 minutes.	—	Causes meningococcal meningitis; occurs under wintry conditions and disappears with the advent of warm weather; the primary seat of infection is the nasopharynx; there may be no apparent symptoms (carrier case). Carriers infect other persons by the spray produced in coughing, and may remain infective for from 4 weeks to several months.	Sulphonamides have superseded treatment by specific sera; virulence of infection and many of the sequelae of the past have been reduced.
Do.	Micrococcus catarrhalis (Neisseria catarrhalis).	Occurs as an oval or spherical coccus, usually arranged in pairs or tetrads.	Grows easily on ordinary laboratory media at 14° C. and 42° C., producing grey or yellowish-white colonies; can be differentiated from meningococcus by its growth on ordinary media.	—	Common saprophyte in the mouth and throat.	May be found in sputum and respiratory infections.	—

PLATE I

1

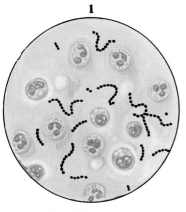

2

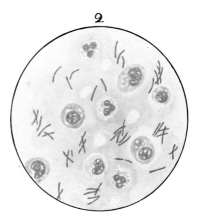

1. Cocci (Streptococcus).

2. Bacilli without spores (Tubercle bacilli).

3

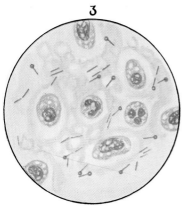

4

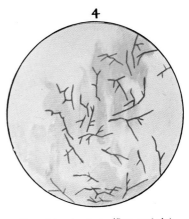

3. Bacilli with spores (Tetanus bacilli).

4. Branching bacteria (Streptothrix).

TYPES OF BACTERIA (A)

Group	Organism	Morphology	Cultural Characters	Resistance	Habitat	Pathogenesis	Chemotherapy
A c i d f a s t organisms. (Mycobacteria—slender rods which are stained with difficulty, but when once stained, are acid fast.)	Tubercle bacillus (Mycobacterium tuberculosis).	Non-motile slender rod, sometimes slightly curved with rounded ends. Size 3μ long and 0·3μ wide. It is more difficult to stain than other bacteria.	Aerobic and facultatively anaerobic, it grows best at blood heat, growth being very slow (4–6 weeks). A pure culture can be obtained by inoculation of tuberculous sputum into a guineapig, the animal showing evidence of disease in 6 weeks.	Survives for long periods in dried sputum; destroyed by heat (60° C.) in milk, by strong antiseptics and sunlight.	In sputum, pus, urine, and milk from tubercular infected cows (bovine).	Causes pulmonary tuberculosis, t u b e r c u l a r glands, tubercular infections of the urinary tract.	No satisfactory results to be recorded.
Do.	Bacillus leprae (Mycobacterium leprae).	Organisms are straight or slightly curved rods very like the tubercle bacillus; may be beaded or may have clubbed ends. Non-motile and non-sporing; bacilli may be found arranged in clumps or bundles.	Improbable that this organism has been cultivated in pure state.	—	In the lesions of leprosy i.e. serum from n o d u l e s, gland secretion and blood during the febrile state. Has been found in most of the tissues and viscera, although it occurs more in the liver and spleen than in the kidneys and brain.	Two types of leprosy 1. the nodular, in which the skin or mucous membrane is infected; 2. the anaesthetic, in which the n e r v e s a r e affected.	—

189

BACTERIOLOGICAL TABLES

Group	Organism	Morphology	Cultural Characters	Resistance	Habitat	Pathogenesis	Chemotherapy
Acid fast organisms Mycobacteria.	Smegma bacillus (Mycobacterium smegmatis).	Rod shaped shorter and straighter than tubercle bacillus. Gram positive.	Grows on agar, forming a granular growth, and in broth, forming a turbid deposit.	—	Prepuce, glans penis, labia minora and around the urethral orifice.	—	—
Spore forming organisms.* Bacilli.	Anthrax bacillus (Bacillus anthracis).	Varies in length from 5 to 6µ, in breadth from 1 to 1.5µ; facultative anaerobe, non-motile; usually a straight rod with characteristic square ends. In cultures, chains of great length are formed. Gram positive. Spores are only developed after death, when the blood discharges come in contact with air.	On agar colonies have appearance of wavy wreath-like locks of hair. In gelatine stabs growth takes place along the needle track with an outgrowth of fine branching filaments, like an inverted fir tree growth. In broth, flocculent growth forms at the bottom of the tube, the broth above being quite clear.	Spores can resist heat at 100° C. for 15 minutes; in non-spore forming state organism is killed at 60° C.	Infected carcases, hides, wool and shaving brushes. Anthrax is primarily a disease of animals, man being infected by the bacilli or spores by handling above.	In man, the chief types of this disease are 1. Malignant pustule, a localised swelling caused by direct inoculation of the skin with the infected material. 2. Woolsorter's disease, a general infection caused by the inhalation of spores from hides, wool and fleece.	Sulphapyridine is most successful.

190

* In this classification, the organisms are now referred to as bacillus when spore forming and aerobic; clostridium, when spore forming and anaerobic.

BACTERIOLOGICAL TABLES

Group	Organism	Morphology	Cultural Characters	Resistance	Habitat	Pathogenesis	Chemotherapy
Spore forming organisms. Clostridia.	Tetanus bacillus (Clostridium tetani).	Straight slender rod 2 to 5μ, with rounded ends. Spherical spores are found at one end and being thicker than the organism, give a drumstick appearance; gram positive.	Strict anaerobe; in glucose gelatine or glucose agar stab culture, feathery growth is formed with slight gas production; gelatine is liquefied and all cultures have a characteristic odour suggestive of a dirty stable.	Spores are resistant to boiling for 1 hour and can survive in a 5 per cent solution of phenol for weeks.	Spores are found very often in cow and horse dung; rarely in human faeces. The bacillus may occur naturally in the intestines of certain animals, e.g. horses, cattle and sheep.	Pathogenic to man. Birds are slightly susceptible. Dogs are immune; cats only affected by heavy inoculation; horses are easily infected. Main symptoms are muscular spasm including lockjaw.	Clostridium tetani is sensitive to penicillin.
Do.	Bacillus Botulinus. (Clostridium botulinus).	Large (4 – 10μ long) with rounded ends and a tendency to form short chains; it exhibits slight motility and forms spores; gram positive.	Strict anaerobe, and cultures must grow in the dark. Stab culture on glucose-gelatine grows white along the stab with lateral offshoots. On agar, greyish translucent colonies. Broth becomes turbid. Sporulation does not occur at blood heat.	Spores are destroyed by moist heat at 100° C. in 5 hours.	In earth, in greatest abundance in virgin soil, especially at high altitudes. May appear in tinned meat and preserved foods in which it forms a poisonous toxin.	Botulism, which has toxic effects on the parasympathetic nervous system, is caused by eating tainted food.	—

Group	Organism	Morphology	Cultural Characters	Resistance	Habitat	Pathogenesis	Chemotherapy
Spore forming organisms. Clostridia.	*Bacillus Welchii.* (*Clostridium Welchii*).	Plump bacillus (4–8μ long, by 0·8–1μ broad) with rounded ends; forms oval spores, generally located at one end. Occasionally found to be encapsulated; gram positive.	Strict anaerobe which grows best at 37° C. In glucose agar, it produces surface colonies, which have round, smooth opaque discs. Broth is rendered turbid. Gelatine is slowly liquefied. In milk a characteristic "stormy" fermentation is produced; in 48 hours a firm white honeycomb curd and a clear watery whey with abundant gas formation, are evident.	—	Occurs chiefly in soil, in excrements, sewage and dust and normally in the large intestines of man and animals.	In children summer diarrhoea is caused. Wound infections, uterine infections (septic abortion), infections of intestinal tract, gallbladder and urinary system.	Sensitive to penicillin.
Do.	*Clostridium septique.*	Large bacillus with rounded ends about 3–10μ long; is a motile rod, with several flagella. Has a tendency to grow in long filaments; stains with ordinary dyes and is gram positive.	Strict anaerobe and can grow on ordinary media. Glucose accelerates growth. Agar stab culture: a white line of growth with short lateral processes. Produces a foul smelling gas in both gelatine and agar stab cultures.	—	Occurs chiefly in soil.	May be the exciting cause of gas gangrene after injuries, especially when the parts are crushed or lacerated and soiled with earth; pathogenic to man, horses, pigs, sheep, guineapigs, rabbits, rats, mice and some birds.	Sensitive to penicillin.

Group	Organism	Morphology	Cultural Characters	Resistance	Habitat	Pathogenesis	Chemotherapy
Gram Positive Non Sporing Bacteria.	Diphtheria bacillus (Corynebacterium diphtheriae: Klebs-Loeffler bacillus).	Slender, delicate, non-motile organism, rounded ends, said to be reservoirs for food and not spores. Not killed by drying ; it can retain its virulence in dust for months under certain conditions. Aerobic and facultatively anaerobic. When stained with Loeffler's stain it shows a "beaded" or "barred" appearance. As confirmatory stains, Neisser's or Pugh's stains are used.	On gelatine, growth is slow and without liquefaction. On blood serum and glycerine agar growth is rapid, but Loeffler's serum is most generally used as the growth is so rapid. Colonies consist of white or cream coloured opaque spots about the size of an ordinary pin head.	Thermal death point is at 37° C.	—	Causes diphtheria of 3 types—1. Gravis, a serious infection; it shows, on culture, a daisy head, grey-black; 2. mitis type, a milder infection which produces smooth black colonies; 3. intermediate type, a moderate grade of infection (small flat colony with defined edge). Virulence test: this may be necessary in the case of carriers and is carried out by injecting a guineapig with the culture. Diphtheria is a disease of the young (2–10), mortality peak being highest at ages below 5 years. Mucous surfaces are most susceptible; here false membranes may be formed.	Sensitive to penicillin.

BACTERIOLOGICAL TABLES

Group	Organism	Morphology	Cultural Characters	Resistance	Habitat	Pathogenesis	Chemotherapy
Gram Positive Non Sporing Bacteria.	Corynebacterium hoffmanni (Hoffmann's diphtheroid bacillus).	Differs from the diphtheria bacillus; shorter, plumper and a somewhat spindle shaped rod; is an aerobe.	Grows well on ordinary media; large opaque colonies.	—	Common inhabitant of the throat and nasal mucous membrane of the town dweller.	—	—
Do.	Xerosis bacillus.	Found on the conjunctiva, similar in staining and morphology to the diphtheria bacillus.	Can be differentiated from B. diphtheriae by production of acid in saccharose.	—	A commensal in the conjunctival sac.	Non-pathogenic.	
Do.	Lactobacillus acidophilus.	Found in the faeces of infants.	Ferments glucose, lactose and maltose with the production of acid.	—	Occurs in faeces, saliva and milk.	—	—

Group	Organism	Morphology	Cultural Characters	Resistance	Habitat	Pathogenesis	Chemotherapy
GramNegative Non Sporing Bacilli.* GramNegative Intestinal Bacilli. Coli-Aerogenes Group.	Bacterium coli (B. coli).	Short rod 2–4μ long, with rounded ends; 3–4 flagella; is feebly motile	On an agar plate, a greyish-whitegrowth is visible in 1–2 days. Broth: general turbidity. MacConkey's medium: red colonies. Fermentation reaction: many sugars are fermented, the most important being glucose, mannite and lactose, in which acid and gas are formed. B. coli produces indole in broth or peptone water cultures, in 2 days.	Resistant to heat but killed at 60° C. and by disinfectants.	Intestinal tracts of man, the lower animals, birds and fish.	In certain situations it may be pathogenic, being one of the commonest causes of acute cholecystitis and infections of the urinary tract.	—
Do.	Bacillus proteus.	Short rod 1 to 2·5μ long, is motile, with lateral flagella.	On agar plates bacillus proteus spreads rapidly, covering the entire surface in 24 hours; it produces a moist translucent whitish-grey growth. Gelatine and Loeffler's blood serum are liquefied.	—	Decomposing matter and faeces, as a saprophyte.	B. proteus may be responsible for acute bacterial food poisoning, septic infections, suppurative wounds. urinary sepsis, otitis media and summer diarrhoea in infants.	Insensitive to penicillin.

195

* These include many important pathogenic and non-pathogenic organisms, the identification of which depends on a knowledge of the source from which the material for examination is derived, apart from the results of other microscopical investigations. For simplicity they are grouped under the following headings: 1. Gram negative intestinal bacilli; 2. Gram negative bacilli from the respiratory tract; 3. Other Gram negative bacilli.

BACTERIOLOGICAL TABLES

Group	Organism	Morphology	Cultural Characters	Resistance	Habitat	Pathogenesis	Chemotherapy
Gram Negative Intestinal Bacilli. Coli-Aerogenes Group.	*Typhoid bacillus.* (*Bacterium typhosus*).	Measures 2-4 µ in length, 0·5µ in diameter, with rounded ends; aerobic and facultatively anaerobic; usually carries 8-12 flagella, arranged round its sides and end; actively motile.	On agar, a greyish-cream layer is produced; on gelatine, a thin whitish growth; in broth, a general turbidity. Organism does not ferment lactose or sucrose, but produces acid with glucose, maltose and mannite. Widal Reaction, see p, 231	Is not killed by drying; its thermal death-point is 55°C. Direct sunlight is fatal to *B. typhosus* in 5 hours.	In carriers it is harboured in the gallbladder. Organism can nearly always be found in blood in the fever stage, in the faeces on the 8th or 9th day, in the urine between the 1st and 3rd week.	Causes typhoid fever. Channels of infection: water-by sewage contamination; shell fish—oysters, winkles, mussels and cockles—stored in contaminated water; milk, handled by infected persons or polluted by infected water in rinsing vessels; butter or ice cream made from infected milk; flies—infected through the excreta; vegetables—watercress grown in sewage polluted stream and vegetables from sewage farms; direct contact; the typhoid carrier.	Insensitive to penicillin.

BACTERIOLOGICAL TABLES

Group	Organism	Morphology	Cultural Characters	Resistance	Habitat	Pathogenesis	Chemotherapy
GramNegative Intestinal Bacilli. Coli-Aerogenes Group.	*Bacillus paratyphoid A, B and C (Bacterium paratyphosum A, B and C).*	Similar to that of *B. typhosus* and *B. coli.*	Cultural characters similar to *B. typhosus* and *B. coli.* Does not ferment lactose, but with glucose and mannite, acid and gas are produced; the final identification depends on the agglutination reactions (see p. 215 and 231).	—	Inparatyphoid fever whether caused by A or B bacilli, the organism may be found in the blood or faeces. Meat and milk are supposed to have conveyed the infection and these organisms have been isolated from suspected water.	Gives rise to paratyphoid fever.	—

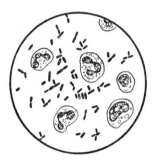

Fig. 68.—Typhoid Bacilli.

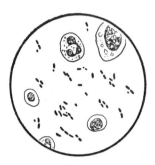

Fig. 69.—Pertussis Bacilli.

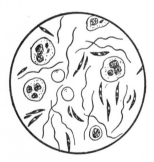

Fig. 70.—Slide from Case of
Vincent's Angina.

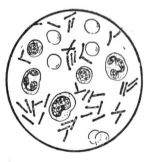

Fig. 71.—Diphtheria Bacilli.

Group	Organism	Morphology	Cultural Characters	Resistance	Habitat	Pathogenesis	Chemotherapy
Gram Negative Intestinal Bacilli. Coli-Aerogenes Group	Dysentery bacillus (Bacterium dysenteriae). Several types, best known being Flexner, Shiga and Sonnei.	Non-motile, similar in microscopical appearance to B. typhosus, B. coli and paratyphoid organisms.	Growths on agar and gelatine are like those of typhoid. There is no liquefaction on gelatine. Aerobe and facultative anaerobe. Flexner type ferments mannite and glucose, with the production of acid but no gas. Shiga bacillus has no action on mannite, while the Sonnei type ferments lactose in a fluid medium. The blood serum of patients gives an agglutinative reaction, if the type of organism causing the disease is used.	Destroyed by heat at 60° C.	—	Found in ulcerative colitis or "asylum dysentery," and in cases of infantile diarrhoea (summer diarrhoea). It is the causative organism of an acute form of dysentery met with in tropical and sub-tropical countries, but sometimes occurring as well in temperate climates.	—

BACTERIOLOGICAL TABLES

Group	Organism	Morphology	Cultural Characters	Resistance	Habitat	Pathogenesis	Chemotherapy
GramNegative Intestinal Bacilli. Food poisoning Group.	Salmonella group (includes *Bacterium enteritidis of Gaertner* and *Bacillus aertrycke.*	All actively motile; in microscopical appearance very similar to typhoid bacillus, *B. coli* and dysentery bacillus.	Agar, broth and gelatine cultures similar to those of *B. coli.* Organisms ferment glucose, fructose, maltose and mannite, with the production of acid and gas; no effect on lactose. Identification as to cause of the disease may be shown by a satisfactory agglutination with the patient's serum.	Similar to that of *B. typhosus* and *B. dysenteriae*	—	The salmonella group causes meat and food poisoning, in which a sudden attack of illness produces symptoms of acute gastroenteritis, accompanied by toxaemia. The salmonella organism also produces epidemic infections in rats and mice, in certain birds, cattle and pigs. Cases of food poisoning have been traced to the consumption of infected eggs (shell and dry).	—

Group	Organism	Morphology	Cultural Characters	Resistance	Habitat	Pathogenesis	Chemotherapy
GramNegative Bacilli from Sputum and Respiratory Tract.	*Friedländer's bacillus (Pneumo-bacillus).*	Short non-motile capsulated rods, with rounded ends 1-2μ in length.	Grows well on ordinary media, either at blood heat or room temperature. Agar: raised slimy colonies. In stab gelatine culture, a nail shaped growth is formed; gelatine is not liquefied. Broth: turbid growth. Aerobic and facultatively anaerobic.	Similar to that of *B. coli* and coliform bacilli.	May be found as a commensal in the throats of normal healthy people.	Organisms may give rise to suppurative conditions including empyema and occasionally septicaemia. This organism was at one time credited with being the causative organism of pneumonia.	Insensitive to penicillin.
GramNegative Bacilli from Sputum and Respiratory Tract.	*Bacillus influenzae (Haemophilus influenzae) (Pfeiffer's bacillus).*	Coccobacillus about 1·5μ in length and 0·3μ in thickness; non-motile.	Strict aerobe. Does not grow on ordinary laboratory media, but must have one containing blood e.g. chocolate agar, or certain growth producing substances present in blood and also in certain vegetable tissues. Cultivated on Fildes's medium (agar medium containing peptic digest of blood) producing round transparent colonies.	Killed by exposure to heat at 55° C. in 30 minutes.	—	The *B. influenzae* is the common cause of purulent catarrh, and is no longer considered to be the primary cause of influenza, even although the organism is found in the sputum and nasal secretions of patients with this disease.	Insensitive to penicillin.

BACTERIOLOGICAL TABLES

Group	Organism	Morphology	Cultural Characters	Resistance	Habitat	Pathogenesis	Chemotherapy
Gram Negative Bacilli from Sputum and Respiratory Tract.	*Bacillus pertussis* (*Haemophilus pertussis*) (Whooping cough bacillus).	Very small oval coccobacillus, slightly larger than *B. influenzae* and is non-motile.	Not strictly haemophilic but it is generally cultivated on media containing blood. Primary cultures are difficult to obtain except on special media, of which the Bordet-Gengou medium (see p. 178) is the best. After 2–3 days' incubation, the bacillus forms small glistening dome shaped colonies like pearls.	—	—	*B. pertussis* causes whooping cough in man; it is found in the sputum and in the spray produced on coughing during the earlier stages of the disease.	Insensitive to penicillin.
Other Gram Negative Bacilli.	*Diplobacillus of Morax* (*Haemophilus lacunatus*).	Rod shaped and arranged in pairs, end to end. Size—about 2 by 1/4; is non-motile.	The diplobacillus is an aerobe and requires blood or serum. On serum agar, it produces liquefaction and pits or *lacunae* are developed on the colonies on the surface of the medium.	—	—	Organism specifically associated with conjunctivitis.	Instillation every 1–2 hours, drops containing 500–2,000 units of penicillin per ml. or the application of penicillin ointment or by ophthalmic tablets containing 250 units.

PLATE II

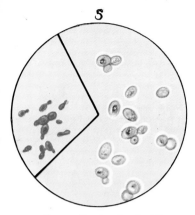

5. Yeast cells, showing budding.

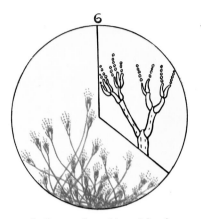

6. Spores of moulds and fungi (Penicillium).

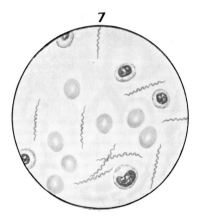

7, Spirochaetes of syphilis.

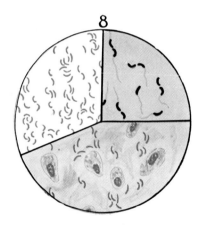

8. Vibrio cholerae.

TYPES OF BACTERIA (B)

Group	Organism	Morphology	Cultural Characters	Resistance	Habitat	Pathogenesis	Chemotherapy
Other Gram Negative Bacilli.	*Koch-Weeks bacillus* (*Haemophilus conjunctivitidis*).	Short slender rod, sometimes found within the cytoplasm of the polymorphonuclear leucocyte.	Does not grow on ordinary medium, but like *B. influenzae* with which it is identical, requires a medium containing blood. On blood agar, it forms minute dewdrop-like colonies.	—	—	Causative organism of acute contagious ophthalmia.	Same reaction to penicillin as *diplobacillus of Morax*.
Do.	*Bacillus pyocyaneus* (*Pseudomonas pyocyanea*).	Small bacillus, size 1·5 to 3μ, motile, with 1–3 flagella.	Aerobe and a facultative anaerobe, grows on ordinary media. Creamy growth on agar, to which it imparts a greenish fluorescence. Gelatine is liquefied and the fluid is coloured in the same way, a greenish blue. Broth: a greenish colour is produced on the surface.	—	Found in polluted water and sewage.	Debility, wasting and diarrhoea result when the organism attacks the alimentary canal. It occurs in suppurative conditions, giving rise to blue pus and is a rare cause of septicaemia.	Insensitive to penicillin.

203

Group	Organism	Morphology	Cultural Characters	Resistance	Habitat	Pathogenesis	Chemotherapy
Other Gram Negative Bacilli.	*Bacillus melitensis (Brucella melitensis).*	The bacillus melitensis is a coccobacillus usually showing a round or oval formation. In size 0.4μ, it may occur singly or in short chains; non-motile.	Aerobic. On agar, small transparent discs in colonies are found. Broth : faint turbidity. Gelatine stab: delicate line of growth occurs along the needle tract, but no liquefaction occurs.	Killed at 60° C., but resists drying for 2 or 3 months.	—	Causative organism of Malta fever. In addition to man, goats, cows, sheep, horses, mules and dogs are liable to the infection; since goat's milk was prohibited to troops stationed in Malta (1906), the disease has almost disappeared from among the troops; these bacteria are found in the blood early in the disease and later in the urine.	Insensitive to penicillin.

BACTERIOLOGICAL TABLES

Group	Organism	Morphology	Cultural Characters	Resistance	Habitat	Pathogenesis	Chemotherapy
Other Gram Negative Bacilli.	*Bacillus abortus* (*Brucella abortus*).	Closely resembles *B. melitensis*: is a small coccus or bacillus occurring singly, in pairs or in short chains.	When cultivated, growth is slow and requires an atmosphere containing 10 per cent carbonic acid gas.	—	—	Causative organism of bovine contagious abortion (bovine type); it may infect pigs (porcine type or *Brucella suis*). It may infect sheep, horses and fowls. Human infection is caused by drinking infected cow's milk, and gives rise to undulant or continued fever.	Insensitive to penicillin.

BACTERIOLOGICAL TABLES

Group	Organism	Morphology	Cultural Characters	Resistance	Habitat	Pathogenesis	Chemotherapy
Other Gram Negative Bacilli.	*Bacillus pestis* or *Plague bacillus* (*Pasteurella pestis*).	Short oval coccobacillus, with rounded ends, occuring in pairs or singly; non-motile.	Grows aerobically and anaerobically on ordinary culture medium. Cultures on agar show small transparent white discs. Gelatine: no liquefaction. Broth: granular deposit on the base and sides of the test tube.	Is very easily killed by disinfectants, and at a temperature of 55° C. complete desiccation destroys the bacillus.	—	Causative organism of oriental plague, of which there are 3 types—bubonic, septicaemic and pneumonic. Organism is found in the buboes, in the rusty sputum in the pneumonic type, in the blood in the septicaemic type. Human infection is conveyed by rat fleas or by direct contact with patients with the disease. Plague is primarily a disease of rats and other rodents. The pneumonia type is communicated from person to person by infection from the respiratory tract.	Insensitive to penicillin.

206

BACTERIOLOGICAL TABLES

Group	Organism	Morphology	Cultural Characters	Resistance	Habitat	Pathogenesis	Chemotherapy
Vibrio. A class of bacteria in which the organism is short, curved c o m m a - shaped.	*Vibrio cholerae (Koch's comma bacillus).*	Curved rod, 2 by 0·3 μ in size. It is actively motile, with a single flagellum at one end only.	Vibrio grows readily on most media; aerobic; abundant growth is seen on alkaline medium (e.g. Dieudonné's medium). Agar: white circular discs about the size of *B. coli.* Gelatin stab: a bubble of lique-faction at the top of the slab in 48 hours. Broth: some tur-bidity. Agglutin-ated by anti-sera known as *V. cholerae.*	—	—	Causative organisms of Asiatic cholera. Symptoms: suppressed urine and copious and watery stools which have the characteristic rice-water appearance due to detached epithelium. The organisms are generally confined to the stomach contents, intestinal contents and dejecta.	Insensitive to penicillin.

BACTERIOLOGICAL TABLES

Group	Organism	Morphology	Cultural Characters	Resistance	Habitat	Pathogenesis	Chemotherapy
Streptothrices: filamentous organisms which show true branching and form a mycelium.	Actinomycosis streptothrix (Streptothrix actinomyces).	Organism grows as a felted mass of branching filaments with terminal clubs, (mycelium) which are comparatively slender (0·8–1μ thick). The filaments are Gram positive, the clubs Gram negative but acid fast.	Both filaments and clubs respond to aerobic and anaerobic cultures, so both reactions are tested. Agar: growth is slow on artificial media, small discrete greyish-white colonies appearing on glycerol agar or glucose agar in 3 or 4 days. Broth: some deposit is present. Gelatine: slow liquefaction.	—	—	The disease occurs in cattle (actinomyces bovis) and may be transmitted to man. In human beings, the lesions usually show a suppurative tendency and the pus contains colonies of the parasite in the form of small granules about the size of a pin head, which are a bright yellow in colour, often known as sulphur granules. This disease may affect the lungs, the skin, intestines and appendix, the commonest avenue of infection being the mouth and throat.	Some strains of actinomyces bovis are sensitive to penicillin.

Group	Organism	Morphology	Cultural Characters	Resistance	Habitat	Pathogenesis	Chemotherapy
The Pathogenic and Commensal Spirochaetes.	Treponema pallidum (Spirochaeta pallida).	Delicate spiral filament (size 6 to 14μ) with 6–12 coils. The ends are pointed and tapering. In the unstained condition, it is best seen by dark ground illumination, which shows a rotatory corkscrew like motility. Staining: the organism does not react to ordinary methods.	Serological reactions are used generally more than artificial culture, the most important being the Wassermann reaction. In this, the diagnosis is found to be negative in the incubation stage, but in from 10–30 days after the appearance of the primary sore, the reaction is positive in 93 per cent of the cases, and remains positive throughout the secondary and tertiary stages, unless antisyphilitic treatment is given.	—	—	Causative organism of syphilis. It is found in the primary sore and neighbouring lymphatic glands, in the papular and roseolar eruptions and condylomata of the secondary lesions; it is also found in the liver, lungs, pancreas, spleen, thymus and adrenals of the syphilitic foetus.	In both primary and secondary syphilis penicillin therapy has proved satisfactory.
Do.	Bacilli and spirochaetes of Vincent's angina (Bacillus fusiformis and spirochaeta Vincenti).	Films of these organisms made from ulcers of the throat, show both types of bacteria under the microscope; the fusiformis bacillus is associated with the spiral threads or spirochaetes. Both are anaerobic.	Organisms are cultivated anaerobically on ordinary media with the addition of human serum.	—	—	Causative organisms of Vincent's angina. Can be isolated from necrotic tissues in the ulcerations of the mouth, throat and gums.	Sensitive to penicillin.

BACTERIOLOGICAL TABLES

Group	Organism	Morphology	Cultural Characters	Resistance	Habitat	Pathogenesis	Chemotherapy
The Pathogenic and Commensal Spirochaetes.	*Spirochaeta of infective jaundice (Leptospira icterohaemorrhagica).*	About 7–14μ long by 0·15μ in size. The coils are numerous and so fine that they are difficult to see in stained preparations, although they are quite apparent when dark ground illumination is used. The hooked ends are a characteristic feature morphologically. Movement is both rotatory and undulant and is visible with a dark ground illumination.	Diagnosis is made by the inoculation of guineapigs, with the blood during the first week of the disease. In later stages of the disease, the urine is used for inoculation. Agglutination test can also be carried out.	—	—	The leptospira occurs in wild rodents, which act as carriers of Weil's disease. It is excreted in the urine of the animals and contaminates food and soil, especially the soil of coal mines. Infection of human being occurs through the alimentary canal or by the passage of the spirochaetes through the skin, which becomes sodden through continuous swelling or through abrasions.	Sensitive to penicillin.

Fungi.—The infections caused by fungi are usually described as mycoses, and the most important of these are due to a group known as *Fungi imperfecti.*

Microsporon or scalp ringworm.—The *microsporon* is the common cause of scalp ringworm among children; it seldom attacks the body and is supposed not to infect the individual after puberty. The mycelium (mass of vegetative filaments) develops in the horny layers of the epidermis of the scalp and in the medulla of the hair. The hyphae (threads or filaments) pass through the cortex of the hair and produce a small covering of spherical shaped spores, arranged in a mosaic pattern on the outside of the hair.

Tricophyton.—This organism is found in ringworm affecting the beard and occasionally on the scalp and nails. Its spores are large, hence the name, large-spored ringworm.

Achorion schönleinii.—This fungus is associated with favus, which affects the scalp and other skin areas and is characterized by the formation of concave yellow discs (scutula) around the hair follicle; it leaves considerable scarring of the scalp owing to the destruction of the skin. The disease affects man, dogs, cats, caged rabbits, mice and rats, and is transmitted from animals to man. The fungus grows on ordinary media; on agar, the colonies appear in 48 hours; they are surrounded by a fine fringe of threads.

Tinea cruris.—This fungus grows in the deeper layers of the epidermis and the skin folds and is the cause of dhobie itch, a parasitic skin complaint common in the tropics. It can be grown on maltose agar, producing branching filaments and spores in epithelium.

Oidium and monilia.—These are fungi which sometimes produce mycelia and at times give rise to free yeast-like cells. Oidia produce free yeast cells by a breaking up of the mycelium.

The moniliae give origin to free cells by budding from the mycelium. *Monilia albicans* grows on the mucous membrane of the mouth and pharynx of babies, causing the condition known as thrush. When the material from the typical white patches has been removed and teased up the filaments and yeast cells can be distinguished.

Moulds.—Moulds belong to the vegetable kingdom and are the fluffy felted masses which grow on food substances e.g. jam or cheese. They may also appear on culture media. They show a more advanced development than bacteria. The commonest type of mould (*penicillium glaucum*) is seen as a pale bluish green fur on jam and damp surfaces. It gives rise to a peculiar musty odour. On bread-pap mould grows at first in the form of white fur which afterwards becomes green. On gelatin plates, fine threads diverge from a point and radiate over a large surface.

The mould, *penicillium notatum*, was discovered by Fleming, who found that it was capable of producing a powerfully anti-bacterial soluble substance; this substance was named penicillin. It was discovered to be non-toxic, and after long and patient research, chiefly carried out at Oxford, it has been found possible to produce pure penicillin on a large scale.

Many organisms including staphylococci, streptococci, pneumococci, the gonococcus and the meningococcus are sensitive to penicillin, growth of these organisms being inhibited by a high dilution of the substance.

CHAPTER 4

THE MICROSCOPE

A SUITABLE microscope and a sound knowledge of its mechanism and use are of primary importance to those engaged in bacteriological work. This science is necessarily a microscopical one, and its birth may be said to coincide with the making of the first good simple microscope by Leeuwenhoek in the seventeenth century. Now, 200 years later, with the final production of the modern compound microscope, bacteriology may be said to have reached maturity as an independent science.

Component Parts.—The mechanical parts of the microscope are concerned with the support and adjustment of the optical parts, the functions of which are to enlarge the image of the object to be seen. The parts are as follows.

1. The base or stand, with the pillar, which gives support to the instrument: both are made of heavy metal in order to minimize vibration as much as possible.

2. The inclination joint in the pillar, which allows the microscope to be tipped back to any distance required by the worker.

3. Arm and body tube: the arm acts as support to the body tube to which the principal lenses are attached.

4. The draw tube, revolving nose piece, tube length: fitted inside the end of the body tube is the draw tube, which may be drawn out to various distances; within the draw tube is fitted the ocular (or eyepiece), and the purpose of the draw tube is to adjust the tube length, i.e. the distance between the upper lens of the ocular above and the attachment of the objective into the revolving nose piece below.

5. Coarse and fine adjustments: the body tube and objectives are moved up and down by means of a rack and pinion termed the coarse adjustment while the fine movements necessary for accurate focusing are performed with the fine adjustments. The use of these adjustments is necessary in order to bring the object into focus so that its outlines are sharp and well defined and great care should be exercised in the use of the adjustments.

6. The stage: this is the part of the microscope on

which the microscopical preparation to be examined is placed, usually some piece of tissue on a glass slide.

7. The mirror: this collects and reflects light up into the microscope; the plain side of the mirror is used in conjunction with the condenser when a bright artificial light is used; the concave side of the mirror is used when a large amount of light is needed as it helps to concentrate light.

8. Substage condenser and diaphragm: below the stage is the substage, which should be provided with a contrivance for raising or lowering it, usually a rack and pinion or a spiral screw. The substage is fitted with a substage condenser (Abbé type) attached to which is the iris diaphragm.

9. The ocular or eye piece is a short tube with two lenses, which fits into the upper end of the draw tube, its main function being to act with the eye itself in order to magnify the image of the object formed by the objective.

10. Objectives: the objectives are the most important items in connection with the optical apparatus, in that they limit the size of the image we require to see; further, they are responsible for the quality of the image.

The Objectives.—Most of the microscopes are equipped with 3 objectives of different magnifying power viz. the low power, the high power and the oil immersion objectives.

The lower power objective is useful for the examination of protozoa and other larger sized micro-organisms, also for the study of colonies of growing organisms. It is the shortest, and has a much larger lens at its end. This lower power objective is marked generally " 3 " or " 2/3 " (= $\frac{2}{3}$ in.) or 16 mm.

The high power objective is used for the examination of living organisms suspended in drops of water or other fluids. It is generally longer and more slender than the lower power objective and the lens at its end is smaller than the one of the lower power, although it is larger than the oil immersion objective. It is usually marked " 6 " or " 1/6 " (=$\frac{1}{6}$ in.) or 4 mm.

The oil immersion objective is one of the most essential needs of the bacteriologist, and is indispensable for the examination of stained smears of bacteria. The objective may be long or short, but it will always have a very small visible lens at its end, usually marked " oil immersion " and the figures 1/12 (inch) " 1·9 mm," or " 1·8 mm," should be engraved on it.

The oil immersion objective differs from the lower and high power objectives, in that the latter are " dry " and the lower lens of the oil immersion objective is immersed in cedar wood oil, which fills the space between the front of the objective and the object slide, and is the special oil for this purpose, because its refractive index or power of bending light rays is the same as that of glass.

CHAPTER 5

IMMUNITY

ANTIBODIES.   NATURAL IMMUNITY.   ACQUIRED IMMUNITY.
SERUM THERAPY.   ANAPHYLAXIS.   SERUM SICKNESS.

IMMUNITY may be defined as the power possessed by the body to resist an attack of some infectious disease or its poisonous products.

In order that the body may resist disease, and especially bacterial invasion, it is provided with certain chemical substances, which are formed in the blood plasma and are known as antibodies; the production of these is the result of reaction to antigens, of which the toxins of bacteria are one example.

Antibodies.—There are several types of antibody, each acting in its own way as a defending force in the attack launched by disease-producing organisms.

1. *Agglutinins.*—These are substances which cause the bacterial surfaces to become sticky, so that they adhere or clump together in masses, thus preventing reproduction and bringing about finally the death of the organisms.

2. *Precipitins.*—These absorb moisture from the bacterial cells, and by this process of dehydration bring about their disintegration.

3. *Bacteriolysins.*—These are substances which are capable of dissolving bacteria.

4. *Opsonins.*—These are substances which prepare bacteria for ingestion, rendering them more susceptible to phagocytosis i.e. acting as a sauce to the palate of the leucocytes. Normal blood contains opsonins, although their number is greatly increased by bacterial invasion.

Natural Immunity.—Immunity may be considered under the following headings: 1. Natural; 2. Acquired. Natural immunity is the inborn insusceptibility to certain diseases as a result of the possession of antibodies; the latter vary in man and animals and depend upon the race, species or individual heredity.

Racial immunity.—This type of immunity is found in man (in which different races appear to show immunity to certain diseases) and is clearly portrayed in the resistance of the native of countries such as Central Africa to yellow fever and malaria, whereas strangers to such parts contract these diseases easily. On the other hand it may be appropriate here to mention that the natives of Africa soon contract tuberculosis and pneumonia on account of the fact that they have no established hereditary immunity or the appropriate antibodies to protect them. Racial immunity is due in all probability to heredity and natural selection, the weaker and less resistant members of the race being thus weeded out.

Immunity of the species.—Cold blooded animals (fish, frogs, turtles) are not susceptible to disease common to warm blooded animals, resistance being due to difference in temperature of the species.

Differences in susceptibility of individual species to the tubercle bacillus is another important point. Fish for example are known to have tuberculous disease, but the organism which affects fish will not cause tuberculous disease in man. Birds are susceptible to the tubercle bacillus, but the avian organism has no effect on man. Many diseases of human beings do not infect certain animals e.g. syphilis, gonorrhoea, cholera, typhoid fever, influenza, measles, mumps and poliomyelitis.

Individual immunity.—Certain members of a family or of a community never contract infectious diseases such as scarlet fever, measles or mumps. This is termed individual immunity; other factors, such as age, habits, general health and occupation, are important in the establishment of individual immunity.

1. *Age.*—Old people, owing to enfeeblement of resisting power, are very prone to acute catarrhal infections e.g. bronchopneumonia.

2. *Habits.*—Many diseases are due to uncleanliness and dirty habits and lead to infections of the skin, so endangering the resistance of the individual to other disease e.g. impetigo.

3. *Occupation.*—Work carried out in badly ventilated and inadequately lit rooms makes the individual more likely to become affected with pulmonary tuberculosis.

Acquired Immunity.—Two types of acquired immunity are recognized viz. 1. *active immunity*; 2. *passive immunity.*

Active immunity.—Active immunity is acquired first from an attack of the disease, which produces antibodies and antitoxins in the blood stream in sufficient numbers to protect the individual from a subsequent attack. This state of affairs may persist for long periods, or even throughout life, as in the case of vaccinated persons. Active immunity may also be acquired by the exposure of the individual during childhood to small doses of an infection, so that eventually a degree of immunity to many diseases is acquired.

Artificially acquired immunity.—This may be developed by (among other things) the introduction of vaccines. A vaccine is a suspension of the dead or attenuated organism in normal saline solution, and is administered by hypodermic injection of small, gradually increasing doses, which, after a lapse of some days, produces reactionary antibodies; these usually appear in the blood and react with the material injected. A toxin gives rise to an antitoxin, and bacteria in a vaccine lead to the production of agglutinins, precipitins, lysins and opsonins, which react only with the particular agent by which they have been created. In conditions such as persistent attacks of boils or acne for instance, organisms are obtained from the patient and are grown on a culture medium. The organisms are then killed and injected into the patient as a vaccine (autogenous) so as to encourage the formation of antibodies and thus raise his resistance to the disease. Dead typhoid and paratyphoid bacteria are injected to raise immunity to these fevers; the antibodies thus formed remain in the blood for about 2 years. Vaccination against smallpox consists in inoculating a patient with the attenuated organism, the lymph being smeared on any small abrasion made by a lancet. Here the activity of the organism is attenuated by transmission through a calf.

Passive immunity.—This term describes immunity which is obtained by the injection into an individual of the blood serum of an animal which has previously been made immune to the disease; thus if a horse is inoculated with small doses of diphtheria organisms, it experiences a mild attack of the disease and substances are formed in the blood (antitoxins) which neutralize the toxins of diphtheria. Increasingly larger doses are given until the horse's blood is saturated with these antitoxins; this immunized horse is then bled from the jugular vein and the serum is separated.

Serum Therapy.—Sera are used therapeutically for two main purposes. 1. Antitoxic : e.g. diphtheria, tetanus, botulism, scarlet fever; 2. antibacterial: e.g. in infections with streptococci, pneumococci, meningococci or the anthrax bacillus.

Anaphylaxis.—Instead of an injection rendering a patient less sensitive to further injections of a serum, it is occasionally found that he may be hypersensitive to the proteins of this serum, producing symptoms of acute shock termed anaphylaxis, especially when the serum is derived from an animal of a different species e.g. the horse. The onset of anaphylactic shock in man may be sudden, and then it occurs within half an hour of the injection, symptoms of restlessness, pallor, dyspnoea, a rapid feeble irregular pulse, muscular twitchings, rigor and convulsions being shown. The face becomes cyanotic and congested, and sometimes the mucous membranes are swollen. An injection of adrenalin (0·5–1 ccm. of 1 in 1,000 solution) is found to be an excellent antidote.

Desensitization.—If the patient has previously been treated with any serum, it should be assumed that he is hypersensitive and he should be desensitized before being inoculated with any large dose of serum.

One of the following 2 methods may be adopted.

    1. A hypodermic injection of 0·5–1 c.cm. of the serum to be used for the treatment is given and an interval of 5–6 hours should then be allowed to elapse before the treatment dose is injected.

    2. An injection of 0·5–1 c.cm. of the serum to be given is injected, and followed by a slightly larger dose every 5 minutes or so afterwards, gradually increasing the doses until the full treatment dose has been injected.

Serum Sickness.—A considerable proportion of persons is affected when a single dose of horse serum is given for the first time. In some cases toxic effects are produced about 10 or 12 days later; the symptoms are fever, an urticarial rash and swelling of the lymph glands and joints.

CHAPTER 6

STERILIZATION OR DESTRUCTION OF BACTERIA

APPLICATION OF HEAT. RADIATION. ELECTRICITY.
STERILIZATION OF LIQUIDS BY FILTRATION. CHEMICAL
AGENTS. DISINFECTANTS AND ANTISEPTICS.

STERILIZATION or killing of bacteria may be accomplished by various methods, including application of heat, radiation, filtration and the use of chemical agents.

Application of Heat.—The following main methods are in use.

Dry heat.—The Bunsen burner or hot air (i.e. dry heat which produces a temperature at or above that of red heat) is used in the laboratory for the sterilization of platinum loops, tips of forceps, needles and knives.

The hot air oven, constructed in copper or iron, is made in the form of a double-walled box heated by a gas flame or electricity, preferably the latter, and can be regulated by means of a thermostat. A temperature of between 160°–180° C. for 1 hour is necessary for complete destruction of bacterial spores. All articles for sterilization, such as test tubes, Petri dishes, glass pipettes and glass syringes must be wrapped in Kraft paper before being placed in the oven; on removal this paper should be charred in appearance, which is a clear indication that the process of sterilization has been thorough. Under no consideration must the oven door be opened until the oven is cool, otherwise the glassware will break.

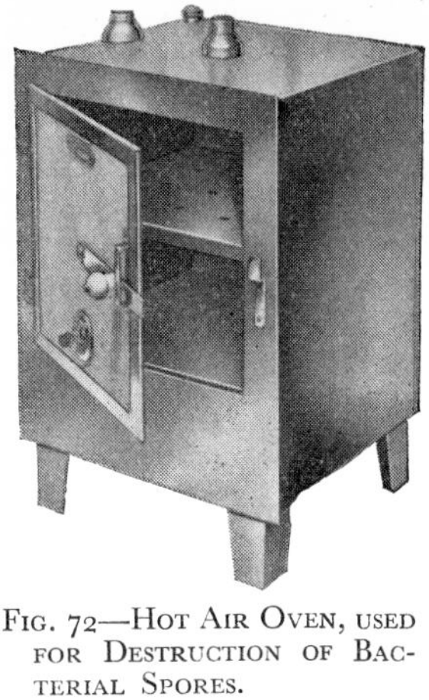

FIG. 72—HOT AIR OVEN, USED FOR DESTRUCTION OF BACTERIAL SPORES.

(*By courtesy of Messrs. Baird & Tatlock Ltd., London.*)

Incineration method.—The method of incineration is used for soiled and infected dressings or articles of clothing which can be destroyed, also for the refuse of the sickroom; nothing is more reliable than a furnace or the ordinary household fire.

Moist heat.—This method includes the application of steam

219

or hot water. A process of boiling in a water bath, universally known as a fish kettle or sterilizer, fitted with a movable tray with a raised rim about 1 in. in depth which prevents any breakable item from falling off, is used for instruments, bowls, syringes and so on.

Moist heat at high temperature.—The autoclave, which consists of a gunmetal cylinder supported by a sheet iron case, is a useful and reliable instrument of sterilization. Its cover is secured by screw clamps and made airtight by an asbestos washer. The cylinder contains water up to a certain level and is heated by a Bunsen gas ring below. Articles such as bouillon, agar, towels, rubber gloves, pathogenic cultures, empty containers and so on can be sterilized by this method.

Koch's steam sterilizer.—This apparatus consists of a metal cylinder supported on legs, and provided with a perforated conical shaped lid, the perforations forming an exit for steam. The sterilizer is surrounded by a jacket of asbestos or felt or some other poor conducting material, and is heated by a Bunsen burner. It is provided with a perforated false bottom which acts as a diaphragm on which the articles to be sterilized may rest, the steam at 100° C. penetrating through this shelf and heating these articles to the required temperature; it is a method very generally used in laboratories.

Sterilization at low temperature.—The sterilization of serum or body fluids is effected by a low temperature (59° C.), the fluid being placed in a water bath or an oven and subjected to repeated exposures. The temperature must be rigidly adhered to, otherwise coagulation will take place. Vaccines may be sterilized in this manner at a temperature of 60° C. for one hour; higher temperatures will diminish their immunizing properties.

Sterilization by hot oil.—This method has been found useful in the sterilization of glass and metal syringes used in the giving of penicillin by the intramuscular method 3 hourly. Oil at a temperature of 120° F. is drawn through the syringe and has been proved to be an efficient method of sterilization in the prevention of the spread of infections, penicillin being so easily destroyed by contact with certain organism.

Radiation.—Sunlight, and to a lesser degree, the electric arc, are very injurious to certain types of bacteria. This action is exerted by the ultra-violet rays, the visible portion of the spectrum not having any effect. Water and milk can be sterilized without any appreciable elevation of temperature by exposure to the rays of a quartz lamp, although fluorescent bacteria are found to be resistant to ultra-violet rays.

Electricity.—The products of electrolysis may destroy bacteria, and currents of high potential may kill bacteria by the heat produced.

Sterilization of Liquids by Filtration.—This process entails the use of filters constructed in unglazed porcelain (the Chamberland type) or in a diatomaceous clay (Berkefield and similar clay filters) the pores of these filters being so fine that ordinary bacteria are prevented from passing through. The Carlson Filter, constructed in the form of an asbestos "disc," is a reliable and inexpensive type of filter, which is fitted into metal holders; after use the disc is destroyed and replaced by a new one for each filtration.

Chemical Agents.—A disinfectant or germicide is a chemical substance which has the power of killing bacteria and their spores. An antiseptic is a chemical substance which inhibits the growth of bacteria, but does not necessarily kill the organisms. A deodorant prevents or absorbs foul smells.

The germicidal properties of a solution depend upon its strength, and a substance which has the power to kill in one strength will only inhibit the activity of the organism when diluted.

Apart from the strength, the antiseptic action also depends upon the temperature at which the substances act, the medium in which they are dissolved and the number and virulence of the organisms present in the substance to which they may be added, thus the properties of these chemical agents may be said to depend upon 1. the strength of the disinfectant used; 2. the length of time to which the organism is exposed to the agent; 3. the temperature of the solution; 4. the substance to be disinfected, whether it be sputum, pus, blood or faeces, all of which are apt to decrease the activities of the agent; further, much depends upon the solubility of the lipoids which form the outside layers of the cell; 5. the resistance of the bacterium, especially if it is a spore forming organism.

Disinfectants and Antiseptics.—Antiseptics most generally used may be considered under the following headings: 1. acids; 2. alkalis; 3. soaps; 4. dyes; 5. coal tar derivatives; 6. solutions of organic salts; 7. oxidizing agents; 8. halogens; 9. alcohol.

Acids.—Acids, because they are capable of destroying living matter, are enlisted under this heading, but have a very limited use on account of their corrosive reaction on tissue.

Sulphuric acid is chiefly used as an antiseptic, disinfectant and parasiticide. Sulphur dioxide in the form of sulphur candles is employed as a gaseous disinfectant for premises in which an infectious disease has occurred. Ample moisture is needed in the atmosphere of the room. A high temperature will assist its action. Sulphur has been used as an ointment to kill the acarus in scabies.

Hydrochloric acid is used medicinally in the treatment of gastric conditions in which there is a deficiency. Normally it is manufactured in the stomach and then it is useful because it kills organisms brought in with the food.

Alkalis.—Caustic potash and caustic soda are both corrosive and destructive to all living matter. Caustic lime may be used in a 20 per cent solution for the disinfection of stools, which must be well broken up in order to allow it to penetrate. Hydration of the lime generates sufficient heat to destroy the typhoid bacillus.

Soaps.—Very few disinfectants are compatible with soap; dioxide of mercury and a few coal tar preparations are exceptions. Apart from removing grease, dirt and pus, soap gets rid of bacteria, many types of organisms being killed by it (meningococci, streptococci, gonococci and pneumococci). Soaps of saturated fatty acids will kill the coli group of organisms, the soap in most general use being a coconut oil soap.

Dyes.—This group of germicides is mainly used in the disinfection of the skin and for the antiseptic treatment of wounds, burns and certain skin diseases e.g. impetigo; it is used also for infections in the mouth, urethra and vagina. A large number of the dyes have a lethal effect but because of the selective nature of their reaction on bacteria they have been classified into two groups: 1. the aniline group; 2. the flavine group.

Those in the aniline group have an inhibitory action on staphylococci and include brilliant green, methyl violet, aniline violet and saffranin. Bonney's blue paint, consisting of a solution of brilliant green and crystal violet in alcohol, is one of the favourite skin disinfectants used in both the obstetrical and gynaecological worlds.

The flavine group has a special inhibitory action on the streptococci, the value of these damp disinfectants being that their efficiency is in no way affected by the presence of blood and that they do not alter the phagocytic function of the leucocytes. Included in this group are acriflavine, proflavine and acridine.

Coal tar products.—Phenol (carbolic acid) occurs in the form of colourless crystals, and is one of the best known among antiseptics. Its chief characteristics are that it is colourless, caustic in action, pungent in odour, has local anaesthetic action and is poisonous. It is an efficient parasiticide against certain vegetable parasites infesting the skin; further it is a reliable disinfectant for infected linen, clothing and so on, the articles being immersed for one hour in a 1 in 40 solution. Phenol is used also for disinfecting all forms of excreta in the nursing of typhoid fever patients, 1 in 20 solution being used for 1 hour. It takes precedence in being the disinfectant used in the Rideal-Walker test, a method adopted in order to determine the efficiency of a germicide as compared with pure phenol; the basis of the test is the amount required to kill the bacillus typhosus in a given time.

Cresol is a coal tar product, usually stored in yellow bottles; it is a better disinfectant than phenol, its action being more rapid in killing bacteria; it is also less caustic. There are many other germicides similar to cresol, e.g. lysol, izal, chinisol, monsol, osyl, cyllin and Jeyes' fluid.

Lysol is a coal tar derivative, a powerful disinfectant when used in its pure state; it is a mixture of tar oil and soap, thus when mixed with water it forms a soapy solution. It is used in its full strength for sterilizing needles and scalpels and other instruments. As an antiseptic it is used for douching or irrigation in a strength of 1–2 per cent solution.

Izal is a coal tar derivative similar in respect of properties to lysol.

Cyllin is a dark liquid coal tar derivative, strongly antiseptic and forming a white emulsion with water; it is purified creolin. It is, like all other coal tar derivatives, more bactericidal in action than phenol, also less toxic and less irritating to the skin.

Trinitrophenol or picric acid is obtained by the action of nitric acid on phenol, and was, at one time, universally used in the treatment of burns and as a skin preparation.

Solutions of metallic salts.—Metallic salts have a coagulating action on protein substances, the most commonly known being silver nitrate, copper sulphate, zinc sulphate, perchloride of mercury and biniodide of mercury.

Silver nitrate is used either in solution or in the solid pencil form as first aid treatment in dog bites as a preventive against rabies. It is also employed as a prophylactic against gonococcal infections of the eye in the new-born infant (in the form of eyedrops).

Zinc sulphate is used in the form of antiseptic eyedrops.

Perchloride of mercury or corrosive sublimate is used in the form of a clear solution which is usually tinted with aniline blue, in order to save confusion with other solutions. It is a powerful poison, coagulating albumin rapidly and corroding metals. In hospitals it is used in varied strengths of 1 in 500 to 1 in 12,000 according to the purpose for which it is required. In a strength of 1 in 1,000 it will kill bacteria in half an hour; a solution double this strength will kill spores in half an hour.

Biniodide of mercury or mercuric iodide is a less powerful germicide than perchloride; it does not have any effect on albumin and does not stain fabrics; it is corrosive to metals; it can be used for the same purposes as perchloride of mercury.

Oxidizing agents.—Hydrogen peroxide is an important disinfectant, because of its property of being an oxidizing agent i.e.

it is able to liberate oxygen in the presence of organic matter. It is very useful for the cleansing of infected wounds, as a mouth wash and in the treatment of discharging ears. Free oxygen is liberated in the form of bubbles and mechanically cleans up the area.

Permanganate of potash, with its well known bluish-purple crystals, is a mild caustic when dry. Its most important action is that when moist it readily gives up its oxygen in the presence of organic matter, and its solutions therefore quickly turn into a dark brown colour; its germicidal action is limited because it so easily gives up its oxygen to organic substances in which bacteria flourish, and very soon it becomes inert.

Halogens.—The word, halogen, means " salt producing " (Greek); compounds of chlorine, bromine and iodine make up the greater part of ordinary sea water. Chlorine is a greenish gas with an irritating odour, used in World War I because of its destructive action on the lungs. This gas has a powerful disinfecting action, but only compounds are used, which readily give up their chlorine.

Bleaching powder or chlorinated lime gives off chlorine at ordinary temperatures and is used in the purification of water supplies.

Eusol (Edinburgh University solution), a solution of calcium chloride, calcium borate and hypochlorous acid compounds, is used in surgical dressings and irrigations. Dakin's solution— consisting of chlorinated soda (sodium chloride and sodium hypochlorite) with sodium bicarbonate—was extensively used during World War I for continuous irrigation of infected wounds.

A solution of electrolytic hypochlorite is extensively used in the treatment of burns and lacerated wounds, in conjunction with Bunyan's bag, which is made in a coated silk fabric in the form of an envelope, its value being the prevention of cross infection.

Iodine, used as a 2 per cent solution in potassium iodide solution or as an alcoholic tincture, is a disinfectant of the first order for the treatment of wounds and for disinfection of the skin previous to operation. It is used in the sterilization of catgut.

Iodoform, an organic compound, yellow in colour and of strong odour, was formerly used as an antiseptic. When in contact with organic matter, it is decomposed and free iodine is liberated, and it is this free iodine which attacks the organism. In the form of a paste known as B.I.P.P., which contains iodoform, bismuth oxynitrate and liquid paraffin, it is sometimes used for packing wounds.

Dettol—a universally popular disinfectant—is a halogen derivative of xylenol prepared by chemical interaction with a coal tar derivative, the halogen content being dissolved in essential oils with soap solution. It is non-irritant and non-toxic, and destructive to streptococci.

Alcohols.—Alcohol is of value as an antiseptic because of its soluble action on fats, and for this reason is used for the purpose of disinfecting the skin before operation, also for cleansing an area of skin before hypodermic injections are given. It is useful in preparing the skin of children because it seldom produces any skin reaction. It also absorbs water from the skin and precipitates albuminous material and so hardens it.

Ether has much the same effect on the skin as alcohol from a cleansing point of view; it has a soluble action on fats.

CHAPTER 7

COLLECTION OF SPECIMENS FOR LABORATORY EXAMINATION

GENERAL RULES. SPECIMENS OF BLOOD. PUS. SPUTUM.
URINE. FAECES. CEREBROSPINAL FLUID. SWABS.
TISSUE.

A KNOWLEDGE of the correct method of collecting specimens is an essential item in the training of every student nurse and one in which she should be carefully instructed so that she may take an intelligent interest in clinical pathology, an important branch of her work.

General Rules.—The essentials, which are of the utmost importance in the preparation of laboratory specimens, and which should have careful consideration, are as follows.

1. To send the correct amount for investigation;
2. To prevent deterioration or contamination of the specimen;
3. To see that the container is scrupulously clean;
4. To cover the specimen immediately after it is placed in the container;
5. To use a sterile container when the specimen is to be examined for bacteria;
6. To avoid contamination of the outside of the container;
7. To see that the specimen is correctly labelled, and that the label is securely attached;
8. To avoid delay in sending the specimen to the laboratory.

Specimens of Blood.—If a large quantity of blood be required, it will be obtained by the intravenous method, and it will be immediately transferred into a culture medium. Special precautions must be observed in order to prevent contamination. The blood can be placed in a sodium citrate " biochemical bottle" which contains the necessary coagulant.

Apparatus.—The apparatus and utensils required are as follows. A sterile all glass syringe of 5 ccm. or 10 ccm. capacity; forceps for handling the different parts of the apparatus; antiseptic solution and swabs for cleansing the skin (iodine or spirit);

tourniquet, rubber band or sphygmomanometer; spirit lamp; sterile test tubes; culture tubes.

Method.—The skin is sterilized with the antiseptic. The rubber band is then applied and the patient is instructed to extend his arm and clench his fist ; when the vein is fully dilated the needle is inserted and the required amount of blood taken. A small amount may be collected either by means of a Wright's capsule or a graduated pipette or on to a glass slide.

Pus.—Films are made on a slide from the pus, dried and fixed by heat; when possible, these are made directly from the lesion, with a sterile platinum loop or sterile capillary tube. The specimen should then be sent to the laboratory in a suitable sterile container. The capillary tube is generally used for the collection of minute quantities and the ends of the tube are sealed in a flame.

Sputum.—When collecting a specimen of sputum, it is advisable to obtain it first thing in the morning before the patient has had any food. It may be collected in a bottle of 2 oz. capacity, in a universal container or specimen tube or a screw capped carton of 2 oz. capacity when the specimen is not being sent away by post. The carton is satisfactory because it has a wide mouth which prevents the fouling of the outside. The specimen should consist of sputum and not saliva.

Urine.—For small quantities of urine e.g. a specimen from a patient with typhoid fever or cystitis, a glass tube with a rubber bung or a universal container can be used. For catheter specimens a sterile wide-mouthed screw capped " bottle " known as a " honey-pot " should be used, which is less likely to be contaminated in the process of catheterization; the distal end of the catheter can be placed in the bottle and the urine withdrawn directly. When possible, catheterization should be avoided; this can be so if an ordinary specimen from a female patient is sent to the laboratory for a preliminary test. If, on testing, no pus cells or bacteria are found, this report should be sufficiently confirmatory, but if presence of pus cells or bacteria is reported, then a catheter specimen should be sent to the laboratory.

Faeces.—Small squat bottles of 2 oz. capacity or a specimen tube 2″ × 1″ fitted with a bark cork, to which is fitted a metal spoon, are generally used, the disadvantage attached to these being that the cork may be blown out in the case of fermentation and cause leakage of the contents with possible contamination, apart from being a source of infection. In the case of small specimens of faeces the " universal container " is safe and suitable because of its screw-on cap. It is provided with a spoon made in tin, with one end bent in a small U-shaped position. The spoons are usually wrapped in Kraft paper and sterilized.

When the specimen is being taken, the spoon is unwrapped and a portion of the faeces is taken with the U-end of the spoon. This is placed in the container and the cap screwed.

Another alternative container which can be used is the capped " pomade pot," with which small cardboard " ice cream " spoons are used. Every care should be used to avoid contamination of the outside of the container, and after the specimen has been collected the hands should be thoroughly washed and disinfected. Rubber gloves should be worn while dealing with a specimen of faeces of a patient with typhoid fever, paratyphoid fever, cholera or dysentery.

So far as the collection of a specimen of faeces from a case of suspected dysentery is concerned, the specimen for examination should be sent to the laboratory as soon as possible after being passed; it should not be mixed with urine. It is collected in a faeces specimen tube which is provided with a cork to which is attached a metal scoop or spoon, which fits into the tube and which is used for the collection of the faecal matter.

Cerebrospinal Fluid.—For the collection of a specimen of cerebrospinal fluid, a strong glass tube $5'' \times \frac{3}{8}''$, with rubber bungs, is provided. The glass tube should be sterilized in the hot air oven; the rubber bungs are boiled for 5 minutes, picked out of the sterilizer with forceps, flamed and inserted into the sterile test tube. The screw-capped universal container is a safe and reliable receptacle for this purpose, due to the fact that the screw cap ensures that the mouth of the container is sterile.

Cerebrospinal fluid for examination is obtained by lumbar puncture, a special long needle being used for this purpose. The puncture is made in the middle line of the back between the 3rd and 4th lumbar vertebrae. The first few drops which flow after the insertion of the needle are almost invariably contaminated with blood which has come from the pierced tissues, and should be discarded. Two test tubes are used, numbered 1 and 2 respectively. Cultures of cerebrospinal fluid should be made for preference at the bedside, or at least within half an hour of taking the specimen, owing to the fact that many of the organisms found in cerebrospinal fluid are of great delicacy.

Swabs.—A swab consists of a thin stick of aluminium or tinned iron wire about 6 inches long; one end is made rough for about $\frac{1}{2}$-inch, a pledget of absorbent cotton wool is tightly wrapped round the rough end and the wire is placed in a test tube of specially hardened glass which is then plugged with cotton wool. If the swabs are to be sent away by post, the cotton wool plug must be replaced by a bark cork. The tube is sterilized in an autoclave.

These swabs are used for taking specimens from certain areas mentioned below:

1. The throat in suspected diphtheria, tonsillitis and pulmonary tuberculosis;

2. Wounds or surgical conditions e.g. a sinus or an abscess which is showing signs of virulent pyogenic infection;

3. Post-nasal or nasopharyngeal space; the wire is bent to an angle which allows it to be conveniently introduced behind the soft palate—used for suspected carriers and for early diagnosis of whooping cough;

4. Rectum; rectal swabs are often taken in the investigation of dysentery, especially in children;

5. Cervix uteri; the swabs are prepared on thin wooden sticks $6\frac{1}{2}$ inches long, which are specially made for this purpose and are known as " Peerless " wooden applicators; a cotton wool pledget is tightly wrapped round one end and the tube is plugged with cotton wool; the swab is used for obtaining specimens of gonococcal and puerperal infections.

Tissue.—Small specimens of tissue can be put into a universal container for laboratory examination, either dry or in a little saline; the specimen should be sent for examination without delay in order to prevent putrefaction.

CLINICAL AND LABORATORY TESTS IN COMMON USE IN THE INVESTIGATION OF CERTAIN DISEASES

WASSERMANN TEST. LUTEIN TEST. SIGMA REACTION. SCHICK REACTION. DICK TEST. SCHULTZ-CHARLTON REACTION. MANTOUX TEST. VON PIRQUET'S REACTION. WIDAL REACTION. BLOOD CULTURE.

It is advisable that the nurse should know not only how to collect and deliver the specimen from the patient to the laboratory, but that she should be at least acquainted with the routine of examination. The main tests in common use are discussed below.

Wassermann Test.—This is used in the diagnosis of syphilis; it is based on immunity reactions and is generally considered to be a reliable method, although even when the reaction is negative it does not mean that the patient is free from syphilis. Despite all the mysteries associated with it, it is without doubt an almost indispensable controlling index in active disease. The blood or cerebrospinal fluid may both be tested by this method.

Lutein Test.—Another test for syphilis is the lutein test, in which an extract of spirochaetes is used. Skin reactions are found in 2–10 days after local injection.

Sigma Reaction.—A third test for syphilis, the Sigma reaction, is rather similar to the Wassermann test and is said to be more simple but quite as reliable.

Schick Reaction.—This test consists of an intradermal injection of 0·2 ccm. of standardized Schick toxin, given on the flexor surface of the forearm; a control injection of toxin which has been heated at 75° C. for 5 minutes is given on the other arm. If the subject be insusceptible to diphtheria infection, the small swelling which occurs at the time of injection is quickly absorbed and no signs of inflammation are visible. A positive reaction shows a red papule, hard and painful, in 24 hours, reaching a diameter of about an inch in 2–3 days. When this reaction fades at the end of a week, it leaves a brownish stain with desquamation of the skin, which can be seen for several weeks afterwards. Many more Schick positives are found among country people.

than in those living in towns, owing to the fact that the latter gain a certain immunity by contact with the diphtheria bacillus which is more prevalent in crowded areas.

Dick Test.—The Dick test is used with reference to scarlet fever and certain other diseases in which the haemolytic strepto-coccus may be active. It is a susceptibility test, and is given intradermally. If the person tested be susceptible, a bright red flush appears at the site of inoculation in 6–12 hours, reaching its peak in 24 hours and then rapidly disappearing.

Schultz-Charlton Reaction.—This is employed clinically in the diagnosis of scarlet fever when there are doubtful signs, generally in fever hospitals. Serum from a convalescent scarlet fever patient's blood (0·2 ccm. of a 1 in 10 dilution) is injected intradermally in an early stage of the disease, which causes blanching at the area of inoculation or extinction of the rash at the site, showing that the rash is a scarlet fever one and not a drug rash or an urticarial reaction.

Mantoux Test.—An intradermal injection of 0·1 ccm. of a 1 in 1,000 dilution of old tuberculin is given to test for the presence of tuberculosis in children showing symptoms of pyrexia and malaise of doubtful origin; a red area about 1 cm. in diameter, appearing in 48–96 hours after the injection, shows positive re-action.

Von Pirquet's Reaction.—In this test, an application of tuberculin to a scarified surface is used. The appearance of a bright red papule in 24–48 hours denotes a positive reaction; it is principally of use in detecting tuberculosis in its early stages in children.

Widal Reaction.—This test depends on the fact that the blood serum from a patient with typhoid fever will agglutinate an emulsion in broth of typhoid bacillus; it is not usually positive until from the 7th to the 10th day. To carry out the test, blood is collected from a puncture in the skin by a small pipette, in which it is allowed to coagulate; the serum is then diluted to a variety of different strengths—dilutions of 1 in 20, 1 in 50 and 1 in 100. Equal parts of these and an emulsion of the germs are then mixed together and the result watched under the micro-scope in a hang-drop preparation or in a small glass tube sealed at one end and set vertically. If the test is positive, agglutina-tion should take place in from half an hour to an hour. A control experiment with healthy serum must be made at the same time. A negative result does not exclude typhoid fever. The sera of persons who have been inoculated against the disease will con-tain agglutinins, and so give a positive reaction to the test.

Blood Culture.—This method, now so frequently used as an aid to diagnosis, is particularly indispensable in the investigation of diseases such as typhoid fever, paratyphoid fever, endocarditis, septicaemia and spirochaetal infections.

The blood required for examination is usually withdrawn from the patient's median basilic vein.   Throughout this procedure rigid asepsis must be observed, otherwise a misleading result may be obtained with the culture.   About 2 c.cm. of blood is collected with a sterile record syringe; this is then transferred to a test tube containing 50 c.cm. of sterile glucose broth, which is then incubated at 37° C. and subjected to daily examination for growth.   If no apparent growth be present at the end of a week, a subculture is then attempted on a solid medium and if it, in turn, should show no growth, the blood is then said to be sterile. If a growth be suspected in the tube before this, a subculture should be made immediately, a positive result being obtained on the 2nd day and the subculture identified on the 3rd day.   Several tubes should be inoculated with varying amounts of blood—1 c.cm., 2 c.cm. and 5 c.cm., until the positive culture is obtained.

THEORY AND PRACTICE OF NURSING (PART I)

CHAPTER 1

THE ETHICS OF NURSING

THE EVOLUTION OF NURSING. EARLY HISTORY. THE
MIDDLE AGES. THE SISTERS OF CHARITY. NURSING IN
THE NINETEENTH CENTURY. THE VICTORIAN ERA IN
NURSING. FLORENCE NIGHTINGALE. MODERN DAYS.
NURSES' REGISTRATION ACTS. THE ETHICAL ASPECTS OF
MODERN NURSING. THE NURSE HERSELF. HOSPITAL
ETIQUETTE. THE NURSE AND HER SUPERIORS.

By ethics we mean a system of rules for regulating the actions of
human beings, a code which includes the doctrines of morality.
In all professions there are certain privileges attached to the
status of the members, and as a result of this more is expected of
them from the ethical point of view. They are, so to speak, the
models of conduct from which others make their copy. In
the medical profession, of which nursing is an integral part, the
etiquette is notoriously rigid and rightly so, since the life of
the doctor and of the nurse is bound up with the confidences, the
intimacies and the private matters of their patients. From the
first day of her training, a nurse is impressed with the necessity
of a very high standard of professional conduct, and while she
may be rather bewildered at the beginning at what she may
think is so much " red tape " and ceremony, nevertheless there
is a meaning for everything; tradition is something which
cannot be gainsaid. In the following pages a few of the main
principles of the nursing profession are dealt with in order that
the nurse may readily understand the why and the wherefore of
the regulations with which she has to conform.

The Evolution of Nursing

The female brain is smaller than that of the male, the hand is
less in size, and generally speaking the physical power is much
weaker, yet from time immemorial the mind, the touch and the
energy of a woman have been associated with the care of the sick.

In certain circumstances a male nurse may be required, but in the normal incidence of sickness as it concerns man, woman and child, it is the female nurse, with the endowments peculiar to her sex, who is called in.

Early History.—Before the birth of Christ there is no record of an organized service of nurses, but in the first century the strong religious atmosphere of the age was reflected in the creation of the Deaconesses, associated with the name of St. Paul. These women, no doubt imbued with the lately demonstrated principles of Christianity, were of strongly religious persuasion, and they naturally turned their minds to the healing of the sick. From that time the church has been more or less closely associated with the care of the sick.   After A.D. 500, the Deaconesses ceased to undertake their visitations as a group of individuals and the Church evidently assumed responsibility for the work.   This was natural, for there were no hospitals as we know them nowadays.   The sick poor sought the nearest abbey or hospice, where they were dealt with kindly and attended by men or women inspired with a strong religious fervour, who thus adopted the profession of doctor or nurse as a matter of course.   In Europe this system was in general operation, as records prove.   The religious aspect of healing became so prominent that ultimately those who were associated with it were superseded by monks and nuns only, or those who had taken strong religious vows.   The first record of qualification of the nursing profession therefore is entirely connected with the Church.

The Middle Ages.—The chief movements of the years 1100 to 1500 were military in character, and such Orders as those of the Templars, the Teutonic Knights, the Béguines and the Hospitallers of St. John of Jerusalem were established to deal with the casualties of both armies engaged in the Crusades.   In England, most interest is taken in the last Order which still flourishes today.   Despite many vicissitudes it succeeded in carrying on its good work to great advantage until it was suppressed, like many other similar institutions, in the sixteenth century.   It was revived later on.   The Béguines are interesting to women, because, started in the twelfth century, their Order was almost entirely a female organization and distinct from the Church, and not only did they found their own hospitals and outpatient departments, but they also accompanied the armies to war, continuing to do so until the present time.   The Béguines have been the inspiration of many other countries, including Great Britain.

The Sisters of Charity.—In 1633 arose the greatest nursing association in the world—the Sisters of Charity of the Order of St. Vincent de Paul.   In the early part of the seventeenth century, it was found that in Europe the organizations associated with the Crusades had broken down. Some new stimulus was wanted, and St. Vincent de Paul, who had formed an association of charity in the country districts, founded along with Mlle. Le Gras a new body to take over the neglected work of the Hôtel-Dieu in Paris. The members were ladies, who although possessed of strong religious motives nevertheless refused to take the veil, and while many were rich and gave their time and possessions to assist the sick, they were hampered by the dictums of the Church, which gradually reduced the Order to inactivity on the practical side, despite its brilliance on the battlefield and elsewhere. The motives were still kept in view, however, and the Order has a great influence in the world today. What it might have done if the Church had not put religious exercise before hygienic knowledge it is very difficult to say. In England, Henry the Eighth, about 100 years before, had brought about chaos by closing the monasteries with their attached infirmaries; these were replaced by hospitals staffed by ignorant and low-bred women : the most retrograde era in British nursing. The effect of this was experienced for about 200 years, and the history of nursing in the seventeenth and eighteenth centuries is a very sorry tale with nothing of a progressive nature to commend it. Plagues and pestilences swept Europe and there was not a representative medical profession to deal with them. It is probable that the Great Fire of London, destroying as it did the cause and source of so much pestilence and disease, was more curative than many physicians' medicine had ever been.

Nursing in the Nineteenth Century.—A new era begins with the visit to England in 1822 of a German pastor named Fliedner. Having consulted with Elizabeth Fry and John Howard about prison reform, he went back to his home at Kaiserswerth, near Düsseldorf, and with his wife established a hostel for discharged female prisoners. Out of this grew an Order providing for the sick of the district. This association had well planned schemes of training for its nurses, who were religiously minded, but who were independent of any religious institutions or political support. It quickly formed branches and subdivisions, dealing with the poor, children and relief to discharged prisoners, and undertaking private and public services of nursing. There was a contract for 5 years to bind the nurse, but otherwise she was possessed of far greater freedom than ever before. For the first time, there was a division of the members into probationers, nurses and sisters. In many ways the organization of the Kaiserswerth Deaconesses was the basis of our present day systems of training and administration. There was a lack of uniformity of education however, and the remuneration was not always assured for the services performed. The Order fell on evil days for some time, but in several countries the Deaconess House is still in vogue, although its system of training is not the same as that of the modern hospital.

The Victorian Era in Nursing.—The reign of Queen Victoria is intimately associated with great advances in the science or healing. The names of Pasteur and Lister are outstanding in the scientific evolution of the profession of medicine, while Florence Nightingale will ever be the ideal to which all good nurses aspire. The imagination is easily stirred by reading the history of medicine at the beginning of the nineteenth century. The healing art was apparently in the doldrums. There was no sign of organization anywhere, and if all reports are true the unlucky invalids were in the hands of inebriate and licentious women. The conditions under which these women worked did not make matters any better for them. Their housing was wretched, their food poor and all their moral standards low—an ample reflection of the attitude of the people towards them. The stigma put on the profession remained for many a long year afterwards, and it says much for the nurses of today when we reflect on the efficiency of the modern service. In the early part of the Queen's reign, the records of three great hospitals show that the sisters were expected to be " from a respectable rank of life," but apparently respectability did not extend to those under them, who were clearly of lower class than the average domestic servant of the time. It was evidently very difficult to get the right type of woman. It is well to hold these unfortunate pioneers of nursing in charitable regard ; they were creatures of circumstance and they deserve a certain measure of praise for the work they did, or tried to do.

Early Nursing Associations.—Elizabeth Fry, the pioneer of prison reform, was also instrumental in founding the English Protestant Sisters of Charity. She was stimulated by what she had seen on the Continent, and secured the patronage of the Church, although she was a Quakeress. This institution, founded in 1840 and still in existence, marked the initiation of district nursing on an organized basis. For ten years after this, rapid developments took place. There were founded in succession the Park Village Community, the Sisters of Mercy, which later joined forces, and St. John's House, London. The last was established in St. Pancras and was closely allied with the Church of England. It was the first attempt to form a real training school, as the nurses attended King's College Hospital in London as pupils. It is now a private nursing association, affiliated with St. Thomas's Hospital. Another centre of activity was in Dublin, where the Catholic Sisters of Mercy had been established. Their work consisted in looking after the sick poor and of district nursing, and they assisted Florence Nightingale in the Crimean

War. In London they now have 2 hospitals fully approved for general nursing courses.

Florence Nightingale.—The greatest handicap to nursing progress was self imposed—the profession would not cast off the shackles of religion, thus advance was constantly prevented by restrictions which survived after centuries of proved error. It needed a crisis to waken the world up. That crisis came in 1854. When Florence Nightingale, who had been trained at Kaiserswerth, was sent to put order into the chaos of the nursing services of the Crimean War, she went through experiences which resulted in a complete revolution in the nursing profession and the beginning of a great modern scientific era. Than Florence Nightingale, a better choice could not have been made. Refined, cultured, imaginative, experienced, courageous, understanding and practical, she had full scope for employing all her gifts, and she seized the opportunity. After the war the public was quick to adopt her ideas. Training schools were attached to great hospitals, conditions of nursing were improved, a better class of woman was recruited. The profession of nurse grew to be the very opposite of what it had been 20 years previously. Many of the principles of Florence Nightingale remain unaltered today. She insisted on sobriety, honesty and truthfulness, cleanliness, quietness and punctuality, efficiency in the hygiene, cooking and routine of hospital life. By 1880, every large centre with a hospital had its nursing school, and was working on the principles enumerated by Miss Nightingale. In 1887 came the first movements towards State recognition and registration.

Modern Days.—With two wars, the biggest in history, to increase the need for nurses, the period from 1901 up to the present day is full of records of progress. In 1893 the Royal British Nurses' Association had been formed, and in 1899 the International Council of Nurses was established with branches all over the world. Its members now number over 200,000. After the South African War (1899–1901), the various Royal Nursing Services were founded. During World War I, in 1916, the College of Nursing was started on the suggestion of Dame Sarah Swift and the late Sir Arthur Stanley, the idea being to enrol fully qualified nurses with general training, and to agitate keenly for State registration.

In 1926 the British College of Nurses was founded, and it now has a large membership also. It keeps in touch with the trained nurse after she leaves her training school, and is interested in all the social and educative needs of the profession.

Nurses' Registration Acts.—After many years of agitation official status was secured for the nurse in 1919. By the Acts, a General Nursing Council was established in England and Wales, in Scotland and in Ireland, its function being to keep a General and Supplementary Register of Nurses. There is a majority of nurses on the Council, which in every way must be regarded as the governing body of the profession. Undoubtedly the education has been improved by its establishment, and there is much more to be done in this direction. Changes are constantly taking place in the syllabus of each course, and this is to be expected if progress is to go on rapidly. A Commission set up under the auspices of *The Lancet* began its sittings in December 1930 and issued its final report in 1932. The whole nursing profession was, so to speak, put through a fine sieve by this select and most representative committee, presided over by the Earl of Crawford and Balcarres. Many of its recommendations have already been adopted by the hospitals and training bodies, and by the General Nursing Council.

It is obvious that the nurse of the future will find her life absolutely different from that of the woman who trained in the late nineteenth century, while she cannot be compared with the Sarah Gamps and Betsey Prigs of the pre-Nightingale days. Increasing changes occur as each year passes. World War II was the means of stimulation of active thought in medical and nursing research. The result has been a multitude of reforms and fresh principles, greater specialization, higher standards and better conditions of life, work and remuneration for the nurse.

The Ethical Aspects of Modern Nursing

The doctrines of Florence Nightingale still hold good today, therefore the moral code for nurses needs little or no revision, but it is a perfect woman who possesses all the qualities demanded by the Nightingale standard. This stipulates the following attributes essential to the ideal nurse : truthfulness ; obedience ; punctuality ; observation ; sobriety ; honesty ; quietness ; devotion ; tact ; loyalty ; sympathy ; humility.

In addition to these moral qualities, however, there is the matter of physical efficiency. It is useless to attempt to preach the gospel of hygiene unless the preacher herself is in good health, and it is one of the main duties of a nurse to ensure that she maintains her fitness by making her leisure time so many hours of real recreation. The type of woman in demand today is not the drudge who has chosen the nursing profession as a last resort, nor is there any need for the surplus woman who feels she might like nursing as a hobby. It is a hard profession, demanding a good education, the exercise of common sense, the possession of a good pair of hands and the use of a level head. Imagination, understanding and adjustment to the mind of the patient will do more good than being theoretically perfect in the sciences which must be learned also.

Politeness and good manners are always attractive and in no place is it more necessary to have gentleness than in a hospital. Tact and persuasion have a place in dealing with contemporaries and fellow workers as well as with patients.

The Nurse Herself.—On duty a nurse has a task that is admittedly difficult. Not only has she to be a social companion, but she must also do her professional work which may or may not be irksome to the invalid. Sometimes it may be difficult to keep the smiling face in the midst of worry, but in no circumstance should the nurse display her emotions to the patient. It is occasionally the good actress who succeeds most in restoring her patient to health. The value of charm is inexpressible in words ; it is the epitome of the born nurse ; it succeeds in completely dispelling the atmosphere of the sickroom. The less disease and all connected with it are mentioned in the patient's presence the better for health. We have already appreciated the necessity cf recreation for the nurse. If she is to meet her patient, when she comes on duty, with a cheerful countenance and a smile which radiates wellbeing and confidence, she must make sure that her mind and body are periodically relaxed by amusements, games, healthy reading and discussion of current affairs. She must realize that she is the medium through which her patient acts, and her reactions are invariably the subject of scrutiny, therefore she can only use her power by having an abundant reserve of positive characteristics. Another very important point is the regular taking of off-duty time. The public is better educated now, but at one time objection was raised to the amount of leisure taken by the nurse ; in the emergency of illness in the household, people were apt to forget that a nurse has working hours like any other person and can work only for a certain spell. It is universally agreed by all nowadays that unless a nurse gets right away from the atmosphere of her patient, she cannot cultivate friendships, have hobbies or indeed have any social life and she will therefore have a very limited outlook and knowledge. The benefits of a few hours of life with her own friends may make all the difference to her. Her own meals are as important as her patient's feeds. She should be able to have them regularly and to take a reasonable time over them. Her sleeping hours should be regular to avoid over fatigue. Her leisure will be spent according to her temperament and her inclinations, but some outside interest should be considered and some leisure time spent in the open air each day.

With regard to the management of her patient, a nurse must remember that nothing else matters but him ; every action should therefore be prompted by a preliminary consideration of what is for the best.   Approach to the patient must always be professional, but the nurse must make her patients feel that they are her chief concern.   If she is thoughtful for them, they will not make constant demands on her and they will have confidence in her. She will need to confide in her patient, as she will require to have his confidence ; thus there will be no mystery about his treatment or high handed action on her part.   It is a good plan to treat sick persons as one might a child and explain as much to them as they are able to understand, and then there should be mutual co-operation.   The mind of a sick person is not the same as in health and a firm kind hand is needed to keep the initiative, and so the confidence of the patient.   Familiarity is not kindly or helpful ; it may lead to many difficulties, therefore a strictly professional attitude must be maintained.   No terms of endearment or familiarity must ever be used on either side.

Of great ethical importance is the question of professional secrecy ; this applies especially to private nursing, which after all is the work of the majority of nurses when they leave hospital. On no account should the circumstances of one patient be discussed with another, or with relatives of the latter.   What the nurse sees, hears or does should be kept to herself.   It is very difficult for a nurse to forbear from referring now and then to patients or houses with which she has had a professional association, but it is not diplomatic to criticize or discuss what went on during her privileged stay.   In this matter, as in others, the handling of the relatives of the patient is a great art.   Private nurses are expected to enter into the routine of a household, and to make themselves more or less at home, but this does not mean that they are to take part in the spread of gossip and scandal.   A good nurse can soon let it be known that she does not encourage the probing of her confidences, and she will soon establish herself in her proper perspective with the members of the family, who will respect her all the more because of her high ideals.   Tact is essential at all times ; the nurse must keep in mind that the relatives of a dangerously ill patient are over wrought mentally and say and do things that they normally would repress.   Unfortunately she finds that much of the oiled machinery of the hospital is lacking in a household and success depends upon her capacity of accommodation to the prevailing conditions.   She may have to look after her own room, to do odd shopping, to give advice about personal matters and to reassure constantly visitors and friends who ask about the patient.   But all these subsidiary jobs are simply the amplification of the code formulated by Florence Nightingale, and the more a nurse fits in with the situation as she finds it the nearer will she approach the high standard set by the pioneer of her profession.

Hospital Etiquette

Every hospital has its own code of rules and every institution has its traditions, so that the individual stamp is put on every one of its graduates. Over and above this, however, there is a general standard of etiquette in hospitals which governs the conduct of those serving in them. Hospital etiquette is the basis of professional manners and is rigidly insisted on because of the need for strictness in dealing with matters of such vital importance to the public.

The Nurse and Her Superiors.—The essence of discipline is obedience. The raw recruit trusts in the established routine of a long existing institution, and therefore does not reason with herself. Admittedly there is a certain sinking of personality to begin with, but once the fundamentals of etiquette are mastered, there is ample scope to use the individual expression to the full. The medical superintendent and the medical officers should be regarded with the respect due to their learning, skill and position. The nurse has to see that the advice of the doctor is taken full advantage of by the patient ; on her report the doctor makes up his mind as to the progress of the case. No matter what the nurse's own views may be, she must not express them to the patient. Her duty is to ensure that confidence of the sick person in his medical attendant is complete, and it is against all the canons of etiquette that she should by the slightest hint or action rouse feelings of doubt. There is no reason to assume that, because the nurse does not feel that the treatment is correct, she should air her views ; sometimes indeed there is evidence to prove that she is wrong in her way of thinking. Whatever the reaction, there must be no jeopardizing of the patient's recovery. Now and then, especially in private practice, a crisis or a situation arises in which the nurse may have to take some action on her own responsibility. The doctor is always very grateful for help and is usually the first to commend the nurse for taking the law into her own hands during an emergency, but when possible, it is best to communicate with the doctor first.

The matron, sisters and senior nurses all have their privileges, and the gestures due to them should be made ungrudgingly. In the ward, the nurse has to mix with patients, other nurses, maids, porters and students, and her conduct should be such that she is above reproach. The policy of working while at work and playing while at play is to be recommended. Slovenly habits and unpunctuality will inevitably lead to censure or to failure to become efficient. If there is a good team spirit in the ward, the capable nurse will take her place and keep it, imbued with the ideals of the captain of the team. The work to be accomplished can be done thoroughly only if each member does her share efficiently and unselfishly ; a helping hand lent today may be rewarded tenfold tomorrow. In all great hospitals the influence of the administrative staff is in evidence everywhere, but more especially does the individuality of the ward sister show itself, and the teaching of a skilful head is always reflected in the work of the whole ward staff, down to the rawest wardmaid. Under such influence, an honest and energetic woman could not fail to succeed in making herself proficient and it must be impressed upon nurses that there is great benefit in being attached to hospitals with a big reputation to uphold.

The little gestures of hospital life stand a woman in good stead afterwards. "Where were you trained ?" the specialist often asks when he finds his advice satisfactorily interpreted by the nurse. Let every nurse be proud to own her hospital. Let her show in her every action that she has been taught the ethics of the profession. Much has been said about the unwritten law, tradition, instinctive actions and the honour of an establishment. When a nurse has fully appreciated what these mean, she will have learned far more than has ever been written about etiquette in books.

CHAPTER 2

DOMESTIC WARD MANAGEMENT

METHODS OF CLEANING. THE DAILY ROUTINE. WORK
IN THE WARD ANNEXES. CARE OF BEDDING, LINEN,
BLANKETS AND WATERPROOFS. SANITARY METHODS OF
CLEANING UTENSILS, CROCKERY. CARE OF THE KITCHEN.
DISPOSAL AND DISINFECTION OF SOILED LINEN AND
DRESSINGS. THE DAILY DUTIES.

EVERY hospital has its own architectural peculiarities, and the
well equipped ward of today may be obsolete tomorrow. Generally speaking, however, the ward in most hospitals, apart from
feeding and some special services, is a complete and self contained
unit, with commonly 20 beds in the main apartment or ward
proper. There are conveniently situated service rooms, including ward kitchen (where special cooking can be done),
linen room, stores room, doctors' room, lavatories and bathrooms, with special apparatus for the disposal of excretions, and
one or two private rooms for special cases. The general methods
of cleaning, ventilating, heating and lighting are dealt with in
the section on Hygiene (pp. 13–26 and 107–123).

Methods of Cleaning.—Not so very long ago, the work of the
average probationer was partly that of a housemaid and partly that
of performing the most menial nursing tasks in the ward. The
beginner of today finds that things have been altered a lot within
recent years. The cleaning of the ward itself is left to the wardmaid, while the nurse has more to do with the personal cleanliness and the hygiene of the occupants. Routine is established
by the sister, who is responsible for the administration of the
ward. If her orders are faithfully carried out the ward should
run without a hitch. Neatness should be one of the main
attributes of a ward, with a place for everything and everything
in its place. The contents of a ward vary according to the government of the hospital, but fundamental articles of furniture are
beds, wire mattresses, bedside tables, chairs, ward tables, sister's
desk and various sundry utensils. The bedding, utensils for
feeding and the other things in use every day usually belong to
the siderooms, and are dealt with later.

A ward is the place where one or many patients live ; they

sleep and eat and are there all day. All their toilet is attended to there and often they have wounds which have to be dressed and changed in the same atmosphere. There is always dust in

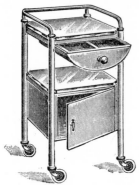

the air, no matter how much care is taken to get rid of it; besides the fluff and dust from bedmaking there may be dried discharges in powder form which will soon make the ward a very dirty place. Besides all this the bacteria which we cannot see are present on the small particles of dust which float in the air. For these reasons the nurse must know how to keep the ward thoroughly clean so that the patients do not get any further disorders by becoming re-infected. A high standard of cleanliness and ample ventilation are essentials.

Fig. 73.—Modern Pattern of Bedside Locker.

(*By courtesy of the Surgical Manufacturing Co. Ltd., London.*)

The Daily Routine.—After bed-making has been done in the morning, the beds should be pulled out from the walls as well as the chairs and lockers so that the sweeping may be done efficiently. This duty may rest with ward orderlies, ward helps or the nurse, but whoever is responsible for it must do it thoroughly, brushing away from her and towards the door. The broom must be kept low so as to prevent the dust from flying about. When this is finished, the dusting must be done most conscientiously, preferably with a damp duster. Glass shelves, marble tops and enamelled locker tops are all washed with soapy water. Ash trays are washed and cleaned and fruit plates are washed and returned to the locker. Any drinking mugs on the lockers should be washed also. The centre of the ward is cleaned and all the things returned to their correct places. The patients' lockers are cleaned out thoroughly once a week but every time the nurse goes to the locker she should remember it is the only place the patient has for all his belongings and should keep it tidy. In the weekly clean, the shelves and inside are scrubbed and the contents are not replaced until the locker is dry. Nothing belonging to the patient must be taken from his locker or thrown away without his permission.

The ward floor is usually the pride of the entire staff who take pains to keep it as nice as possible. Wooden parquet floors are polished with special mops or electric polishers and composition floors are also polished. This is to prevent the growth of organisms which do not thrive on a dry shiny surface ; in order to preserve the latter, the staff must be careful not to spill any liquids on the floor. If this accident should happen the floor may be made dangerous to walk upon, hence the need for prompt mopping up and drying. So far as composition floors are concerned, these require to be swept, but are also scrubbed to keep them clean ; this is done usually once a week but any area can be done at any time when conditions demand it.

The main electric lights of the ward are usually kept clean by the porter staff but the hand lamps and bed lights must be included in the daily routine of the ward staff. The chairs and tables must be dusted carefully and thoroughly, including the legs and ledges. The sinks and basins in the ward as well as the taps require to be washed with cleansing powder and a soft cloth. When there is any brass in the ward it requires a daily rub over with one of the well known liquid polishes.

Flower vases need to be washed daily and filled with clean water ; flowers should be freshly arranged each morning. These should have a little trouble and thought spent on them as in most cases they have been brought in by the relatives often at great sacrifice and any wishes regarding them should be taken into consideration when arranging them.

A neat and tidy ward has a good moral effect on the patients and the staff ; the cleanliness of it reflects on the staff and the wellbeing of the patients.

Work in the Ward Annexes.—The small rooms attached to the ward and used as stores, lavatories, kitchens and for other purposes may now be dealt with in turn.

The sluice room, when it exists apart from the lavatories, is usually tiled on floor and wall, and generally made to stand the application of a hose if necessary. It is fitted with special sluices for washing out urine bottles and bedpans, and may have a slate-covered table for the washing up of various sanitary utensils employed in the wards. This room requires to be specially treated with strong disinfectant daily, and with the lavatories may be dealt with by a trained male staff, which deals with each ward in turn. The utmost care should be taken to keep the floor, walls, furniture and fittings free from germ-carrying material, and the sinks should be maintained clear of any material likely to choke the traps (Figs. 74 and 75).

The lavatories and bathrooms are usually constructed on much the same principle as the sluice room, and therefore require the same system of cleansing. All urinals for males, and w.c.s, should be thoroughly cleaned as often as necessary. The more these offices are flushed out the better, a strong disinfectant like lysol, izal or other phenol product being employed. It is wrong to put things other than excrement down the closets; cotton wool, dressings, lint and similar fabrics should be incinerated.

The kitchens, linen rooms, stores rooms, and doctors' room need not have the same disinfection as the above. They generally conform to the plan used in the ward.

Care of Bedding, Linen, Blankets and Waterproofs.—In any busy ward, there is a constant changing of bedding and other linen, and the linen cupboard is one of the most important depots of the establishment. The stock depends upon the resources of the hospital; a certain inventory is supplied to each sister, and she sees that it is maintained. It is therefore the rule to stamp each article clearly with marking ink; sometimes distinctive emblems are embroidered on the hems. It is impossible to lay down any fixed scale of linen supply. In the store for the whole hospital, a certain reserve is kept of beds, wire mattresses and covers, hair mattresses and covers and pillows. In the linen room of a 20-bed ward, we might expect to find 70 pillow covers, 120 pillowcases, 50 counterpanes, 80 blankets, 100 sheets, 100 drawsheets and 30 waterproof sheets. Towels both for bathing and washing might amount to 130, while the regulation clothing for patients usually consists of half a dozen dressing-gowns, 30 face flannels, 80 nightgowns, the same number of vests and 50 bed jackets. In addition to this list there may be certain personal articles of clothing belonging to patients. It will be understood that a large proportion of this stock is either in use, or at the laundry or sewing room, where all the repairs are carried out, and the whole stock can never be reviewed at one specified time. Therefore it is an important duty to see that the linen is efficiently distributed, kept in good condition and replaced when worn out. The above stock list is not laid down as a fixed supply ; it may be that in some hospitals the linen is reduced to a minimum at the wards, but as a guide to equipment of a 20-bed ward it will suffice to indicate roughly how many of each article are necessary for efficient service. In many special cases, more sheets, waterproof sheets and patients' clothing are essential. For instance a surgical ward, or a ward dealing with children or with bladder cases obviously requires an almost unlimited store. Nowadays the difficulties of supply are extraordinary, and greatest care has to be taken to conserve every article. The nurse in charge of the linen is responsible that each article when it is taken from the laundry basket is checked with the list sent out, that it is in good condition and repair, or if not, that it is condemned and replaced. She should be able to account at any time for the whole inventory in her possession.

Blankets are washed only at intervals, as they tend to shrink. During the summer, spare blankets are usually stored away and carefully protected against moths.

Mackintoshes (waterproof sheets) require to be specially cleansed. They should be well washed with tow, hot water and

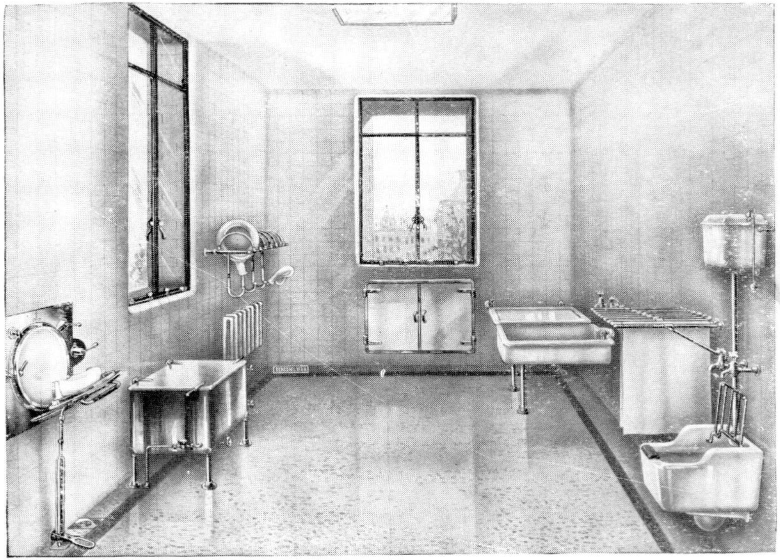

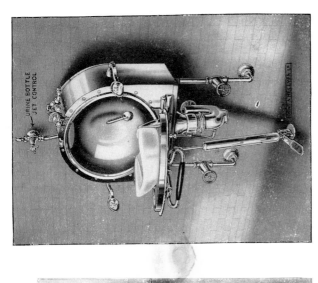

URINE BOTTLE
JET CONTROL

FIG. 75.—MODERN BEDPAN WASHER ("PROTEC-
TOR")

This is devised to cleanse the utensil both outside and inside with water at any temperature required, and in a sealed chamber. Urine bottles may be washed when the hinged door is open by placing them over the central nozzle.

(By courtesy of Messrs. Dent & Hellyer, Ltd., London.)

FIG. 74.—A MODERN HOSPITAL SLUICE ROOM.

The appliances illustrated include built-in "Protector" bedpan washer for scouring bedpans and urine bottles; bedpan sterilizer; hot water circulating bedpan and urine bottle, drying and warming rack; specimen cupboard; mackintosh scouring sink with hinged scrubbing slab, mackintosh rail; and hospital slop sink fixed clear of floor.

(By courtesy of Messrs. Dent & Hellyer, Ltd., London.)

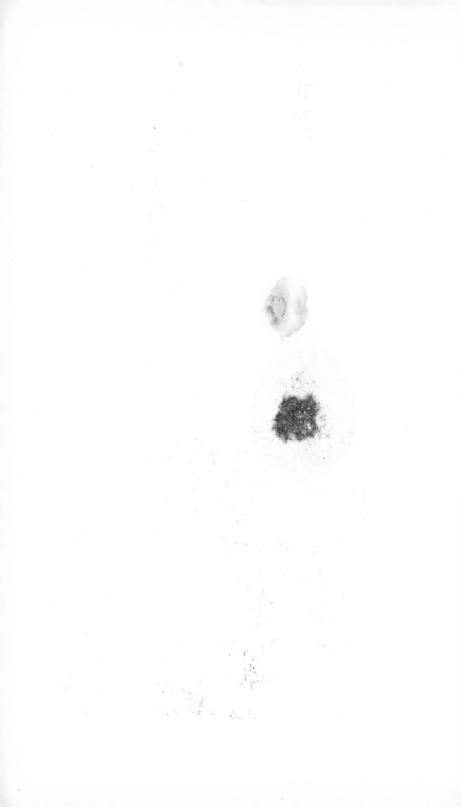

soap on a smooth scrubbing board, and then rinsed with phenol solution (1–40) and dried by hanging up. They must never be folded, therefore after drying they should be put away rolled on a wooden roller. It is advisable to dust them inside with fine talcum powder.

The general principles governing the care of linen, bedding and similar fabrics are established in order to effect economy as much as need be. When possible, stains should be immediately removed otherwise they may become a permanent disfigurement; all linen should be kept dry, in specially aired and heated cupboards ; if a patient is sick or incontinent, the sheets and bed-covers should be protected by waterproof sheeting ; at intervals mattresses must be brushed or cleaned by a vacuum machine. Linen may be stained by various things. Fresh blood is best dealt with by soaking in cold water and gently rubbing the fabric. When all the colour has gone, wash with soap and water and rinse well. Dry blood is dissolved by cold water ; it should be washed out carefully afterwards. Iodine is perhaps the commonest stain. A solution of phenol is often used to remove it, but it can also be diluted by surgical spirit applied at once. Often blankets show evidences of the yellow picric acid, which cannot be removed from wool, but other textile fabrics may be dealt with by ordinary washing. Anything of a greasy nature such as vaseline or ointments can be absorbed by the old-fashioned use of a hot iron and a layer of blotting-paper. The stains must be well rubbed, otherwise a circular " tide-line " is left. Tea, coffee, and cocoa stains are frequently found on the tops of sheets and down the front of bed gowns. If steam is forced through the stain, the latter will disappear.

Sanitary Methods of Cleaning Utensils, Crockery.— When utensils and equipment are removed from the ward, if they are not expendable they must either be disinfected first and washed afterwards, or simply washed and put away. A summary of the things dealt with in either or both ways includes feeding cups, mugs, spoons, forks, knives, cups, saucers, plates, porringers, sputum cups, kidney trays, urinals, bedpans, urine specimen glasses, glass and porcelain dishes, teapots, feeding bottles, brushes and combs, instruments, glassware, crockery, milk jugs, milk pails, condiment dishes and many other sundry articles in constant use. Sometimes feeding utensils are grouped on a tray and separately disinfected by boiling or simply washed. The instruments and other dressing utensils are kept by themselves and specially washed after being disinfected. Their disposal is fully dealt with later on at various suitable points. If a disinfectant is used with glass or crockery, it must be completely removed especially when feeding utensils are being dealt with. In most hospitals there is an abundant supply of boiling water, and even of steam, so that we are assured of proper sterilization and cleaning of every article. In the sluice room, the bedpans, urinals, urine test glasses, sputum mugs, kidney basins, enamel basins for vomited matter and other enamel ware soiled by use can be cleaned first, then washed well with washing soda and water.

The feeding utensils, after careful washing and drying, should be put away neatly in their respective places in the kitchen.

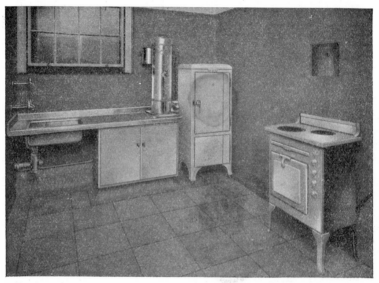

Fig. 76.—An All-Electric Ward Kitchen with Electric Stove and Oven Refrigerator, and Hot Water Apparatus.

(By courtesy of the British Electrical Development Association, Inc., London.)

Special attention should be paid to the spouts of feeding cups ; a small wire brush is useful. In some cases, steam cleansing of crockery and drying by placing the utensils in a rack is the rule. Babies' feeders should have the teats and valves removed, and first the cold and then the hot taps should be applied at one end, the water pouring out at the other. It is better to keep these feeders in an enamel basin containing sterilized water, in which also the cleansed teats and valves are kept.

In many wards, a check is made of the above equipment once a week; this is in addition to the annual stocktaking.

Care of the Kitchen.—As a general rule, the ward kitchen contains a slate covered table, gas cooker and cupboards. Adjacent may be a pantry and larder. All foodstuffs should be kept free from flies and should be carefully covered up. The food is supplied from the main kitchen of the hospital, but there may be special little things for certain patients, and these belong to the ward. The dry stores are supplied once a day. Bread should be kept in an enamel bin, which as a daily routine, should be cleared of crumbs and scraps; the latter are collected as pigs' meat. After that the bin should be thoroughly washed with soap and water, then carefully rinsed with boiling water and dried before the fresh bread is put in. Special care must be taken with all milk jugs and pails, as milk is easily tainted and is one of the most important articles of diet. All such receptacles should be thoroughly rinsed with cold water in the first place, a special hard brush being used, so that not a particle of the old milk remains, then boiling water should be used to wash them out. After that they can be turned upside down on a drying rack. No towel is necessary. All fresh milk should be stored in the larder. Most of the milk is supplied in glass bottles and is pasteurised. The ideal method of storage of food or milk is in a refrigerator and most hospitals have complete refrigeration installation. It should be the aim of every good nurse to see that the food is delivered to the patient in an attractive way. The trays should therefore be scrupulously clean and the utensils bright. (See also p. 154.)

Disposal and Disinfection of Soiled Linen and Dressings.

—All soiled dressings are put into a special enamel bucket with lid, and when this has collected the discarded lint, gauze, cotton wool and so on for the day, it is taken away by the porter staff to be incinerated. The bucket is disinfected in the usual way, and kept in the sluice room (Fig. 77). Infected linen should be placed in a bath or pail of phenol solution (1 in 20) for an hour, then rinsed and dried before being sent to the laundry. The mackintosh is treated as already described. Crockery should soak for an hour in phenol or lysol solution, and then be rinsed and boiled for 20 minutes. The blankets, mattress and pillows are placed in a strong canvas bag and sent to be sterilized by steam.

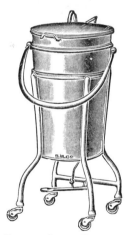

FIG. 77.—SOILED DRESSINGS BUCKET ON WHEELS.

(By courtesy of the Surgical Manufacturing Co., Ltd. London

The Daily Duties.

—One of the most important duties of a ward sister is to see that a routine is established. This is necessary in view of the fact that nurses have intervals of off-duty time, periods for meals and certain duties commensurate with their experience, and the complex and comprehensive nature of the work is such that it requires careful planning. Once the night nurse has gone off duty, the sister decides how the day is to be occupied, but the routine performance of various duties is simple, because each nurse knows her job and is able to carry it out. A sister possessed of good administrative powers will see that the hygiene of the ward is sound and that the morning "toilet" of the ward proceeds apace. Any abnormal development is reported to her and receives her attention. Meanwhile the ward is prepared for the house doctor's visit, which is usually at 10 a.m. The allocation of duties in the morning is a matter of the rule existing in various hospitals; in some cases, the night nurse does a certain proportion of the patients' toilet, bedmaking and so on, but this may be left until after breakfast, which is usually one of the first events of the day. Before the arrival of the house physician or surgeon, the sister makes herself acquainted with the condition of each individual patient and preparations are made for dressings, special examinations or other procedures. The information collected by the sister should be such that she should be able to tell the doctor anything of note that has happened since he last visited the ward. She, or the senior nurse, is expected to assist at any dressing. In training schools for doctors, the medical students help by doing dressings and by acting as clinical clerks. By dinner time, which is usually noon or 12.30, the most important work of the ward ought to have been done. The patients are washed after dinner, which is served by the nurses from the kitchen, the sister supervising the distribution of the food. Probationer nurses take urinals and bedpans to those who require them. The afternoon should be spent quietly; operations may be done, which certain nurses attend, or visitors may call on approved days. The ward never ceases to be a hive of industry, and description falls far short of the impression conveyed by actual experience. The successful sister is one who has reached a stage at which, although she holds many reins in both hands, she must yet be ready for more ; she must be ready to accommodate herself to the slightest breakdown and she requires to have the patience of a saint. Tea for the patients is a simple meal, followed by recreation for those who can take it. Wireless is a great benefit in wards. After tea, patients newly admitted may require to be put to bed; their particulars must be taken and arrangements made for the complete investigation of their case as soon as possible. It is convenient to give baths at night both in the bathroom and in bed. Supper should be over before the night nurse comes on duty at 8 p.m.

The first thing the night nurse gets is the day report. This tells her in full the events of the day, each patient being mentioned personally. Special details are given about new patients and about those critically ill. One of the great functions of the night nurse is to get her charges settled down for the night. Between 8 p.m. and 10 p.m., inmates of a ward are always restless; some cannot sleep and require drugs ; others are in pain ; helpless patients must be watched in case they slip too far down in bed or disturb dressings, bandages or splints. The night nurse acts in a conservative way if possible, leaving all unnecessary work to the day staff. Sometimes she has to deal with emergencies such as acute abdominal inflammation or with haemorrhage. By the time the house doctor calls round for his last visit, the night nurse should have obtained a good idea of the condition of each patient, and she should have a list of questions to put to the doctor about anything that has struck her as abnormal. During the night the nurse may have to attend to the sanitary arrangements, to mark the 4-hourly charts and to prepare dressings and other materials for the stores room. She should make sure that the temperature of the ward is maintained all night at a regular level. During the night she is periodically visited by the night sister and her assistant, to whom she may apply for any help in deciding on any unusual course of action. Nurses should remember that they are not expected to take any responsibility outside their own sphere of work.

The above is a mere outline of the day's work in a ward and no doubt there are hundreds of variations in routine. It must be stressed that the only way to appreciate the work of a ward to the full is to play an integral part in its activities for a long spell. A nurse at the end of her training will have amassed an amount of knowledge by experience alone that cannot be imparted by a textbook, however complete the treatise may be.

CHAPTER 3

GENERAL CARE OF THE PATIENT

RECEIVING A NEW PATIENT. ADMISSION TO THE WARD.
LIFTING AND TURNING PATIENTS. BATHING. IN THE
BATHROOM. THE BLANKET BATH. FINAL DETAILS.
SPECIAL AREAS OVER WHICH CARE MUST BE EXERCISED.
CARE OF THE BACK. HANDS AND FEET. HEAD AND
HAIR. TREATMENT OF THE HAIR AND SCALP WHEN
VERMIN ARE PRESENT. MOUTH AND TEETH.

EVERY nurse must know something about psychology. She
must have imagination and she must be able to make a correct interpretation of other people's minds. Only by putting herself
in the patient's place will she gain the full understanding of the
real science of healing. Every newcomer to a ward should be
the object of careful study, and that study should be conducted
without arousing the suspicion in the patient's mind that he is
under review. Yet he must have complete confidence in the
n terest that is being taken in him, so that there will be no nega-
itive thought to retard his progress. How should a nurse approach and deal with the new patient? How is she to ensure
that the first impressions are good ones and that the patient is
made to react at once for his own good to the environment in
which he has been placed? Hundreds of questions like these
arise and the answers are not always easy because each nurse
has her own way of thinking, her own attitude to life, her own
methods. The success of a nurse's work very often depends upon
the possession of that quality which is given to some and denied
to others, which has as much power as the remedies of the
pharmacopoeia and which is often uncanny in its achievement—
personality. It is by personality that a nurse may achieve her
purpose when all other efforts have failed.

Receiving a New Patient.—Patients are admitted to hospital
from different places. Doctors may recommend medical cases
for observation, acute abdominal emergencies may result in the
rushing to hospital of a person who is seized suddenly with
dangerous disease at any hour of the day or night. Accidents
continue to grow in frequency. The out-patient department—
that sorting room of the hospital—sends daily its quota for the

252

in-patient department. Generally the patients are accompanied by notes from their private practitioners, but the nurse may not see these. In the reception department, however, there is always a system, variable though it may be according to the hospital, of filling up several admission forms which are distributed to various administrative groups. When the patient has been examined by the doctor who is responsible for allocating him to a ward, he is provided with certain personal papers, including an admission card, which are taken to the ward by the porter who conducts him there. Sometimes all the documents referring to his previous recent history accompany the card, but in many cases the nurse simply gets the card, with a few brief particulars stating the type of case.

When she goes to look at the new arrival on the wheeled stretcher, she may have to think rapidly and make up her mind what to do. If it is a case of serious accident, with haemorrhage temporarily stopped, and the clothing torn and covered with mud, she must make some arrangement to cleanse the patient before he is put into an ordinary bed. On the other hand, if the case is one of pneumonia, she must see that the bed is ready as quickly as possible and all prepared for a severe chest case. The system of dividing the hospital into wards of surgical, medical, gynaecological, special and children's diseases makes a certain amount of limitation of the type of case, but even with this subdivision, there is no saying what may have to be accomplished, and nurses must be ready for everything.

The first thing to be done is to demonstrate to the patient and to his relatives who may accompany him the spirit of homeliness and the attitude of a friend. A few kind words spoken quietly and confidently to the mother of a child with a broken leg make a splendid first impression which is never forgotten. This matter of the manner of the nurse cannot be overstressed. So many times has it been discovered that wrong thinking and acting have spoiled the whole atmosphere of the case by the unfortunate attitude of the nurse, that we must get it deeply rooted in our minds that no matter what strain of work or anxiety or personal feeling may affect the nurse, she must put aside all these in the desire to create the proper impression. It is admittedly often very hard, and on certain days a nurse may be exasperated by the activities which almost overwhelm her, yet she must never expose her worries to outsiders and she must not on any account appear to be too busy to attend to the newcomer. The more interest, indeed, that is taken in him the better for all concerned.

Admission to the Ward.—In the absence on the admission card of any instructions about early treatment, preparations should be made to give the patient a bath. Usually the sister of the ward issues her orders about this on being informed of the arrival of the new patient. Some people may not be in a fit state for immediate bathing and may be put to bed as they are, the bed being covered with an old blanket and mackintosh until emergency treatment has been done to enable the patient to be properly washed. In most cases, however, the patients arrive with night clothes on, and can be put to bed, where they are given a blanket bath (see below). The other possibility is that the newcomer may walk in and that he may be able to have an ordinary bath under supervision. While the bath is being prepared, the nurse can take the temperature, the pulse and the respirations, and make a general survey of the case. Anything unusual should be reported to the sister. When the patient has been settled comfortably in bed, there are certain formalities to be carried out. If he cannot give particulars himself (e.g. in critical illness or unconscious states), he must not be troubled. The usual procedure is to keep one of the relatives—wife, mother or father—waiting outside the ward, then when the patient has been left in the charge of another nurse, the admitting nurse takes a note of the following particulars : 1. The personal effects, keep-sakes, valuables brought by the patient ; 2. the address of the next of kin ; 3. the full name, address, age, occupation, of the patient; 4. the history of the case, including family history, the personal history (noting the previous illnesses, kind of work, habits and so on) and the present illness, with details of the symptoms in series. In other words, the nurse should try to get as many details as possible about the case which will help the doctors in their diagnosis. In many instances the writing down of the details is not insisted on, except for the making out of a case-sheet and temperature chart. The rest is left to the clinical clerk or house surgeon. In the case of an expected operation permission must be obtained from parents for children under a certain age, which varies according to the hospital. When the patient is critically ill, the relatives must be treated with every consideration; to them it may be the most difficult time of their lives and sympathy must be shown for their grief, anxiety and distress. When a patient is put on the danger list, his relatives must be informed through the central office of the hospital, from which a telegram or police message will be sent. In some cases, an " S O S " message may be broadcast by radio.

No nurse should commmit the breach of etiquette involved in giving an opinion about a case to the relatives. She is often asked searching questions, but in all her replies she must be frank but non-committal. Let her never forget that since she is not in possession of a medical degree she is not expected to take the responsibilities which rightly belong to a qualified doctor.

Lifting and Turning Patients.—One of the first things that must be remembered by the nurse at the beginning of her career is that unless she is of unusually fine physique and strength it is unwise to attempt to lift a patient single handed. Lifting should always be done by two nurses, one at each side of the bed. The way a patient is handled makes a big difference to the ease of lifting. The best way to lift is to carry out the following routine. A nurse stands close to the bed at one side and her assistant in a similar position on the other. Both look towards the head of the bed. Together they link their proximal arms under the axilla, their free arms being round the lumbar region, with the hands supporting the small of the back. The patient is then told to cross his arms firmly over the sternum and to put his chin as near to the chest as possible, in the middle line. His knees should also be drawn up, so that he avoids by his whole attitude any looseness of limb and makes his body a compact unit for lifting. He can then be set up as far as is convenient in the bed.

When the patient is helpless, a type of cradle should be made by the nurses. They face each other on either side of the bed, pass the hands below the patient and firmly clasp them at the levels of the scapulae and the pelvis. The patient can then be slowly lifted to any other position. The same principle holds good when the position is changed from the sitting position to the recumbent one.

When a paralysed, unconscious or otherwise helpless patient has to be moved from his bed, say, to another bed, a pole-stretcher is used (Fig. 78). This consists of a canvas sheet, with

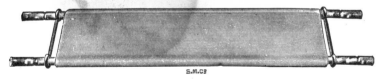

S.M.C?

FIG. 78.—STRETCHER, WITH REMOVABLE BAMBOO POLES AND IRON SUPPORT.
(By courtesy of the Surgical Manufacturing Co., Ltd., London.)

the long edges made into a hollow hem, forming a channel for two stout poles. The sheet is carefully placed under the patient who is rolled over on his side for the purpose, then he is rolled back and when the sheet is adjusted properly underneath him, the poles are pushed in and the patient is thus easily carried off. In an emergency, the drawsheet can be used, but a third nurse must support the head while the patient is being transported.

Turning.—Stand at the side of the bed to which you wish to turn your patient. Loosen the bedclothes. Stretch out your hands towards the patient, one passing well over the back at the level of the scapulae, and the other just over the buttocks, and with great care and deliberation, gently pull the patient towards

wheeled chair or stretcher to the bed and he is quickly undressed. The clothing on the sound side is removed first and since there is usually extensive damage by tearing, dirt, blood and other stains in the region of the injury, it is no sacrifice to cut off the sleeve on the injured side.   The seams may be ripped open on the outside and inside of the jacket ; this allows the garment to be removed easily.   The shirt may have to be cut open down the middle.   When a leg is injured, the trouser seam can be cut up on the outside.

In all these cases there is shock, and plenty of heat is required —hot water bottles, hot blankets, hot water in abundance. The sooner the patient is settled down thoroughly warm and as comfortable as possible between warm bedclothes, the better the outlook for his future.   The clothing may require to be destroyed or it may be worth putting through the Thresh disinfector.   In either case it must be laid in a compact bundle on a sheet spread out at the side of the bed.   During these operations, the nurse should wear an overall outfit which covers her from head to foot and it is better to wear rubber gloves which overlap the cuffs of the sleeves.

After the clothes have been removed the other warmed blanket is kept over the patient; it is usual to slip it over the shirt and pants, and to remove these from underneath it; this prevents undue exposure of the patient.   The body is then washed thoroughly, bit by bit; in the case of the patient we have taken as our example, the affected part must be carefully protected, and left to the last.   The face is washed first, the ears, neck and eyes being carefully cleaned.   The sound arm is brought from below the blanket and washed, the nails being scrubbed and trimmed if necessary.   In succession, the chest, the abdomen, the right leg and the left leg are taken for treatment; then if possible, turn the patient over and wash the back.   A little methylated spirit should be well rubbed in, then the back should be powdered to prevent bedsore.   In some cases, the groins and the folds of the buttocks are cleaned by the patient, but in many instances he is so helpless that the nurse must do it herself.   In washing the groins, or indeed any folds of skin, it is well to use plenty of soap, especially if it has a tarry basis, then after the lather has been dried gently off, powder should be applied.   In the female, the skin under the breasts is very often red and may be broken.   Great care is therefore necessary in order not to irritate the condition further.

The injured arm can now be dealt with ; it should be disturbed as little as possible, and the washing done thoroughly as close to the dressing above and below as may be practicable : the surgeons will look after the affected area.   The water may require to be changed several times.   The hair should be examined and a note made of its condition with reference to pediculosis or other skin lesions.

The above method equally applies to non-accident cases; the only difference in the routine is that in doing the washing the farthest away arm is taken first, then the chest, then the nearest arm. The patient is also able to help to a certain extent. But it will be understood that the more helpless the patient, the more work there is to do for the nurse, because not only may a paralysed or unconscious person be unable to give assistance but he may have incontinence of urine and faeces, and may also have been vomiting.

In the example we have taken, we assume that the new patient is infested with pediculosis. It may therefore be necessary for the nurse to shave the axillary and pubic hair, to search for nits or lice, and to finish by rubbing in some antiparasitic ointment supplied by the sister. If the head is badly affected, it may be covered with a protective cap as a temporary measure, since it will undoubtedly require to have intensive treatment later on.

Once all the toilet is finished, the bed garments, which have been well warmed, are put on the patient, and the mackintosh and under blanket are removed while the bedclothes are replaced and the upper wash blanket removed. All these articles are potentially verminous so they should join the heap of clothing in the bucket. Ultimately, the nurse's overall, together with the washing flannels, towels, blankets removed after washing and the pail with its contents should be put into a special bag of linen or canvas and carried straight to the sluice room, from which it is removed for disinfection as quickly as possible.

Final Details.— In leaving a patient after bathing it is advisable to test the hot water bottle to see that it is not too hot. There should be a flannel cover on the bottle and it is wise to place the hot water bottle a sheet and a blanket away from the patient. Many serious accidents have occurred through the placing of very hot bottles against insensitive feet. Another essential in the case of new arrivals is to ask about the bladder and bowels. The availability of the urinal and the bedpan should be explained, also the method of summoning the nurse. Special arrangements have to be made for incontinent persons. The test of a capable nurse is a patient who feels the better for his blanket bath—relaxed but not worn out with over-exertion ; warm, but not overheated.

Clothing which belongs to the patient can be returned to his relatives, together with any possessions not required ; if it has been found to be necessary to disinfect clothing the fact should be mentioned to them. In some cases, the hospital can store the clothing and the nurse responsible should see that an inventory is made and the list signed before the clothing is put away.

All new patients must be kept under observation for the first few hours. If they are coughing or spitting, an enamel sputum mug should be put on their locker, with the instructions that sputum must be expectorated into the mug and the top quickly closed. The mug should have some cold water in the bottom. The first sample of urine should be kept, as well as the stool, and when vomiting occurs the vomited material should be retained until the medical officer has seen it.

Special Areas over which Care Must be Exercised.—In dealing with personal hygiene (pp. 74–78) we found that a routine toilet is necessary. The following paragraphs give the essential procedures from the nursing point of view.

1. *Care of the Back.*—The daily routine of washing may be observed in the form of blanket bathing every morning, the toilet of the hands and face after dinner and a final washing of the face and hands at night. Every patient has different problems according to the type of his ailment and the stage of his progress. The skin of the folds of the body and of the scalp has already been mentioned as important; liberal powdering of the folds will prevent irritation, while the scalp is treated with the hair. If there is any sign of poor circulation, or of pressure of bone, or of waterlogging of the skin of the back, especially in the lumbar region, the nurse must be very careful, as this condition, both from the patient's and nurse's point of view, is a heart breaking and most obstinate defect. The slightest ra strain on the skin may cause a bedsore; this can usual y prevented by good nursing, but it is sometimes inevitable i very difficult cases. The subject is fully discussed later and at present we are concerned only with the prevention. To make efficient defence against the starting of an ulcer, the nurse must keep her eyes open for the preliminary reddening of the area on which pressure is put. When she carries out the routine skin hardening, however, there may be no question of bedsore at all. If the skin of the back is well washed with soap and water twice daily, and the area carefully dried and then dusted with talcum powder, there may be complete immunity to bedsore. Generally some methylated spirit is well rubbed in, or some other strong alcoholic extract such as eau de cologne, brandy or whisky if cheaper things are not available. This not only hardens the skin; it stimulates the circulation and keeps the area well nourished. The alternative is the use of some very soft, oily ointment, possibly containing zinc oxide. By rubbing this into the pressure areas, the nurse can make the skin pliable and free. If done twice a day with the palm of the hand in a rotatory motion, the " dangerous areas " can be protected against degeneration. The other methods are those of air beds and water beds, both of which are fully dealt with later (pp. 276–278), and of variation of the posture. Constant pressure is the great danger, therefore the position of the

patient should be changed regularly every two hours or so, and thus he is saved from a prolonged irritation of one portion of his back.

2. *Hands and Feet.*—Special attention should be paid to the hands and feet, making sure that the nails are cut and trimmed that all dirt is removed and that cleanliness of the webs of the feet and of the toenails is assured. Corns should be pared. Bedsores should be prevented on elbows and heels.

3. *Head and Hair.*—There are various accepted methods of dealing with the head and hair of the female patient confined to bed. In the case of the male patient all that is necessary is thoroughly lathering with soap or any of the simple shampoo lotions available.

For females with long hair the equipment necessary comprises 2 bath towels, a small shoulder blanket, one hand towel, one large mackintosh, waterproof shoulder cape, cotton wool plugs for the ears, hairdresser's neck wool, one large deep washing basin, a pail for waste water, 2 large jugs or ewers (one for cold, one for hot water), 2 half-pint jugs (one for soap solution, one for vinegar), a brush and comb, 2 face cloths, hot water bottles (or an electric hair drier) and safety pins.

All equipment should be checked before the nurse starts to shampoo the hair; this will avoid leaving the patient in the middle of the procedure. There are 3 main methods, each of which is outlined b

Method 1. Expl   to the patient what she is expected to do. Fold the upper end of the mattress under, so that the hair projects well beyond it ; alternatively the mattress may be drawn down over the foot of the bed sufficiently to allow the basin to rest on the wire mattress at the top of the bed, which is protected by a mackintosh. The pail is placed in a position conveniently near to the bed. When all preparatory details have been completed the patient's nightgown is removed and is replaced by a small shoulder blanket and waterproof cape; cotton wool is inserted between the neck and the neckband as a seal, and ear plugs are put into the ear passages. The long mackintosh is arranged round the patient's shoulders and is allowed to extend over the wire mattress. The patient is then gently drawn to the top of the bed and her head is supported over the basin by the nurse's hand, which is applied at the occiput. The nurse, with her free hand, then proceeds to soak the hair with warm water, adding small quantities of the soap solution, this being rubbed well in until a good lather is produced ; after the first lather has been rinsed out the process is repeated once more. A final rinsing is done with diluted vinegar when need for this exists. The hair is then squeezed dry and wrapped in a warm bath towel. The mackintoshes are removed and the bed is remade. The patient is put into a comfortable position and her hair is rubbed dry with a fresh warm bath towel or dried by the electrical dryer when one is available. Finally the hair should be well brushed and combed to remove any tangles and in the case of very long hair, 2 plaits should be made.

Method 2. This method has now been superseded almost entirely by Methods 1 and 3, although it is sometimes still employed when the patient has long hair. Preparations are similar to those described above. The pillows are removed and the patient is drawn to the side of the bed with her head resting on the edge of the bed. A large mackintosh is arranged to form a trough below the head, the trough leading to a small enamel bath on the floor. The washing basin is placed on a chair, protected by a mackintosh and in line with the patient's head. The hair is then allowed to hang into the basin, which is half full of warm water ; the whole head is soaked by having additional water poured over it. The shampoo is rubbed into the hair with the tips of the fingers until a good lather is produced after which thorough rinsing is carried out, with the head over the basin; the process is repeated. Finally the hair is squeezed free of all water and is made into a coil on the top of the scalp, with a warm bath towel as a head wrapping. The mackintoshes and blanket are removed and the patient is clothed and comfortably settled in bed. If an electric dryer is not available, the hair should again be uncovered and arranged over rubber hot water bottles protected by a bath towel.

Method 3. In some hospitals in which the beds are provided with a movable back which can be lifted off, shampooing of the hair in bed is a comparatively simple procedure : the bed is drawn away from the wall, the headrail of the bed is lifted off, a chair is placed between the nurse and the head of the bed, and the basin is set on the chair. The patient is raised so that the head is extended over the top of the bed and supported under the occiput. The details of shampooing are similar to those described above.

4. *Treatment of the Hair and Scalp when Vermin are Present.*—On admission to hospital a patient may be discovered to have a verminous head. Several cleansing methods may be adopted, some so efficient that they have abolished the need for cutting the hair, a custom seldom supported these days and indeed one which in certain districts can be observed only when a written order has been obtained from the local Medical Officer of Health. Remedies most commonly used are oil of sassafras and medicated lethane hair oil.

Oil of sassafras may be applied as follows. Unless the patient is an infant, she should lie on her back, the bed being well protected by a red rubber mackintosh and the patient's shoulders by a cape and white towel; the neck of the cape should be padded out with barber's wool. The margins of the skin round the hair should be smeared with soft paraffin or other similar preparation with a view to protection. The hair is then parted in the middle and taken up in small separate sections, the oil being applied thoroughly to each with a cotton wool swab. The whole of the hair is treated in this way. The head should then be covered completely by a piece of lint over which is put a layer of jaconet and a firm bandage. The head should be left thus all night and first thing next morning the scalp and hair should be shampooed as described above.

So far as medicated lethane oil is concerned, this is the favourite nowadays and undoubtedly the most efficient remedy. The treatment should be carried out rigidly according to instructions. The hair is parted and a few drops of the oil are applied to the scalp, 4 areas being thus treated ; the scalp and hair should be massaged with the fingers until it is certain that the oil is properly incorporated. Another 4 areas may be dealt with, making a total of 8. The hair must be left afterwards in an unwashed condition for 10 days; at the end of this period the vermin will have disappeared.

5. *Mouth and Teeth.*—From what has already been said about the mouth in the Hygiene Section, it is clear that the greatest importance rests in the daily cleansing of the mouth and teeth. Especially is this so in patients who are paralysed, who have affections of the mouth or who suffer from fevers like scarlet fever, or diphtheria or pneumonia. In these special cases, it may be the regular duty of a nurse to see that the toilet of the mouth is carried out every 4 hours or oftener. In long continued and debilitating fevers, the tongue becomes dry, furred and brown; sordes (a condition of soiling of the teeth owing to the mixture of dry saliva, epithelial debris, germs and particles of food) collect on the teeth and the breath is foetid. It is a wonderful tonic to the patient to have his mouth " done out " frequently. The tongue is dealt with by winding round the handle of a toothbrush a few strips of gauze soaked in sodium bicarbonate solution, and then using the contrivance as a " squeegee," from the back of the tongue to the tip. The inside of the mouth, edges of the gums and the surface of the teeth can also be dealt with by pledgets of cotton wool soaked in sodium bicarbonate and fixed in the teeth of small artery forceps (a spongeholder will do equally well). The teeth may be cleaned with a soft toothbrush and any of the well known dentifrices. The mouth should afterwards be well rinsed out with one of the following solutions: sotol, borax and glycerine, lemon and borax, thymol, glycothymoline, listerine or hydrogen peroxide. In many cases, the patient likes to have his mouth rinsed out with copious draughts of ordinary water, which is both cooling and refreshing, as his

mouth cells are very dry. Syphon soda water is also refreshing and cleansing.

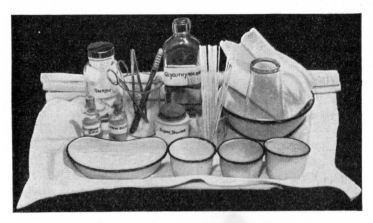

FIG. 80.—TRAY PREPARED FOR MOUTH WASHING.

A serviceable tray may be made up for cases requiring constant mouth lavage. On it should be kept ready lint, gauze, solutions for the mouth, artery forceps or sponge holders, a feeding cup for holding the mouth wash, cotton wool, small enamel basin for expectorated matter and a kidney basin for the dirty swabs. The greatest care must be taken to sterilize each instrument and utensil after use.

CHAPTER 4

BEDS AND MAKING OF BEDS

THE HOSPITAL BED.   MAKING OF BEDS.   SPECIAL BEDS.
OPERATION BEDS.   FRACTURE BEDS.   PLASTER BEDS.
AMPUTATION BEDS.   RHEUMATIC BEDS;   RENAL BEDS.
BEDS FOR HEART CASES.   ADJUNCTS TO BEDS.

THE bed is all important to the patient.   In it he is forced to remain for nearly all of the 24 hours of the day ; he is limited by its confines; he is peculiarly susceptible to the slightest changes in its composition; his progress of mind and body depends intimately on the comfort of the place in which he spends his period of treatment.   Therefore it is essential that the patient should be absolutely free from all possible discomfort, and that every effort should be made to adjust the bed to suit the person in it.

Fortunately the era of military precision and uniformity in wards is nearly over.   At one time the index of a sister's good management was a row of beds evenly spaced and carefully " dressed."   Except in very special cases, the bedding was arranged according to one pattern only, and the clothes were tucked in securely as if it were intended to imprison the patient and not to alleviate his indisposition.   Anyone who has spent a few weeks in the atmosphere of such discipline can appreciate how a period in bed in such circumstances becomes almost unbearable and how the moral effect of the restriction is bad for recovery.

Today, while we all strive to keep the ward tidy, we are not so hard on those who are restless in bed and who thus upset the applecart of uniformity.   We regard bed making as being carried out on the principles—in order of importance—of comfort, cleanliness and appearance.   It is quite easy to make a proportionate estimate of all three and to act according to it.

The Hospital Bed.—The usual hospital bed is 30 inches from the ground, 6 feet long and 3 feet wide.   The best patterns are the simplest (Fig. 81). Cast iron frames with several coats of enamel or paint, and with open ends surmounted by hollow rails, make cleansing and disinfection very easy.   A wire mattress is fixed to the top of the frame, either by straps or by small catches and slots.   On the top of the wire mattress is a thick hair mattress but in some cases, two " biscuits," each 3 feet by 3 feet are interposed, making the bed firmer, and to some, more comfortable.   If there is not any cover provided for the hair mattress

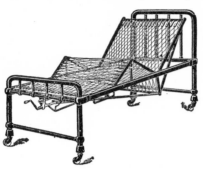

when it is used without the underlying biscuits, the wire mattress should be covered with a sheet of hessian. On the top of the hair mattress it is usual to place an old blanket which has shrunk so that it occupies an area of the bed roughly 4 feet by 3 feet—the part on which the main weight of the body is put. In many cases however, a waterproof sheet becomes necessary owing to the nature of the illness; and

FIG. 81.—" LAWSON TAIT " BEDSTEAD, WITH
FOWLER POSITION ADJUSTMENT.
*(By courtesy of the Surgical Manufacturing
Co., Ltd., London.)*

when there is any question of urinary or bowel weakness or other possible soiling of the mattress, this takes the place of the old blanket.

The foundation of the bed having been built, the bedclothes proper must be put on.   First comes the bottom sheet, which should be laid with its edges straight, and the same amount of overlapping at the top as at the bottom.   It cannot be too strongly impressed on the nurse how essential it is that this sheet should be drawn tightly, and firmly tucked in below the mattress all round.   The slightest crease may cause all kinds of discomfort and probably a bedsore.   It is customary in cases of acute illness to add a drawsheet, which consists of a piece of old soft sheeting, about 30 inches wide, and fixed over the bottom sheet at the part of the bed upon which lies the part of the patient's body extending from the shoulders to the knees. It is a method of ensuring that the portion on which the patient lies is perfectly smooth, as it is a simple matter to pull each end of the drawsheet at intervals and tuck it below the mattress.

The top bedclothes consist of a sheet and several blankets with a counterpane.   For those who do not object to it, and who may be susceptible to cold, a thin, narrow blanket may be put on next to the patient.   The fixing of the top bedclothes is a very important matter, as stated above.   When patients lie on their backs, their toes stick up in the air and it is most uncomfortable to have the top bedclothes tightly drawn over the feet.   Another point is that although the sheets and blankets should cover the chest as far up as possible, they should not be such that the patient is hemmed in. He must have freedom of movement. Naturally, however, the clothes should be arranged so that the maximum heat is retained. Too much weight of top bedclothes should be avoided. Every nursing school has its own way of finishing off the bed so as to make it neat. In most hospitals the blankets are tucked in with the sheet below the mattress at the bottom, while by making an " envelope " fold, the clothes hang down neatly at the sides of the bed. In some instances the sides of the sheet and blankets are tucked below the mattress as well. At the top of the bed, two or three pillows are put or a firm bolster and a soft pillow, which act as a support and pad for the head, neck and shoulders. Generally speaking, the sheet should be folded back over the blankets at the lower edge of the bolster, allowing 18–24 inches of an overlap. When a counterpane is in use, it is laid over the bed, tucked in at the bottom and folded back with an overlap like the top sheet; the sides are allowed to hang down, the bottom being made neat by envelope tuck. Sometimes the counterpane extends right over the pillows and thus covers the entire bed.

All the above directions are subject to modifications, but they serve as a standard pattern. During the night, patients, in sleeping, adopt the postures they instinctively know to be the best for sleep and they should never be prevented from doing this. If they want to pull the bedclothes over their shoulders, they should be allowed to do so. Restless patients who throw off the clothes should naturally have their beds adjusted, but they need not be aroused from their sleep.

Making of Beds.—The daily routine of bed making generally consists of a complete re-making in the morning, and a general tidying at bedtime. In the morning, when the beds are stripped, the nurses should work in pairs. The most convenient way to make the bed is as follows. First put the bedside chair in the passageway at the foot of the bed ; the counterpane is folded neatly and put on the seat. In succession follow the blankets and sheets, each being folded lengthways so as to reduce the length to one-third, the top flap being covered by the bottom flap. These can then be placed neatly over the back of the chair, and arranged so that none of the bedclothes touch the floor. Drawsheets and the bottom sheet usually contain debris and crumbs, and therefore they must be shaken ; the waterproof sheet must be laid over the chair unfolded. If the patient can be placed for a moment on another chair or on the next bed, the mattress should be turned, shaken up and quickly set in position.

Now and then the wire mattress requires to be brushed

in which case the hair mattress is rolled successively to the top and to the bottom while each half of the wire is being cleaned. After the mattress has been turned, the rest of the bottom clothes are laid on, the patient is put back to bed and the clothes are quickly spread over him in the approved fashion.

When the patient cannot leave the bed.—This condition calls for somewhat different treatment. The best that can be done is a changing of the bottom sheet, with adjustment of the mackintosh and drawsheet. Two ways of doing this are described below.

1. Have all the clean linen handy, properly aired and warm. The nurses prepare the new sheet by making it into a roll of cloth on its long axis. Make sure that the windows are closed. One nurse stands at one side of the bed and the other at the other side. Take away pillows and top coverings. Loosen the bottom sheet, drawsheet and mackintosh. The assistant then helps the patient to rise on his elbows and as he does so, the old sheet is rolled down while the new sheet is rolled into its place, the whole direction being from the top of the bed to the bottom. The drawsheet presents no difficulties, as it is only about 30 inches wide. If a mackintosh is used, it can be rolled on the outside of the bottom sheet and it falls into position with the sheet. The disadvantage of this method is that it puts too much strain on certain patients.

2. A much more popular method is the side-to-side method. In this the sheet which is to be put on, together with a new draw-sheet inside it at the proper position, and the mackintosh outside it, is rolled lengthways on its short axis. The assistant gently draws the patient, covered by a short blanket, to the extreme ₁edge of the bed. Two-thirds of the bed are thus left vacant, and the undersheet, drawsheet and mackintosh are rolled towards the patient. Immediately afterwards, the new sheet is rolled out to two-thirds of its width, and the remainder of the roll lies close to the patient's back. The assistant then lets the patient roll over on his back to the clean sheet, and immediately afterwards pulls away the soiled clothes and rolls out the remaining third to the edge of the bed. The patient is then lifted to the centre of the bed, which is adjusted in the usual way. Occasionally the draw-sheet is fixed separately, as it is an easy matter. In cases in which the mackintosh sheet is not removed, it can be sponged and quickly dried, smoothed and adjusted ; the mattress can also be beaten up, the whole procedure occupying about a minute. With skilled nurses the complete change should be done in less than 5 minutes.

In all these procedures, the nurse's last act must be that of ensuring that the bottom bedclothes are without a wrinkle and that the patient is placed comfortably over the middle of the drawsheet.

Special Beds

In various types of illness, accident, post-operative conditions and other abnormal states, a special form of bed must be devised. The main varieties of special bed are discussed in the following pages.

Operation Beds.—When a patient is in the operating theatre, the bed he is to occupy on his return must be prepared. It is usual to strip the bed of its top coverings; the bottom coverings are examined to make sure that the sheets and mackintoshes are perfectly smooth. The pillows are removed, except in special cases, and in their place is put a tightly drawn mackintosh covered by an old bath towel. On the locker is a sickness basin, with squares of cloth for swabbing out the mouth and a small sickness towel. Three hot water bottles are put on the bed and they are covered by a blanket doubled from side to side. Three methods of preparation are then possible. In the first, the top clothes are fixed in all along one side, and halfway along the bottom. When the patient arrives, it is a simple matter to take out the bottles, to cover him with the hot blanket, and then to tuck in the rest of the clothes. In the second way, the clothes are left loose except at the bottom. When the patient returns, the whole of the top layer is rolled down and the above procedure then carried out. The third method consists in putting the bottles all together in the centre of the bed. The top clothes are arranged in the same way as for an ordinary bed, but instead of being tucked in under the mattress, the sides are brought up as flaps over the middle, the bottom third being folded on top of them and lastly the top third over the bottom third. A blanket is heated over the hot pipes or at the fire. It is a simple matter to lay the patient on the bed—one nurse having lifted up the packet for a moment—to cover him with the hot blanket and to unfold the coverings in the reverse order to that in which they were made into a packet.

It is not considered necessary to keep the hot water bottles in the bed in cases in which the bed and bedclothes have been properly warmed. When necessary an electric blanket is placed over the blanket next to the patient to counteract shock.

Fracture Beds.—In these, wooden fracture boards are put below the hair mattress to prevent any sagging. A fracture bed is used for amputations, plaster cases and any injuries which demand a firm basis. In certain circumstances, the biscuit method of mattressing is used, so that for toilet purposes the portions can be moved apart, and the bedpan put in their place. For cases of fracture of the spine and for incontinence and senile cases, a very fine arrangement can be used. The fracture board has a circular hole in it, about 9 inches in diameter. A straw mattress, also constructed on the same plan, is placed over it, and on the top a water bed, furnished with a small funnelled aperture passing through its middle and ending in a rubber pipe. This pipe passes through the hole in the mattress, and in the board, and is received into a bucket. By this method, the patient can be kept reasonably dry. The buttocks lie over the circular aperture, and may be padded by an air ring.

Plaster Beds.—After a limb has been put up in plaster, the plaster may take some time to dry, and a shock cradle provided with electric bulbs is used. Another method of dealing with such cases is the suspension of the limb from a wire cradle or cage over which the bedclothes can be placed. This type of cage is very useful in many cases of injury or illness when the pressure of the bedclothes cannot be tolerated.

Amputation Beds.—The lower half of the bed should be covered with a draw mackintosh and drawsheet. The stump is raised slightly on a small pillow or sandbag and kept steady with two sandbags and an extension cloth. A cradle is placed over

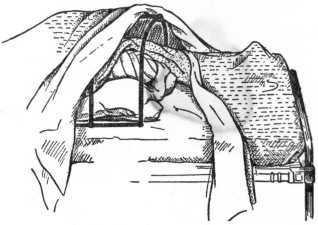

FIG. 82.—AMPUTATION BED.

this. The other leg is covered with a blanket or long theatre stocking and a divided bed is made over the cradle. The lower half may remain over the cradle or may be tucked under.

Rheumatic Beds ; Renal Beds.—For acute rheumatism and acute nephritis (infection of the kidney) the beds are very similar. Owing to the great amount of perspiration it is necessary to retain as much heat as possible and to absorb the moisture. Blankets are therefore put below and above the patient and exchanged for dry ones when necessary. The draw mackintosh and drawsheet are narrow (only 18 inches in width). In acute rheumatism either no pillow is given, or one small one only, as it is necessary to nurse the patient as flat on his bed as possible. In renal conditions pillows may be given for comfort.

Beds for Heart Cases.—Heart cases are always difficult to nurse. In the beginning, the inflammation of the lining of the heart is so acute that the patient must have absolute rest on his back, and therefore pillows are often dispensed with. In advanced heart disease, the back pressure on the lungs is so great that there is difficulty in breathing, a condition called dyspnoea. The patient becomes very restless and requires constant attention because he

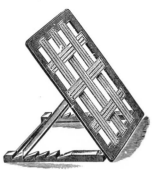

Fig. 83.—Wooden Back Rest with Web Centre.
(By courtesy of the Surgical Manufacturing Co., Ltd., London.)

seeks a new position of possible greater comfort every few minutes. He should be put into a half sitting posture with

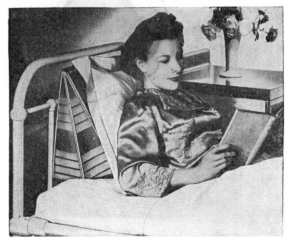

Fig. 84.—Dunlopillo Bolster used as a Back Rest.
(By permission of the Dunlop Rubber Co., Ltd., London.)

stiff pillows at his back, or better, a bed rest (Fig. 83). The adjustable Dunlopillo bolster can also be used, the most suitable arrangement being as shown.

At one time Fowler's position was used in cases requiring special drainage (empyema, acute abdominal abscess and similar conditions) but nowadays this is regarded as out of date.

Some patients like to let their heads fall forward on a pillow, and in this position only can they get any sleep. If a bed table is covered with a small pillow, it forms a very satisfactory rest (Fig. 86). The nursing of advanced cases with great swellings due to dropsy is very hard work ; some patients end their days propped up in armchairs as they cannot lie in bed.

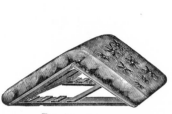

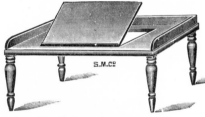

Fig. 85.—Adjustable
Leg Rest.

Fig. 86.—Wooden Bed Table with
Reading Desk.

(By courtesy of the Surgical Manufacturing Co., Ltd., London.

Adjuncts to Beds.—Air rings, air cushions, air beds and water beds are all special methods of giving support while causing the least pressure, and are much employed. These are discussed in the next chapter. In addition to these, other helpful comforts are special bedside tables, reading tables, foot rests and the cradles or cages already mentioned. In an emergency, a foot rest can be improvised from a three-legged stool or a hard pillow (this is often used in midwifery), while a bed rest can be extemporized out of a kitchen or deck chair.

CHAPTER 5

BEDSORES : SPECIAL TYPES OF BEDS AND PILLOWS : HEATING OF BEDS

BEDSORES. CAUSES. PROGRESS OF BEDSORES. SYMPTOMS
AND SIGNS. TREATMENT. SPECIAL TYPES OF BEDS AND
PILLOWS. AIR BEDS. AIR PILLOWS AND RINGS. RUBBER
MATTRESSES. HEATING OF BEDS. HOT WATER BOTTLES.

SOMETIMES a bedsore occurs despite the greatest care and attention on the part of the nurse. While this condition can be prevented in the majority of cases, it does not follow that the nurse should be blamed for carelessness when it does occur; often circumstances are such that a bedsore is produced on account of difficulties associated with the patient's environment or with the disease from which he is suffering. As a general rule, however, every nurse, provided she has the facilities for efficient nursing, should make a special point of preventing bedsores. This may involve the use of water beds, water pillows, air pillows and many other appliances devised to take the pressure off the skin. These are all described below; in addition the subject of heating of beds is conveniently discussed.

Bedsores

When a bedsore breaks out, it is a complication which adds further load to a case already burdened with difficulties. The nurse's task is increased tenfold; the condition means almost constant work and often the most skilled treatment fails to improve the lesion. The difficulties are most marked in out-of-the-way places, where the usual hospital appliances and facilities are not available.

Causes.—These can be divided into general causes and local causes.

General causes are those associated with old age, with general debility, with chronic heart or kidney disease, with excessive fat, with advanced emaciation and with many nervous diseases. An old person usually suffers from poor circulation and is not able to change his position in bed ; therefore he tends to keep the pressure on one spot.   Weak persons e.g. after typhoid fever or peritonitis are in a similar category.   Those with heart and kidney complaints suffer from waterlogging of the tissues with fluid and the skin is soft and easily broken down ; added to this there is frequently the irritation of certain parts of the skin by incontinence of urine.   People who are too fat are also prone to develop a boggy condition of the skin and underlying tissues; on the other hand, thin people have little or no fleshy or fatty pads on their bony prominences, and so the skin is worn through. In nervous diseases, usually accompanied by paralysis, the sensation is lost and the general nutrition of the part is affected. This results in a characteristic abrasion called trophic sore.   In certain types of paralysis it is almost impossible to avoid this variety of bedsore, the occurrence of which makes the nursing very difficult.

Local causes include all conditions in which the local blood supply to the part is deficient, this being the exciting cause of all bedsores. Thus, as we already know (see p. 260), a bedsore may be looked for at certain special areas where the patient, in his recumbent position, inevitably rests the weight of his body i.e. the bony prominences.   The occipital part of the head, the shoulders, the elbows, the rounded knobs marking the line of the spine on the back, the sacrum, the spines of the ilium, the great trochanters, the heels—indeed any part exposed to constant pressure—are the commonest sites.

In addition to the above local causes, however, there is a class which comprises the bedsores resulting from irritation or rubbing of a susceptible part.   It is well known that those who are confined to bed for any length of time become restless and irritable.   The frequent rubbing of the elbows on the sheet, or the rubbing of the ankles against each other, or the rubbing of folds of skin made unbearably itchy by sweat or urine (e.g. the folds of the buttocks) ultimately passes from redness to inflammation, accompanied by irritation, smarting and excessive tenderness, and finally to ulceration.   In the pressure sore there is not so much pain; redness may precede the breaking of the skin surface, but the most characteristic feature is the soft, pulpy appearance of the skin, which looks like lard covered by a thin membrane.

Progress of Bedsores.—In a very short time after the abrasion has occurred, the skin begins to slough, which means that there is actually local death of the tissues, which are cast off. A mild form of circumscribed gangrene is presented.   The rate of development of the bedsore depends upon many contributory factors.   For instance, a patient who is allowed to remain lying on bedclothes soaked with urine or who is so situated that the toilet of the body can be carried out only at infrequent intervals, is in the ideal environment for further stagnation of the circulation, and his bedsore advances rapidly. Moist heat, wrinkles in the sheets or clothing, crumbs allowed to lie under the patient's back, the pressure of appliances and other apparently trivial agents are all contributory factors in the development of the condition.

Symptoms and Signs.—To begin with, the patient may complain of a slight ticklish sensation in the affected part, but the observant nurse will always, in her routine examination, anticipate the appearance of the blush on the skin, which is the sure sign of weakened circulation to a part. If the bedsore is allowed to develop, the irritation will become a real difficulty to the patient. The burning heat is much the same as the pain of neuritis. The patient may or may not rub the skin. If he does, it hastens the abrasion of the part and ere long a small circular ulcer is seen, the circumference of which rapidly increases. In those who have nervous diseases of the spinal cord, the absence of sensory impulses from the part affected may delude the patient—sometimes the nurse—into the belief that all is well. Let the efficient nurse keep in mind therefore that signs and not symptoms are of chief importance to her. She should really take it for granted that in paralysed patients a bedsore will threaten, and she should be ready, on the appearance of the faintest blush, to apply pads of cotton wool.

The bedsore which has gone beyond control is a very unsavoury sight. Deep ulcers, the size of a crown piece, with evil smelling sloughs at their base, and with unhealthy edges surrounded by angry looking skin tissue, give the impression of disease of a very callous type. In very severe conditions the underlying bone may be exposed.

Treatment.—The preventive measures have already been discussed (see p. 260), and even after the first signs of irritation and reddening, they may be applied and used to ward off further development.

In the established bedsore, a state of affairs exists which demands the cooperation of the doctor ; the slightest break in the skin should be reported without delay, therefore, so that appropriate measures may be taken to apply the proper treatment. There are various remedies. Usually the first dressings aim at removal of all dead tissues and other sloughing matter. This can be accomplished by cutting pieces of boracic lint exactly the shape of the ulcer and making a moist dressing by soaking the lint in boiling water, and when cooled app'ying it to the sore with a guttapercha tissue cover. Other weak antiseptics may be used, incorporated in fine gauze. Monsol or dettol solution is soothing and yet very powerful, and acts very satisfactorily.

Once the ulcer is clean some stimulating lotion must be used to help the healing process.   Ointment of zinc oxide, alone or combined with sphagnol ointment, ichthyol, tannic acid, magnesium sulphate, zinc sulphate or gauze incorporated with bismuth, is very efficient.   The sulphonamides and penicillin may be used.   But the most important thing to maintain is reduced pressure on the affected part, and the utmost care must be taken to ensure that all the factors productive of the condition are eliminated.   The use of beds specially constructed as described below, the addition of air pillows, rings, cushions and so on and the efficient padding of a wide area round the sore will hasten recovery.   A very good pad can be made by taking several thin squares of cotton wool, " fluffing " each one out, so that it is full of air, and laying one layer over another in a succession of pads.   The cushion so formed is fixed at the edges either with wound varnish or with strips of adhesive plaster and forms a sound pad which takes all the pressure from the ulcer. In moving patients with bad bedsores, and especially in providing them with bedpans and urinals, the greatest care must be taken that the affected area is not aggravated by the procedure.   Bedsore cases demand all the patience, ingenuity and attention of the nurse in charge.

Special Types of Beds and Pillows

Air Beds.—Massive rubber bags partially filled with air, or divided up into transverse tubes, each filled with air, are the best known forms of air bed, which is never at any time so satisfactory as the water bed.   In the tubular type of air bed it is possible to arrange the air in each compartment according to the needs of the case—thus to a certain extent this form is handy as a mould for the body as well as a support, and it allows for careful and accurate adjustment.   A special pump usually is provided for all air beds and pillows.   Success depends upon the introduction of just the right amount of air—not too much to make the patient roll off the bed and not too little to allow him to sink down in the middle and expel all the air to the edges.

Air Pillows and Rings.—We are all familiar with the common types of air pillow and air ring.   These are of great use, as they are smaller than the air beds or water beds and they can be moved easily and fixed according to the special circumstances of the case.   They are used for the head and for the buttocks, the ring pillow being frequently employed to take the strain off the sacrum in those who are sitting up in bed or who are in the semi-recumbent position.

In filling all air-containing appliances, nurses should remember that they should never commit the outrage against asepsis by blowing up the bag with their own breath; on all occasions the pump should be used. When not in use all such appliances should be left dry, and hung up (not folded) with enough air inside to keep the inner surfaces from touching, and in a dark cupboard away from the light, which has a deleterious effect on rubber.

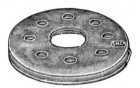

Water Beds and Pillows.—Water beds are very commonly used; they are heavier and more unwieldy than air beds and must be safely fixed on the bed. In most cases the base of the

Fig. 87.—Circular Air Ring.

(By courtesy of the Surgical Manufacturing Co., Ltd., London.)

bed must be strengthened with boards similar to those used for spinal fracture cases. When a water bed is ordered, the following should be the order of the bed from the wire mattress upwards: wire mattress; fracture boards; hair mattress; mattress cover; mackintosh sheet or old blanket; water bed; blanket well fixed over the water bed by tucking in the sides carefully; waterproof sheet; bottom sheet; draw sheet. The rest of the bed is as usual.

Before putting a patient on a water bed, see that it is of the proper size, that it does not leak and that it contains the right amount of water, so that the patient is comfortably suspended. The most practical way to install a water bed is to test its freedom from small holes or other damage, and then to place it in position on the bed. There is a nozzle at one corner (Fig. 88). See that

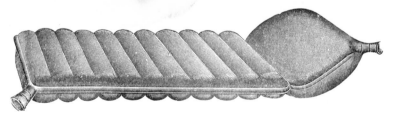

Fig. 88.—Combined Air Pillow and Water Bed.
(By courtesy of the Surgical Manufacturing Co., Ltd., London.)

this is freely accessible at the foot of the bed. Have several jugs of water at about 80° F. by the bed. A little formalin may be added to the water to prevent decomposition. Carefully pour in the water, using a funnel (some beds have rubber funnels fixed). There are various ways of testing the efficiency of the bed. Some press firmly with both hands and make sure that they cannot touch the underlying hair mattress; others use the unofficial method of employing the healthy human being (nurse or porter) as a test weight. If a patient is on a water bed for many weeks the water will require to be added to and 2–3 pints may be needed. This should not disturb the patient.

As with air beds, water beds should be stored in a dark place. It should be ascertained that the rubber inside is clean. Most authorities recommend that a little air be left in water beds to keep the internal surfaces apart, but in some cases enough water is allowed to remain in order to prevent the lining becoming adherent. All oils or greasy preparations should be avoided, but talcum powder can be used with advantage in dry water beds.

Rubber Mattresses.—Various types of solid and partially aerated rubber mattresses are now increasingly supplied. The

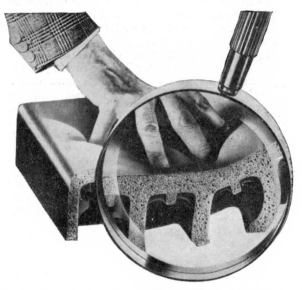

FIG. 89.—STRUCTURE OF AERATED RUBBER MATTRESS (DUNLOPILLO).
(By courtesy of the Dunlop Rubber Company, Ltd., London.)

basis is generally of the spongy rubber which gives buoyancy to the mattress. These mattresses have the advantage of being strong, efficient, comfortable, easily cleaned and of long usefulness.

Heating of Beds

Electrical devices for the heating of beds are now in common use, and it cannot be long before electrically heated blankets or cushions are universally employed (see Figs. 90 and 91). Meanwhile if steady heat is required, a cage can be introduced, as described elsewhere, and the heat from an electric bulb used.

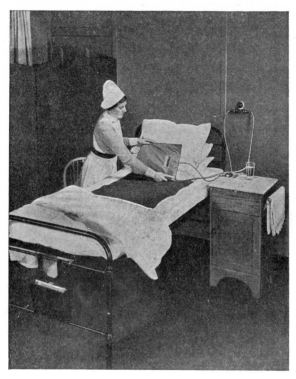

FIG. 90.—ELECTRICAL HEATING OF BEDS.
Both pillow and blanket are heated from a two-way switch at the bedside.
(By courtesy of Thermega, Ltd., London.)

Apart from these special methods, however, the old established and well tried hot water bottle is the chief means of keeping a patient warm in bed.

Hot Water Bottles.—The earliest type is the earthenware bottle. Of similar shape and size is the aluminium or tin bottle. These stand boiling water well, and retain their heat for a lengthy period, but they are hard and clumsy, and even dangerous from the point of view of cracks, breakages and burns inflicted on the patient, so the hot waterbag of rubber is the most popular. One of the most elementary accomplishments of the nurse is the correct method of filling a rubber hot water bag. A jug and funnel should be used, with the bag lying on a flat surface. The water should not be boiling and should have been poured into the jug some minutes previously. The bottle should be half filled only, then the air is pressed out and the stopper screwed in. The bottle should be held upside down and shaken a little to ascertain that it is not leaking anywhere and then completely covered in a flannel bag and fastened in. It should for safety be placed a sheet and a blanket away from the patient.

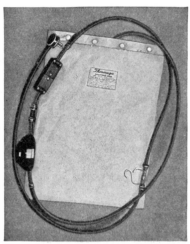

Fig. 91.—Electrically Heated Pad, useful for Many Forms of Rheumatism, as well as for General Comfort of the Patient

(*By courtesy of Thermega, Ltd., London.*)

If a burn should occur as a result of want of care on the nurse's part, it is a black mark against her for the rest of her career; indeed, in some cases it has led to legal action being taken. The greatest pains should always be taken to prevent all possibility of burns by hot water bags.

A patient who is unconscious for any reason does not feel the heat or pressure of the bottle and may develop a burn or pressure sore from it. Those who are paralysed may feel but may be unable to remove the limb from the bottle. It is therefore much wiser not to use hot water bottles in these cases.

CHAPTER 6

RECORDS ; TEMPERATURE ; PULSE ; RESPIRATION

INFORMATION : HOW TO COLLECT IT. THE STATE OF THE
PATIENT. HOW DOES THE PATIENT LOOK? THE CON-
DUCT OF THE PATIENT. THE IMPORTANCE OF PAIN.
CHARTING. THE TEMPERATURE. THE CLINICAL THER-
MOMETER. THE FAHRENHEIT SCALE. HOW TO TAKE THE
TEMPERATURE. THE NORMAL TEMPERATURE. ABNORMAL
TEMPERATURE. TYPES OF FEVER. THE FEBRILE STATES
SUMMARIZED. RIGORS. TERMINATION OF FEVER.
TIMES AT WHICH TEMPERATURE SHOULD BE TAKEN.
THE PULSE. HOW TO ESTIMATE THE PULSE. PULSE
RATE. VOLUME. TENSION. RHYTHM. OTHER TYPES
OF PULSE. RESPIRATION. RATE OF BREATHING.
VARIETIES OF BREATHING. DYSPNOEA. ORTHOPNOEA.
STRIDOR. STERTOR. ACCOMPANIMENTS. APNOEA. CHEYNE-
STOKES BREATHING. CYANOSIS. COUGH AND SPUTUM.

It is the nurse's duty to find out all she can about her patient so
that the doctor may be enabled to make his diagnosis and give
orders regarding the treatment. The doctor is with the patient
for only a short time, the nurse all day, and so she has greater
opportunity to see and hear more of her patient. The patient
will complain of various pains, sensations and states—these are
termed symptoms; the nurse sees things for herself—these are
referred to as signs. The patient may complain for example of
shivering and of feeling thirsty. The nurse takes the temperature
of the patient and sees that the mercury denotes a rise. The
patient complains of pain on coughing ; the nurse notes that
there is distress when the patient coughs. Facts must be given
clearly and simply and without any opinion being expressed.
A notebook is handy and more reliable than many memories.

When the doctor arrives, therefore, whether it be in the ward
or in the sickroom of private practice, the nurse should have all
the important occurrences of the previous 24 hours marshalled
in her brain, and in addition to having ready the details and
written statement of the various essential records, she should be
ready to answer any questions about the conduct or appearance

of her patient which may add some constructive evidence to the case. It is a waste of time to make observations in an abstract and indefinite way. What the doctor wants is not the opinion of the nurse, but a clear cut, exact statement of the facts observed by her during her period of duty, and these facts should neither be embellished nor belittled by language stimulated by the idea or the imagination of the person making the report.

Information: How to Collect It.—All symptoms should be substantiated by signs, and the nurse should use all her powers of examination and deduction in the quest of abnormal demonstrations in the various systems of her patient. For instance a patient may complain of pains shooting down from the small of the back to the bladder; this may be a symptom of many ailments, but when the nurse notes that in addition there is frequency of passing urine, coupled with a smoky or reddish appearance of the urine, she is bringing the diagnosis to a much more accurate basis which will probably become definitely one of small stone in the kidney. Aware of the normal from her knowledge of anatomy, physiology and hygiene, the nurse must therefore be ready to discover any deviations from it, however small they may be ; this is the whole art of diagnosis. On pp. 252 and 253, reference was made to the details required from the patient on admission, most of which were concerned with the historical aspect of the case ; the routine of the day in the ward also involved close observation and record. It is now necessary to outline the main principles which must guide the nurse in her personal investigation of the patient's condition.

The State of the Patient.—It is very difficult to know how to begin the examination of a sick person. Confusing factors are the complaints of the patient, the excited and worrying attitude of most relatives, the alarming conditions of the disease and so on. Below is given a list of the main things to be noted in all diseases.

How Does the Patient Look ?—This question must be answered as clearly and concisely as possible. The face is the chief register of abnormal sensations. From its expression we can deduce pain, sickness, depression, exaltation, weakness or distress. The lines of the mouth, the state of the eyes, the complexion, the colour of the lips, the condition of the skin, all have their meaning. The wide eyed, highly flushed and restless head of acute lung trouble can be distinguished from the narrow eyed, pale faced and stiffly held head and the pursed lips usually indicative of abdominal inflammation. Again, the ivory pallor of anaemia, the dusky white of wasting disease, the yellow of jaundice and the purple of congestive chest troubles are all important signs which lead us to the real seat of the disease at which the remedy must be applied. There is no limit to the information an observant nurse can provide if she keeps her eyes open. For instance, a transient jaundice may appear in the evening or a hectic flush on the cheek at night. The doctor may not be on the spot to observe these himself, therefore he trusts to the nurse to tell him exactly how the change comes on and how it passes off. In these matters the nurse may indeed provide the key to the whole situation.

The Conduct of the Patient.—Another very important aspect of observation is the attitude of the patient. A casual visitor to a ward sees patients lying in various positions presumably because each invalid selects the posture of his body and limbs according to the comfort and freedom from pain produced by doing so. But in 24 hours the position may change markedly; it is an unfortunate, but nevertheless undeniable, fact that the patient makes a supreme effort in the majority of cases to appear at his best when the doctor is making his call. The latter must be told of any unusual attitudes adopted by his patient. As a general rule, abdominal pain causes the patient to lie in bed on his back, with his knees drawn up, since this position takes all the tension from the abdominal muscles. Intermittent pain in the abdomen, caused by colic of digestive or renal origin, makes the patient unsettled, apprehensive and restless ; during an attack he will double himself up and press his hands on the abdomen as if to squeeze out the pain. All people affected with acute lung ailments or with chronic defect of the heart adopt the upright position in bed, as it gives the accessory muscles of respiration more scope to do the extra work entailed and minimizes the pressure of superfluous fluid in the thorax. In very severe heart disease, the patient may not be able to remain in bed at all ; frequently the nurse has to report that he has spent the night sitting up in an armchair. When severe pain exists in the side of the chest, the patient usually likes to lie on the affected side for two reasons. First it gives the sound side the maximum range of movement and secondly it puts the affected lung or pleura in the position of greatest inactivity and so reduces the pain to the minimum. Unconsciousness is a condition which results from numerous physical states, and the behaviour and attitude of the patient in the state of coma are in a category by themselves. The nurse should note all the evidences of rigidity, twitching, convulsions or the passive, almost lifeless condition of grave collapse which may be found.

The Importance of Pain.—Pain is a symptom, but it is too dramatic to be unheeded, therefore it is perhaps the outstanding subjective demonstration of the patient which requires careful investigation. Of the varieties of pain, nothing need be said at this point, since in the general diseases each symptom is fully described, but the nurse should bear in mind that pains vary in intensity and patients vary in sensitivity, so that there is a

284 *RECORDS; TEMPERATURE; PULSE; RESPIRATION*

wide range of variety in the sensation of pain. She must be on
the alert for the casual and mild complaint of the impassive
person. The slightest pain may mean a serious complication, but
the converse is equally true. Real pain is upsetting to all the
sensory sides of the patient's system ; when it recurs at regular
intervals, and with unvarying characters, it is a sure sign that it is
a proper interpretation of the defect which prompts its occurrence. Experience of acute appendicitis is one proof of the
fallacy of concluding that relief of pain means recovery ; often
when pain passes off in this ailment it is the sign of abscess
formation.

Charting

In addition to the case sheet filled up for each patient, there is
the familiar so-called temperature chart which must be kept

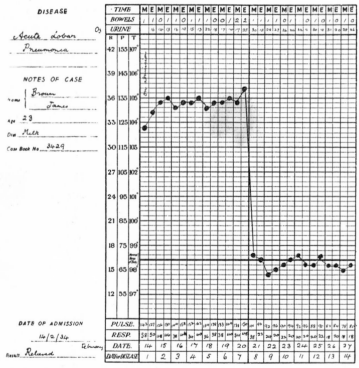

FIG. 92.—DAILY CHART OF A TYPICAL CASE OF ACUTE PNEUMONIA, SHOWING
HOW THE CRISIS MAY OCCUR WITHIN 12 HOURS.

Note gradual decline of rate of pulse and respiration, also increase of
daily amount of urine.

up to date by the nurse. While the notes of examination, treatment and progress are entered almost invariably by the qualified medical man or the advanced student, the entering up of the details on the temperature chart is in the nurse's province, and therefore a knowledge of correct charting is essential to the proper conduct of the case. The ordinary temperature

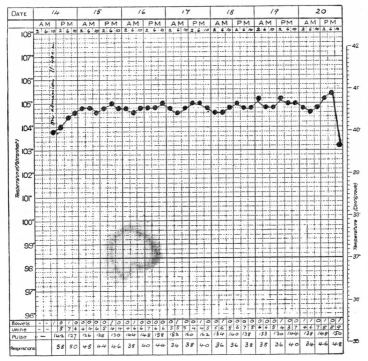

FIG. 93.—4-HOURLY CHART OF THE CASE OF PNEUMONIA
SHOWN ON FIG. 92.

chart is of two varieties, the 4-hourly chart and the " morning and evening " chart. But, as mentioned above, the temperature chart is not a document which registers the fluctuations of the temperature alone. In Figs. 92 and 93 are reproduced 2 typical charts and it will be observed that the following details must be entered up, in addition to the name, age and disease of the patient.

1. The date.
2. The pulse rate, morning and evening.
3. The average rate of respiration, morning and evening.
4. The day of the disease.

5. The daily amount of urine passed.
6. The number of bowel motions for the day.

The temperature chart is made up of vertical and horizontal lines. The former divide the chart into days and weeks by thin and thick lines respectively ; the latter indicates the level of temperature by degrees, which are marked on the left hand margin of the sheet. A dotted or heavy black line indicates the level of the normal temperature. In some cases there is a line for every two-tenths, so that very accurate recording is possible. This is done by making a small neat dot in the appropriate column and at the proper level. By joining these dots with fine lines a very clear graph is obtained which has peculiar characteristics according to the disease. Experience soon teaches the nurse to recognize anything unusual on the chart at once, and therefore it is a most useful and almost indispensable record in her work.

The Temperature

The physiology of the heat regulation of the body has already been discussed (Vol. I, pp. 225 and 226). The normal temperature of the body is an index registering the amount of heat in the tissues maintained as a result of the action of all the influences which heat or cool the blood.

The Clinical Thermometer.—The expression, taking the temperature, is commonly used to describe the process of ascertaining the heat of the body at a given time. The instrument in use, the clinical thermometer, is a small glass tube with a bulb

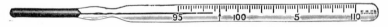

FIG. 94.—CLINICAL THERMOMETER.
(By courtesy of the Surgical Manufacturing Co., Ltd., London.)

at one end. In this bulb is mercury, a substance which is so sensitive to heat that it expands as soon as it is warmed by the slightest amount of heat. The level of the mercury in the bulb is so adjusted that when heat is applied to it it rises into a narrow canal formed by the glass tube. Naturally the mercury will rise to various levels according to the temperature of the substance with which it is in contact. By grading the glass tube in degrees, we obtain a scale which is a register of the heat. Three kinds of thermometer are in use—the Fahrenheit, the Centigrade and Réaumur ; but since the Fahrenheit type is in universal use in Great Britain, it is the only one fully described in this work. The Centigrade thermometer is much used by scientists, and ranges from 0° (freezing point) to 100° (boiling point), or much higher according to the need. The Réaumur thermometer is used in France ; its freezing point is 0°, but its boiling point is 80°. The thermometer registrations can be compared and expressed in terms of each other by doing simple calculations which need not be dealt with here.

The Fahrenheit Scale.—The Fahrenheit thermometer is used by every nurse, therefore it is essential that its mechanism should be fully understood. The lowest point is 95°, a level very close to the bulb. At equal intervals, the levels above are marked by narrow lines cut into the glass and painted black. In this way the indices of temperature are engraved from 95° to 110°—in other words, the range likely to be met in dealing with the heat of the human body under varying conditions of health. Each division on the glass is further subdivided into 5 other small equal divisions by very fine grooves on the glass ; these represent fifths of a degree and are spoken of as ·2, ·4, ·6 and ·8. A small black arrow is cut into the glass with the point at the line indicating the level of 98·4°. This clearly defines the level of the normal temperature. Other markings on the thermometer, apart from the name of the maker, are indications about the length of time the thermometer should be left in the site at which the temperature is being taken. We read the words, " ½ Min.," " 1 Min.," " 2 Min.," and this means that the thermometer must be left, at least, for the period stated. As a matter of fact, it is always best to err on the safe side and to leave thermometers in for several minutes. This is usually the routine in most hospitals. Certain thermometers are more expensive than others, and are very accurate. Those tested at the National Physical Laboratory are marked "N.P.L." and are absolutely trustworthy in all respects. Great care should be taken with thermometers at all times. If they are carried on the person, they should have a stout metal case with a small pledget of cotton wool soaked in disinfectant, preferably lysol ; when belonging to the ward or sickroom, they should be kept in a small glass jar containing glycothymoline or biniodide of mercury solution, 1–4,000. (It should be noted that phenol and certain similar solutions wash off the lettering and make the reading difficult.) In order to sterilize the thermometer after use it should be rinsed well in cold water and left for 5 minutes in a strong solution of mercury perchloride before it is returned to its jar. The bottom of the jar should be padded with several pieces of lint or with cotton wool.

How to Take the Temperature.—The first thing to do is to rinse the thermometer in cold water. It should then be held with the bulb pointing outwards and flicked vigorously several times until the mercury is steady at a level of about 96° ; this procedure usually dries the glass sufficiently. Four well established sites have been adopted for temperature estimation ; the commonest is the mouth, under the tongue ; the others in order of popularity are the axilla, rectum and groin. The choice of site depends upon the type of patient. If there is any danger of biting through the thermometer e.g. in nervous, convulsive or mentally afflicted adults or in young children, the groin or axilla should be used. The rectum is chosen in certain diseases, and usually for a specific reason known to the physician. Within recent years in certain cases the temperature has been taken in the vagina, and interesting variations have been recorded which have caused some controversy. In a series of temperature records, it is essential that they should be the readings at the same time and in the same place each day, as otherwise errors are allowed to come into the chart which alter the true history of the case.

Temperature of the mouth.—The ideal conditions for taking the temperature of the mouth are those in which there has been no possibility of extraneous heat for about half an hour previously. Obviously if a patient has been lying in bed with a poultice on his cheek, the mouth is not the place for the thermometer, but in ordinary cases all hot drinks, exposure to the fire in the room and even smoking should be forbidden for the period stated above. Excessive cold must also be prevented. It will be found most satisfactory if the patient is told to put out the tongue with the mouth half open. The thermometer, checked and prepared, is then placed with the bulb well under one side of the tongue, passing over the lower bicuspid teeth. The patient is warned to avoid closing the teeth, but told to press on the thermometer with the tongue, while keeping the lips firmly closed ; he must be reminded that speaking is forbidden.

Temperature of the axilla and of the groin.—These two sites can be discussed together, as the procedure is much the same in both. The longer the thermometer is left in position the better ; at least 5 minutes should be allowed. Before inserting the bulb, make sure that the axilla is not wet with perspiration, and that there has not been any source of heat (such as a fomentation, a hot water bag, or a poultice) near the axilla for at least 20 minutes ; the same precautions apply to sources of cold e.g. the ice bag in pneumonia cases. All washing and dressing of wounds should have been completed at least half an hour previously. It is essential to make sure that the bulb and as much as possible of the stem of the thermometer are covered by the folds of the skin, which should be closely in contact. In the axilla, therefore, it is best to place the bulb deeply in the angle between the arm and the chest wall, avoiding the danger of breakage by laying the stem paralle to the arm and keeping it in position by carrying the arm across the chest, with the hand over the opposite shoulder, while the elbow is better supported by the patient's other hand. In the groin, the thermometer should be laid in the furrow at the top of the thigh, while the thigh is flexed on the abdomen or the legs crossed above the knees.

Temperature of the rectum.—Although not very often used, this method gives the most accurate reading, as there is the minimum chance of heat loss. It is the approved method for very young children, for unconscious patients and for those emaciated by chronic disease or injury. Unless the rectum is clear of faeces, the method is useless. The patient should be placed on his left side with the knees drawn up. The thermometer is lubricated with olive oil and passed through the anus for about $1\frac{1}{2}$ inches ; it is retained steadily for about 2 minutes, the nurse holding the free end during the process. The patient must never be left alone with a thermometer in the rectum.

In all the above methods, if the same thermometer is used for successive registrations, it must be very carefully cleansed and checked before it is inserted. If there is any doubt about the reading, it should be again made by another thermometer and a second opinion is always advisable. Certain patients take a delight in interfering with the thermometer, and even " cook " the instrument by putting it for a moment on the hot water bag, or by rubbing it vigorously. The strictest discipline must be observed during the period when temperatures are being taken; in all doubtful cases subjects should be watched.

The Normal Temperature.—This expression is used to denote the level on the Fahrenheit scale which is reached by the mercury when a thermometer is in contact with the healthy tissues. As stated on the thermometer, the normal reading is 98·4°. This does not mean that a reading a little above this or a little below it is not compatible with health. Indeed, there are many factors which vary the reading. The rectal temperature is about 1° more than that of the axilla, but it is not so great as that of the blood, which may be taken as about 101°. A reading of 97·4° in the mouth may not mean anything serious ; as a matter of fact, it is often found in those who enjoy robust health. At the other end of the scale, it is different ; any registration above 99° should be regarded with suspicion. An important point is that the temperature varies during the 24-hour day. It is highest in the evening about 5 p.m. and lowest at 2 a.m., when all the bodily functions are universally depressed. There is thus a peak and a valley in the chart when the accurate hourly figures are plotted on paper ; the rise and fall are very gradual. Normal temperature is affected by all the influences of heat and cold discussed in Vol. I, pp. 225 and 226. Sensitive people may

N. II—10*

therefore demonstrate greater diurnal variation than those of stouter constitution, although it may not be found that any disease exists. Common causes of slight rise are exercise, eating and excitement. Temperatures in a ward are notoriously elevated after the visitors have gone.

Abnormal Temperature.—Wide deviations from the 98·4° mark, either above or below the arrow, indicate some abnormality. A subnormal temperature is associated with extreme debility, the collapse of shock, general failure of the circulation or the very weak condition following severe diseases such as enteric fever, diphtheria or dysentery. The readings are always below the 97·6° mark, but in extreme cases a figure as low as 95° may be registered. Death occurs when the temperature falls below 93°.

Above the normal level, the readings vary according to the disease or fever causing them. The amount of temperature is not invariably an indication of the seriousness of the signs and symptoms. A temperature of from 98·8° to 99° may be found in many so-called mild diseases and " low fevers " which make the patient very miserable. A reading of 99° should never be referred to as " only 99." Any temperature above 99° is referred to as pyrexia. The subfebrile state (low pyrexia) is that between 99° and 101°, the moderate pyrexial state between 101° and 103°, while high pyrexia is said to exist when the temperature runs from 103° to 105°. Above 105° the state of hyperpyrexia is established, and it may be found in heat stroke or in very acute fever, indicating that the mechanism of heat regulation has been seriously affected. In life a temperature of 110° F. has been known, but death has soon followed.

It is obvious that with all the above variations of temperature, the taking of the temperature in certain diseases is a very important matter, as certain ailments are associated with fixed levels, and the progress of the disease can be gauged from the temperature chart. Fundamentally, the heat regulating mechanism, apart from extraordinary external influences such as an excessively heated atmosphere, is affected by the reaction of the blood to the invasion or excessive activity of micro-organisms. The condition of fever, with its high temperature and all its other signs, is one resulting from the efforts of the body to overcome foreign germs or their toxins, and the higher the temperature the more is it an indication that a brisk fight is in action.

Types of Fever.—Fever can be recognized in several varieties according to the daily variations. First there may be an increase in the ordinary nightly elevation and a register of some degrees lower in the morning temperature ; an examination of the temperature chart gives the impression that the whole curve of temperature has been moved from the region of the black line to a level farther up. There is often a variation of 3° between morning and evening temperature, but the state of fever never allows the curve to fall below 99°, or higher. This type is called remittent temperature, and is found in acute septic infections, in bronchopneumonia, and in typhoid fever during the second week.

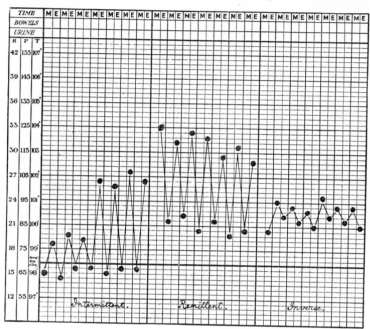

FIG. 95.—THREE COMMON VARIETIES OF FEVER (SEE TEXT).

In certain diseases the fever is high and almost continuous, so that the chart shows a line on a parallel with the normal line, usually in the region of the 103° level, and is characterized by slight, if any, daily variation. To this type of temperature, the name, continuous temperature, is given; it is found in pneumonia, scarlet fever and other diseases (see Figs. 92 and 93).

A third type of temperature is known as intermittent temperature. In this there is a period of normal or subnormal temperature lasting for a few hours or a few days. The temperature "swings" widely, and indicates serious disturbance of the blood. We expect to find it in acute septicaemia, pyaemia and malaria, in which the charts demonstrate high peaks at night and deep valleys in the morning. In certain types of malaria the valley may last for 2 days. This type proves the necessity of taking the temperature at least twice a day. If we were to depend upon the morning temperature only in these acute conditions, there might be very little to record in the way of fever, and the signs would be puzzling. Lastly there is a somewhat rare type of temperature, which is found now and then in phthisis ; instead of a rise of temperature at night and a fall in the morning, the opposite occurs ; this is called inverse temperature (see Figs. 92, 93 and 95).

The Febrile States Summarized.—Correctly speaking, fever is rise of temperature accompanied by marked disturbances of the con titution, as shown by headache, perspiration, dry mouth and tongue, constipation, muscular pains, quick pulse, shivering i.e. the reaction of the whole body to the attack of a mass of micro-organisms. Pyrexia is concerned with rise of temperature alone, but the two terms, pyrexia and fever, are often spoken of as one and the same thing, and it is rare that the state of pyr xia is unaccompanied by fever.

The table given below shows the various ranges of temperatures.

Degree.	*Name.*	*Occurrence.*
96–95	Collapse	Extreme debility; shock.
98–96	Subnormal	Cold; hunger; debility; sometimes natural to the individual.
99–101	Low pyrexia	Chills, colds, influenza.
101–103	Moderate pyrexia	Pneumonia, infectious diseases.
103–105	High pyrexia	Malaria, septicaemia, acute infection.
105 upwards	Hyperpyrexia	Heat stroke, terminal stage of blood poisoning.

Rigors.—When the patient is suddenly attacked by a new or fresh crop of microbes, there is first a flooding of the tissues with the poisons made by the organisms. The body is temporarily depressed by them, and a great and dramatic effort is made by the tissues to neutralize the toxins. This is the condition of rigor, which may occur as the starting point of an illness or as an incident during the course of an illness. It rarely lasts more than half an hour. To begin with there is a feeling of cold, the patient turns pale, and the whole body is seized with a shivering fit which can be heard and felt by those in the vicinity; it is almost a convulsion. The temperature usually shoots up to 104° F. After about 10 minutes, the face becomes red with a dry flush: the patient is restless and thirsty and complains of headache; this is relieved almost immediately by a vigorous perspiration, which may rapidly soak the patient's clothing and even the bed. At this stage the temperature falls as rapidly as it rose, leaving the patient in a weak state almost as bad as that of shock. The whole action goes on so quickly that often the rigor is over before any treatment can be applied, but the after treatment is

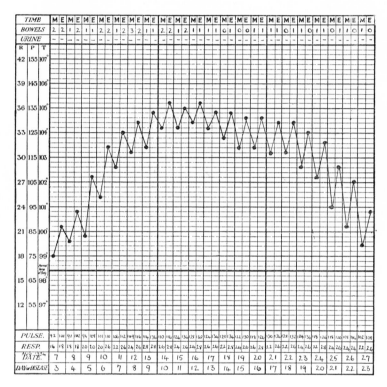

Fig. 96.—Temperature Chart of Typhoid Fever, showing the Typical Ladder Pattern and Lysis in the Third Week.

the most important and should never be missed. The patient requires to be carefully sponged and dried well, and hot water bags should be placed at his sides and feet. Stimulants may be ordered by the doctor. Obviously, a rigor occurring with frequency causes a rapid debility of the patient, and such sharp and sudden strain is one of the gravest dangers in disease.

Termination of Fever.—Fever can end in two ways—by crisis or by lysis. An example of the former is provided by pneumonia which runs the normal course. After 7 days of continuous moderate or severe pyrexia, the temperature suddenly falls to normal or subnormal level. There is a rapid change in the appearance and condition of the patient—from the restless uneasy state to one of comfortable fatigue—and he desires only to sleep. Care must be taken at this very critical juncture, however. A crisis may be accompanied by marked sweating and even diarrhoea and collapse, so that although the temperature has fallen, the patient is not out of the wood. Lysis is a more gradual descent of the temperature level and may occupy 3 or 4 days, with an accompanying steady improvement in the general condition ; it is common in many infectious diseases.

Times at which Temperature should be Taken.—In a 4-hourly chart, the usual hours at which the temperature is recorded are 2 a.m., 6 a.m., 10 a.m., 2 p.m., 6 p.m., and 10 p.m., but in critical or acute cases, observation of the temperature may be necessary at more frequent or more irregular intervals. The ordinary morning and evening chart should be based on the temperature before breakfast and before supper, taken some time between 7 and 8 (a.m. or p.m. as the case may be).

The Pulse

The physiology of the circulation, and the relation of the pulse to it, together with the discussion of blood pressure, are fully described in Vol. I, pp. 168–175. Students are advised to revise this chapter before making a study of the pulse as it applies to the person suffering from a disease.

First and foremost, let it be said that experience helps greatly in the estimation of the pulse. As with physicians, years of practice in this important branch of physical diagnosis give the nurse a peculiar and indefinable power of summing up the general condition of the patient by the palpation of the radial artery at the wrist. It is not the impression of one single factor, but the coordinated reactions of all upon the trained fingers which result in the accurate estimation and appreciation of the situation.

How to Estimate the Pulse.—Every time the heart beats, it sends a wave through all the arteries, so that they are momentarily expanded and enlarged as the increased volume of blood passes through. This causes pulsation, which in the human subject can be observed in any part at which an artery lies superficially. Thus the phenomenon can be observed in the temporal artery, in the carotid artery of the neck and elsewhere. But, a we already know, the classical area for the investigation of the pulse is at the wrist. Here, the radial artery runs down just medial to the lateral aspect of the radius, and will be found very superficially placed at a point about an inch above the junction of the hand and wrist.

The estimation of the pulse should be made with the index, middle and ring fingers of the right hand. The middle finger should be used to make the count of the beats and at least half a minute should be allowed as the unit of time. It is best to approach all patients, but especially those very ill or very nervous, without ceremony or preliminary. When the fingers are placed on the patient's wrist there is, to begin with, an emotional or excited response by the nervous system and the rate is increased, therefore it is an established custom to talk to the patient and to ensure that there is no worry in his mind about the examination. Once it is certain that the pulse is at its normal, usually after about a minute, the official count can be taken and all the other points noted. It is best to make sure that there is no constriction or compression of the arm interfering with the circulation at the wrist. During the pulse test the patient's hand should be placed with the back uppermost, while the examining hand passes over the back of the wrist to allow the tips of the fingers to feel the artery from below ; it can then be pressed against the radius bone. The essential tests are discussed in turn below.

Pulse Rate.—This is stated as the number of beats a minute, the normal rate being 72, but a little less or a little more is quite compatible with sound health. It must also be remembered that, as mentioned previously, digestion, exercise, heat, cold, excitement, the taking of alcohol and so on all tend to raise or lower the rate slightly.

A frequent pulse is one between 80 and 120. It is evidence of the condition of tachycardia, which occurs in very nervous persons, in those suffering from exophthalmic goitre, in bloodlessness, in indigestion, in pyrexia and in those who have been over indulgent in tea or tobacco.

A rapid pulse is one between 120 and 160, and is found in all very acute infections such as blood poisoning, scarlet fever and rheumatic fever.

A running pulse may exceed the 180 mark and its rate may be so fast that it is impossible to count the beats ; it is always a sign of great danger. It is associated with shock, collapse and impending death.

Bradycardia is the condition of slow pulse, and means anything below 60 beats a minute. It may occur as a natural phenomenon of old age, but usually it is found as a serious sign of brain injury or disease, of comatose states and of advanced heart disease.

Generally speaking, if the temperature rises there is an increase of pulse rate with it. A rough method of estimation in use allows about 10 pulse beats for every degree of rise. Thus in a fever with a temperature of 102°, we should expect the pulse to be about 110. There are notable exceptions to this rule, however. When a person is suffering from an overwhelming attack of virulent organisms, the pulse may be very fast while the temperature is moderate ; the thermometer may register only 100°, but the pulse may be 130. This is common in blood poisoning, acute rheumatic fever affecting the lining of the heart, peritonitis and scarlet fever. On the contrary, a group of diseases, including pneumonia, typhoid and paratyphoid fevers, is characterized by high temperature and a rate of pulse which is comparatively slow. For instance, a common chart entry in pneumonia is a temperature of 103° and pulse of 100. If the pulse begins to increase in rate, it is a very bad sign, especially when the temperature is steady or shows signs of falling ; heart-failure is indicated in such circumstances.

Volume.—The examining fingers, in rolling the radial artery beneath the skin against the radius, obtain impressions of the state of the vessel wall, of the size of the vessel and of the tension of the contained blood.

Thus the pulse may be bounding and full, and apart from excitement, may be evidence of a fevered condition. The heart is making its biggest effort to pump the maximum supply of blood at each beat.

The opposite condition is one in which the pulse is small. This may be due to weakness of the heart's action, especially when there is poor muscular tone in long and debilitating disease. The term, thready pulse, is applied to a pulse which admits the minimum volume of blood through at each beat. It may be due to weak heart action, falling blood pressure and congestion of the veins.

Tension.—This is not a very good term, although it is a very old one. It involves two conditions. The first is one in which there is hardening and thickening of the walls of the radial artery as part of a general disease known as arteriosclerosis. The artery may even run a tortuous course, easily appreciated by the fingers. When an attempt is made to stop the pulse, great compression is required, and according to the facility with which the vessel can be closed, the amount of compressibility is defined. A pulse is soft or hard according to the state of the vessel walls. The second condition is one in which the pressure of the blood in the vessel is so great that the power required to overcome it is considerable ; this is the true state of high tension. The methods of testing the blood pressure by the sphygmomanometer are described in Vol. I, pp. 173–175. The common cause of increased tension is inflammation of the kidney, which increases the peripheral resistance. In some cases the volume is very small and the vessel difficult to compress. This very unsatisfactory condition is found in well established abdominal sepsis and inflammation.

A compressible pulse results from loss of tone of the arterial muscles, which are soft, and it indicates flabby heart muscle and general weakness of the central pump. This type of pulse is found in typhoid fever, diphtheria, phthisis and other fevers ; as well as in the semi-collapsed state of prostration after a few weeks of serious illness. Sometimes also in these states the elastic recoil of the aorta sends the secondary dicrotic wave bounding along with much bigger volume, and thus not one, but two, beats are felt at the wrist, a large one followed by a small one.

Rhythm.—Normally the pulse should be regular in time and force i.e. there should be the same strength in each beat and unvarying intervals between the beats. The pulse can be irregular in time, the intervals between the beats being long and short in haphazard fashion. It can also be irregular in force, one beat being much more forcible than the next. When a combination of both occurs it is a serious matter and indicates some fundamental breakdown of the valves of the heart or of the compensating mechanism, or overdoses of certain drugs, or the terminal stages of exhausting infections such as diphtheria. The most advanced type of irregularity is found in auricular fibrillation, a condition in which there is complete disorganization of the heart rhythm, and the radial pulse shows every deviation from the normal—unequal intervals, uneven beats, sudden increase of rate and phases which are frequently imperceptible.

Other Types of Pulse.—Intermittent pulse is the apparent missing of one beat, but it really indicates the crowding of one beat on another, due to premature or extra systole of the heart. The consequence is that there is feeble power in the extraordinary beat, which is not felt at the wrist. A beat is thus apparently missed. It is not a dangerous sign, and is always associated with a slow pulse. Excessive smoking may lead to the condition.

Corrigan's pulse, also known as the water hammer, or collapsible pulse, is found in cases of marked failure of the aortic semilunar valves, which cannot hold the volume of blood issuing from the ventricle. The result is a rapid fall in volume and force after each beat. The pulse is regular and strong, but quickly falls away after each impression is made on the tip of the examining finger.

Capillary pulsation is associated also with aortic regurgitation. The terminal arterioles, full as they are of blood forced suddenly into them, get rid of their contents with a minor wave which is easily observed by closely watching the skin ; this is known as capillary pulsation, and amounts to a sudden blush followed by momentary pallor, the cycle coordinated with the beat of the heart.

Heart block pulse is a pulse as slow as 25 per minute. It results from defect of the atrioventricular bundle (Vol. I, pp. 172 and 173), and may be said to indicate the contractions of the ventricle partially or completely free of its pacemaker. It is a serious condition, often accompanied by fits.

Lastly it should be remembered that there may be differences in the radial pulses of each side; this is very marked in aneurysm of the aorta ; often it is advisable to compare the pulse of one side with that of the other.

Respiration

A revisal of Vol. I, pp. 185–194, is recommended before the nurse goes on to the investigation of abnormal features of breathing discussed below.

Normal breathing is quiet, regular, painless and at the rate of about 18 respirations per minute. It is increased when the carbonic acid gas is in excess of the blood, and in any condition in which there is a demand for more oxygen e.g. in exercise, in taking food and digesting it, and in excitement or worry. It is diminished when a person is at rest or very tired.

Rate of Breathing.—In the first year of life the respirations gradually diminish from 36 per minute to 25 per minute ; from the age of 4 the normal respiration slowly approaches the adult level of 18 per minute, reached about the age of 16. In examining for rate of breathing, we can adopt 2 methods. The first one consists of looking at a fixed point on the chest wall (e.g. at one of the upper intercostal spaces, in the nipple line), and, if possible without the patient's knowledge, taking a count of the total number of rises or falls per minute. The other method is only to be used in special cases in which the visual examination is not satisfactory ; it consists of laying the palm of the hand flat on the upper part of the thorax and of actually feeling the rise of the chest wall.

Normally the ratio of pulse to respiration should be 4 : 1. An increased rate of respiration is found in pneumonia, phthisis, bronchitis, fevers, haemorrhage, shock, abdominal inflammation, heart disease, pleurisy, anaemia and nervous troubles. A decrease occurs in all comatose states resulting from disease or injury to the head, fracture of the skull, concussion, compression, cerebral haemorrhage, poisoning by alcohol, opium or uraemia ; it is found in the dying and emaciated.

It should be also noted that one of the infallible signs of the onset of vomiting is markedly increased respiration.

Varieties of Breathing.—Breathing may vary according to rate, to depth, to rhythm, to type and so on. The chief abnormalities are discussed below.

Dyspnoea.—The meaning of this term is " difficult breathiug." The picture of dyspnoea is not easily forgotten ; the patient usually is very disturbed, sitting up in bed, restless and anxious and changing his position every minute in an attempt to get the proper amount of air into his lungs. Dyspnoea is to be expected in all diseases which involve obstruction to the air passages. Thus it is the chief symptom in asthma, bronchopneumonia and bronchitis, and occurs in heart disease accompanied by congestion of the lungs with fluid. Air hunger is a special variety of dyspnoea, in which the patient makes desperate in hing efforts to get his blood properly oxygenated. It is found updiseases such as uraemia and diabetes, in which the blood is toset in composition by foreign substances which circulate as poisons instead of being broken up and excreted, and in cases in which much loss of blood has occurred.

Ortiopnoea.—The degree of dyspnoea which occurs when the patent is at rest varies with the disease. In very severe illnesses affecting the heart or the lungs, dyspnoea may develop into an extreme condition of orthopnoea, in which the patient may adopt most unusual methods of getting relief from the laboured breathing. Orthopnoea is usually a terminal sign of heart failure ; when the tissues are swollen with fluid and the lungs the encumbered by it almost to the point of strangulation, the most extreme efforts must be made to get air. The patient finds that his only relief is obtained by adopting the upright position in an armchair ; sometimes he will lean forward with his head bd a pillow. Cases have been known in which the patient found relief by kneeling on the pillows of his bed with his face to the iron bars at the top of the bed, and his arms over the bed rail. The idea is to take as much extra strain from the lungs as possible, and since the abdominal organs, themselves suffused with fluid, press heavily on the diaphragm, the more they are allowed to stoop towards the pelvis the better. The state of orthopnoea is on of the most difficult to nurse, and demands special methods quite out of the usual run of ward routine.

In other chest diseases, dyspnoea is a dramatic symptom, but it is not so desperate as orthopnoea, although it alarms those unaccustomed to it. In asthma, for instance, the seizure is sudden the patient sitting up in bed, with bluish congestion of the face, with noisy, wheezy, breathing, and with all the accessory deucles of respiration in full play. The sighing and prolonged and strained respiration adds a pathetic character to the attack, which is not really so bad as it looks, since the spasms often disappear as quickly as they come.

Stridor.—An obstruction of the larynx by a foreign body, by pressure of a new growth, by the spasm of croup or by the diseased membrane of diphtheria causes a type of respiration in which there is a long " crowing " phase. Sometimes the efforts to breath are so marked that the intercostal spaces seem to be sucked in like bellows. To this type of breathing, with its harsh, grating quality, the name, stridor, is given, while stridulous breathing is the term used to designate any breathing with the quality of stridor present.

Stertor.—Stertorous breathing arises in the soft palate, which is sometimes paralysed as a result of injury or nervous disease ; it is akin to the snoring of those in a profound sleep, and occurs when there is unconsciousness resulting from head injury, cerebral haemorrhage, renal and diabetic coma. As the air passes backwards and forwards, it causes a vibration of the curtains of the palate, and stertor is produced.

Accompaniments.—In bronchitis the dyspnoea is not marked, but the respirations, with their characteristic wheeze, and their numerous whistling and cooing accompaniments, advertise the diagnosis of the complaint from the far end of the room.

Pneumonia, on the other hand, although much more serious than bronchitis, is characterized by quiet respiration, which is increased in rate. Standing at the bedside of a pneumonia patient, the nurse will be able to appreciate the soft crackling noise of the respirations caused by the moisture in the alveoli, but the patient exhibits none of the desperate methods of, say, the asthmatic. Sometimes breathing becomes very shallow and almost imperceptible, owing to the onset of painful pleurisy, which forces the patient to make as little effort as possible in breathing. The greater the number of respirations, the shallower they become.

Apnoea.—Apnoea simply means a stoppage of breathing for a temporary period. It is found in cases in which the balance between the oxygen intake and the CO_2 output is disturbed. The breathing suddenly stops, resuming its cycle when the CO_2 has adjusted itself.

Cheyne-Stokes Breathing.—As this is a very dangerous sign, often preceding death, and occurring frequently in unconscious persons, all nurses should learn to recognize it. This is not a difficult matter ; after a few months of night duty, a nurse can train her ear to pick up the characters of Cheyne-Stokes breathing from a long distance ; indeed it is a good way to study the phenomenon. For a few seconds, the breathing is apparently normal. Then the respirations seem to become faster, while the patient takes deeper and deeper breaths ; a certain crisis is reached, like the end of a crescendo, after which there is a gradual inversion of the process, ending in a stoppage of the breathing for a few seconds, and a restart of the whole process. There are various explanations for this peculiar rhythm ; probably it is due to the stimulating effect of lactic acid, which needs more oxygen to split it up into water and carbonic acid gas. The pause is a result of excessive respiration sending out too much CO_2 ; when the latter again accumulates, respiration is once more stimulated.

Cyanosis.—We can grow blue in the face from several causes ; when the latter are serious, the complexion is typical. If the blood is deficient in oxygen and contains too much carbonic acid gas, the capillaries are full of blue blood which shines through the mucous membrane and the skin of the face, showing itself especially in the tip of the nose, the lobes of the ears, the lips and the cheeks. Blue asphyxia is the most marked variety; it is found in sudden cases of obstruction to the breathing (choking, acute diphtheria). In very advanced heart disease, the whole face becomes plum-coloured and cold. The fingers and toes are also affected. Cyanosis is always a fatal sign in such states.

Cough and Sputum.—All respiratory diseases are accompanied by cough and usually a sputum, or spit, is found. These are discussed later under diseases of the respiratory system. The methods of collection of sputum have already been dealt with and are also described later in Section VIII.

CHAPTER 7

THE GIVING OF DRUGS

PRESCRIPTION WRITING. THE FORM OF THE PRESCRIP-
TION. A TYPICAL PRESCRIPTION. COMMON ABBREVIA-
TIONS IN PRESCRIPTIONS. THE MEASURING OF LOTIONS
AND SIMPLE DRUGS. THE IMPERIAL SYSTEM. COMPARISON
BETWEEN WEIGHTS AND MEASURES. COMMON HOUSEHOLD
MEASURES. MAKING UP LOTIONS.

ALL the drugs used in Great Britain are governed by the *British Pharmacopoeia*, which is published by the General Medical Council and which is the official manual in use. Another (unofficial) volume is called the *British Pharmaceutical Codex*, published by the council of the Pharmaceutical Society of Great Britain. While many of the preparations used in the latter are not included in the *British Pharmacopoeia*, and are therefore unofficial, they are, nevertheless, frequently employed by doctors in general practice. The *British Pharmacopoeia* was last revised in 1948, and many changes were made. It is now customary to write the letters, B.P., after the official drugs, while the expression, B.P.C., is used to denote drugs which are taken from the *British Pharmaceutical Codex*.

In hospitals there is invariably a dispensary which is presided over by a qualified dispenser, who has assistants; in this department all the drugs for the hospital are stored and many mixtures, lotions and preparations are made up. It is customary to send out to each ward various types of containers, large and small, filled with the special medicines, general medicines and the lotions and other solutions used in ward routine.

It sometimes happens that the physician or surgeon of the ward may choose to write his own prescriptions in a book specially kept for the purpose in the ward, and, as every nurse should know what these prescriptions mean, a detailed description of the formulas used must now be considered.

Prescription Writing

Whether the doctors' prescriptions be entered in the ward book or whether they be written on the familiar piece of paper which is taken to the chemist by patients treated in private practice, the method of writing out a prescription is established by long years of custom. Properly speaking, all prescriptions should be written in Latin and in full. The reason for this is not to keep the patient from the knowledge of what is being given to cure his ailment nor is it to add any air of mystery to the treatment. A prescription may be utilised all over the world (for example, by travellers) as the names of all elements and drugs are the same for every country. Latin is a universal language which is understood by all dispensing chemists and therefore it has remained the official language on all prescriptions.

The Form of the Prescription.—Generally speaking, the prescription begins with the writing of the symbol ℞ at the top of the paper towards the left hand margin. This is called the superscription and is a shortening of the Latin word *recipe* or " take." A little lower down, and still farther from the left hand margin, is written the inscription, which is a list of the various drugs used in the mixture, pill or powder, as the case may be. Each drug is given a separate line, and the genitive case is used, as it is governed by the word, recipe ; the exception is the vehicle in which the drugs are contained ; this is written in the accusative.

There is a definite order of putting down these drugs. The first drug on the list is usually the most important and the most active agent. This is called the basis. Usually the second drug, sometimes the third as well, assists the action of the basis and is called the adjuvans. Next comes the corrigens or corrector of the action, and finally, the excipient which is also known as the constituens—something which flavours the mixture and makes it more palatable.

The third part of the prescription concerns the directions which are given to the dispenser and is known as the subscription, written immediately below the inscription. It should be written in Latin, although nowadays it is becoming quite common, especially in America and France, to write the subscription in the language of the country.

The signature is the name given to the fourth portion of the prescription, and deals with the directions to the patient. The term actually used is the Latin word *signetur*, which means " let it be labelled." When the dispenser makes up the mixture or other preparation, he writes a translation of the signature on the label and affixes the latter to the bottle.

Many doctors still continue to use Latin as the language of the signature, but this should properly be written in English where English is the prevailing language.

Finally the prescription is concluded by the addition of the initials or name of the doctor who has written the prescription, these being put at the right hand bottom corner, while the patient's name is affixed at the left hand bottom corner, with the date immediately below it.

A Typical Prescription.—

R

Ammonii carbonatis	.	.	.	gr. xl (Basis)
Tinturae scillae	.	.	.	fl. dr. iss. (Adjuvans)
Syrupi tolutani	.	.	.	fl. oz. ss. (Corrigens)
Infusum senegae	.	.	.	ad. fl. oz. vi. (Excipient)
				Fiat mistura

Signetur,

One tablespoonful to be taken three times a day after meals.

Mr. John Brown.

15.1.48.   X.Y.Z.

If this prescription were abbreviated, as prescriptions frequently are, it might be written as follows :

R

Ammon. carb.	.	.	.	.	.	gr. xl.
Tinct. scill.		.	.	.	.	fl. dr. iss.
Syr. tolut.	.	.	.	.	.	fl. oz. ss.
Infus. seneg.	.	.	.	.	.	ad. fl. oz. vi.

Sig.   F.M.

One tablespoonfu ,to be taken three times a day after meals.

Mr. John Brown.

15.1.48.   X.Y.Z.

Common Abbreviations in Prescriptions

It must be confessed that very few doctors are immaculate in the writing of prescriptions, and as it is a well known fact that doctors' writing is frequently almost illegible, the nurse must be prepared to decipher many mysterious hieroglyphics. Druggists and dispensers and all those accustomed to reading abbreviations on ordinary prescriptions, soon become used to the contractions and symbols employed by the medical profession in general; a nurse, after careful study of the common abbreviations, may find that she is equally expert. The following is an alphabetical list of the terms likely to be found on prescriptions given either for a hospital patient or for one treated in general practice :

aa.	.	.	.	Ana	of each
A.C.	.	.	.	Ante cibos	before meals
Ad.	.	.	.	Adde	add
Ad lib.	.	.	.	Ad libitum	according to the desire
Æq.	.	.	.	Æquales	equal
Alter. hor.	.	.	.	Alternis horis	every other hour
Aq.	.	.	.	Aqua	water
Aq. dest.	.	.	.	Aqua destillata	distilled water

Common Abbreviations in Prescriptions—*Continued*

B.d. or B.i.d.	Bis in die	twice a day
c̄	cum	with
Cap.	Capiat	let him take
C.cm. or c.c.	——	cubic centimetre
Co.	Compositus	compound
Collyr.	Collyrium	eye wash
Collut.	Collutorium	mouth wash
Conf.	Confectio	confection
C.m.	Cras mane	tomorrow morning
C.n.	Cras nocte	tomorrow night
Dil.	Dilutus	dilute
Emp.	Emplastrum	plaster
Ex. aq.	Ex aqua	in water
Ft.	Fiat	let it be made
Ft. mist.	Fiat mistura	make a mixture
Fort.	Fortis	strong
Garg.	Gargarisma	gargle
Gutt. gtt.	Gutta	a drop
Hor. decub.	Horâ decubitus	at bedtime
H.n.	Hac nocte	tonight
Linct.	Linctus	a linctus
Lin.	Linimentum	liniment
Liq.	Liquor	solution
Lot.	Lotio	lotion
M. prim.	Mane primo	early in the morning
Mist.	Mistura	mixture
Mit.	Mitte	send
M. & n.	Mane et nocte	morning and night
Ol.	Oleum	oil
O.m.	Omni mane	every morning
Omn. bih.	Omni bihorâ	every two hours
Omn. hor.	Omni horâ	every hour
O.n.	Omni nocte	every night
P.c.	Post cibos	after meals
P.r.n.	Pro re natâ	occasionally; when required
Pulv.	Pulvis	powder
Qq.	Quaque	every
Q.q.h.	Quarta quaque horâ	every four hours
Q.d.s.	Quater die sumendum	four times a day
Q.s.	Quantum sufficit	sufficient quantity.
Rep.	Repetatur	let it be repeated
Ss.	Semisse	one-half
S.o.s.	Si opus sit	if necessary
Stat., st.	Statim	immediately
Sum.	Sumendum	let it be taken
S.V.G.	Spiritus vini gallici	brandy
S.V.R.	Spiritus vini rectificatus	alcohol
T.d., T.i.d., T.d.s.	Ter in die (sumendum)	three times a day
Ung.	Unguentum	ointment

The Measuring of Lotions and Simple Drugs

Two systems of weights and measures are in use—the Imperial and the Metric. In Great Britain both of these are used, but for the present only the main aspects of the Imperial system will be considered, since for the preliminary examination nurses require to know only the elements of the subject, which is fully dealt with in Vol. III, Sect. 7. The standards of these weights and measures are as laid down in the Weights and Measures Act.

The Imperial System.—*Avoirdupois Weight.*—The unit of mass is the grain (*granum*) which is the smallest weight convenient for ordinary use. 437·5 grains = 1 ounce (*uncia*), the symbol of which is " oz." 16 ounces = 1 pound (7,000 grains), represented by the symbol " ℔," a contraction of the Latin word *librum*.

Capacity.—The unit of volume or capacity is the minim, the symbol of which is " min." 60 minims = 1 fluid drachm (fl.dr.). 8 fluid drachms (480 minims) = 1 fluid ounce, which is represented as " fl. oz." 20 fluid ounces = 1 pint (*octarium*), the symbol of which is " O." 8 pints = 1 gallon, represented in short by the letter " C " (*congius*).

Notes.—Many of the former signs and symbols have been abandoned, and the intention of the *British Pharmacopoeia* is to make the weights and measures as simple as possible. The old apothecaries' weight is not used much nowadays, as it is very confusing, the ounce being equivalent to 480 grains. The scruple, ℈, which is one third of a drachm, or 20 grains, is very seldom used, and the drachm, which is equal to 60 grains and which has the symbol ℥ , is rapidly going out of use, but many doctors still employ it.

Similarly, the symbols ℔ for the minim and the ℥ for the fluid drachm, also ℥ for the fluid ounce, are commonly found in prescriptions, but they are not official. In many cases ℥j and ℥j are used to represent avoirdupois weight as 60 grains and 1 ounce respectively, but while medical men are constantly advised not to employ these symbols, the nurse must be prepared to encounter them very often in the course of both hospital and private practice.

Half an ounce is often represented as a double " s " (semisse = one-half). The Greek letter ς (sigma) is often placed first ; the abbreviation for ½ oz. is often incorrectly taken to be " f.s." Actually it is 2 letters " s," the first Greek and the second English.

Comparison between Weights and Measures.—Water is used as the standard liquid in the assessment of all weights and measures. 1 minim is the measure of 0·911 grain of water at a temperature of 62° F. Thus, 100 grains of water at this temperature would measure about 110 minims. As the temperature used is the normal temperature of a comfortable room, it follows that in doing ordinary dispensing the factor of temperature can be neglected ; therefore, a 1 per cent solution of any drug would be made by taking 110 minims of water and dissolving

1 grain of the substance in it. The percentage of mixtures may mean a comparison of weight to weight, of weight to volume, or of volume to volumes.

Common Household Measures.—In general practice, the doctor writes on the prescription the accurate amount of medicine which is to be given to the patient. The druggist, therefore, in writing the instructions on the label, translates the signature of the doctor into language which is easily understood by the patient. Since spoons, wineglasses, tumblers and cups are the common domestic utensils, the doses of medicine are usually expressed in teaspoonfuls, dessertspoonfuls, wineglassfuls and so on ; unfortunately, as is proved by all general practitioners of experience, the size of the teaspoon and of all other domestic utensils is one of the most variable things in the world; therefore a teaspoonful in one household may be equivalent to a dessertspoonful in another. So far as the nurse is concerned, whether she be in hospital or in private practice, she must make a point of always using the standard glass measure which can be purchased either in a surgical instrument maker's shop or at a drug store.

Domestic Equivalents.—As a general rule the following are the domestic equivalents of the official measures, but as stated above, there is no standardization :

1 minim	= 1 drop (approximately)
1 fl. dr.	= 1 large teaspoonful
2 fl. dr.	= 1 dessertspoonful
4 fl. dr. or ½ oz.	= 1 tablespoonful (represented on prescription by ℥ ss.)
2 fl. oz.	= 1 wineglassful
5 fl. oz.	= 1 teacupful
8 fl. oz.	= 1 breakfastcupful
11 fl. oz.	= 1 tumblerful

Making up Lotions.—Most lotions in ward use are represented by percentages ; that is to say, ordinary solutions, such as phenol lotion, may be found in several strengths, varying from 1 per cent to 10 per cent. Knowing that 1 per cent solution is for all practical purposes 1 grain of a substance dissolved in 110 minims of water, it is a simple matter to make up lotions of various strengths. If a 10 per cent solution is required, then 10 grains must be added to 110 minims of water and so on. Solutions may be increased or decreased in strength according to the directions of the sisters in charge of the ward. As a general rule, the stock solutions required in the wards are delivered in a fixed strength. If it is necessary to decrease the strength of the solution, from, say, 10 per cent to 1 per cent, more water must be added to the concentrated lotion ; in this case, nine times as much as the original amount to make the 10 per cent solution.

In the same way, if we have 8 oz. of a 20 per cent solution of phenol, and we wish to make a 5 per cent solution, we must add 3 times the quantity of water present i.e. 24 oz. The total then becomes 32 oz. and the strength of the phenol is 5 per cent. In making a solution stronger, the weight of the material to be dissolved must be calculated according to the amount of increased strength; for example, if we take a 1 per cent solution of any drug and wish to make it a 10 per cent solution, nine times the original amount of drug used must be added to the existing liquid to bring it up to 10 per cent strength.

Nurses frequently have to make these calculations and it is essential that no mistakes occur, otherwise grave consequences may result. This is especially important with strong disinfectants and other poisons. There are various formulas which are intended to help the nurse in remembering how to calculate the quantities required of lotions and solutions, but it is better to take each case separately and to work the problem out, as by this method mistakes can be avoided.

CHAPTER 8

SPECIAL APPLICATIONS AND METHODS OF GIVING DRUGS

INHALATIONS. THE USE OF THE INHALER. OXYGEN ADMINISTRATION. METHODS OF ADMINISTRATION. TUDOR EDWARDS FRAMES. Y-SHAPED TUBE. B.L.B. MASK. OXYGEN TENTS. FOMENTATIONS. HOW HEAT AFFECTS DISEASED TISSUE. MEDICAL FOMENTATIONS. APPLICATION OF COLD. COLD COMPRESS. ICE POULTICE. ICE BAG.

THERE are various ways of introducing drugs into the body, apart from the ordinary method of giving medicines by the mouth. A remedy may be inhaled and therefore taken into the small chambers of the lungs, or it may be absorbed from the skin, or function by its reaction on the skin e.g. in fomentations, ice bags and similar applications. The other methods of giving drugs—by injection or by the rectum—are discussed later.

Inhalations

There are 2 types of apparatus for giving inhalations : 1. the inhaler ; 2. the steam kettle.

The Use of the Inhaler.—All methods of inhalation depend upon the intake, with every inspiration, of a certain amount of a drug, which is very finely distributed in hot vapour. When this specially treated vapour reaches the alveoli, it is spread out on the surface of the small chambers and is thus easily absorbed by the blood. Inhalations are therefore useful in all bronchial conditions, especially in cases in which there is congestion of the fine bronchioles. The method of inhalation is also used largely in inflammations and in catarrhal conditions of the upper parts of the respiratory tract e.g. in inflammation of the larynx, in ordinary sore throat, in diphtheria, in croup and in all irritations due to the effects of microbic activity. Inhalation is not only soothing to the patient ; it is also a very effective way of producing the maximum action of the drug over a given area. There are two methods of giving inhalation treatment—the moist method and the dry method.

The Moist Method.—The commonest and most popular method

of giving an inhalation is by using an earthenware jug (Fig. 97), known as Nelson's inhaler. As shown in the illustration, this consists of a fairly stout, glazed earthenware pot, fitted with a cork, through which a glass tube protrudes. To make the inhalation mixture, a pint of water at a temperature of about 180° F. is poured into the jar, and to it is added one of the well known inhalants, the commonest of which is Friar's Balsam, but crystals of menthol, oil of eucalyptus or pine oil are occasionally employed. Great care must be taken that boiling water is not used, as the steam may scald the mouth of the patient. Although the printed instructions on the inhaler may say that boiling water should be used, experience shows that water at a temperature of 180° F. is sufficiently hot to give off enough vapour. It is advisable to have the container not more than half full, and to make sure that the glass tube protrudes for about half an inch only through the cork into the jug. The nurse must ascertain, before giving the patient the inhaler, that the solution is not too hot, and that there is no possibility of drawing any fluid into the mouth when the glass tube is placed there. In order to maintain the temperature as long as possible, it is customary to wrap up the inhaler in a flannel bag and place it in a bowl. A bath towel may be wrapped round. A piece of gauze should be wound round the mouthpiece so that the mouth cannot be scalded. By doing this more comfort is ensured for the patient, since the lips need not grip the mouthpiece so tightly. The treatment can be applied every hour if necessary in acute cases, and it brings great relief, the patient absorbing a considerable quantity of the drug with each inspiration. Each inhalation should last for about 10 minutes.

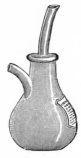

FIG. 97.

NELSON'S INHALER.

(By courtesy of the Surgical Manufacturing Co., Ltd. London.)

Another method well known as a homely remedy for sore throat, laryngitis, tonsillitis and similar conditions is the use of a moderately sized enamelled jug into which boiling water is placed, with a certain quantity of the drug to be inhaled. The steam rises up very copiously, but it cools very quickly, and the inhalation is carried out by the patient holding his head, with his mouth wide open, about a foot above the enamelled jug, while a towel is draped all round his head and round the edge of the basin. In this way the patient's head is enclosed in a sort of miniature tent, and the steam passes both by the mouth and by the nostrils.

A more elaborate method is employed in hospitals, especially when serious cases are being treated. The steam kettle and tent are sometimes used in bad cases of bronchitis or other lung troubles of children. The aim of those prescribing this treatment is to create a constant atmosphere charged with curative drugs, so that the patient, who is enclosed in the tent, breathes medicated air continuously. In some cases pure steam is used when the effect of the warmed air only is required. Usually every large hospital has a special tent frame, which fits over the head of the bed, but in some cases the child's cot is converted by fixing poles at the four corners and draping sheets over the framework so formed. At one side an opening is made, through which the long spout of a kettle is placed. It is possible to im-

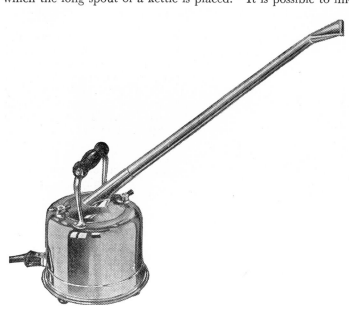

Fig. 98.—Electrical Bronchitis Kettle.
(By courtesy of Messrs. Allen & Hanbury, Ltd., London.)

provise a tent by using screens over which sheets are hung. In all cases of employment of this method, care should be taken that the bed is well protected from draughts which would soon cool the atmosphere.

The steam kettle which supplies the vapour should be set at one side of the bed (Fig. 98). Electricity or spirit may be used for heating the kettle. The former method is modern, and presents little or no difficulty, but the latter, which is the old-fashioned method, demands certain precautions.

In the first place, the kettle must be far enough away from the bed to obviate all possibility of the bedclothes catching fire. Secondly it must be anticipated that there is a danger of the spirit lamp leaking or bursting. The approved method of setting up the spirit lamp and kettle is one which stipulates that an old enamelled basin or other metal container should be put on a chair or stool about the height of the bed ; the spirit lamp is placed on the container and stands in sand. It is also advisable to have a bucket of sand handy in case the fire should spread. The tent is so arranged that the spout of the inhalation kettle passes through an opening which should preferably be on the side farthest away from the door or window. It should also be ensured that there is no possibility of the patient being able to touch the tip of the spout, and that the spout is not in such a position that the fumes will scald the patient in any part of the body. In the case of the child, restrainers or arm splints should be used in order to prevent him from getting down the bed to the spout. Provision should also be made so that there is not too much condensation of the steam. Since there is usually a steady drip from the spout of the kettle, it is advisable to make some arrangement to catch the water as it falls. The temperature inside the tent should never exceed 75° F. The nurse in charge of the steam kettle should see that it is regularly replenished ; to begin with, it should never be more than half filled, and it should be made up with fresh boiling water or a solution of Friar's Balsam, or whatever has been ordered by the physician, at least every 2 hours. This is emphatically a matter for constant watching and adjustment. What must be maintained is a regular and evenly distributed supply of moisture at a steady temperature; a good nurse should always keep an eye on the steam kettle, therefore, making sure that it does not evaporate to dryness, or that it does not splutter and thus sprinkle boiling water on the patient.

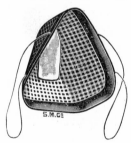

FIG. 99.—BURNEY YEO'S RESPIRATOR.

(By courtesy of the Surgical Manufacturing Co., Ltd., London.)

The Dry Method.—Steam is not used in this method. The drug, which may consist of creosote, chloroform, ether or amyl nitrite, can be placed on a gauze pad or on an anaesthetic mask, which, when fixed over the patient's mouth and nose, allows the drug to be inhaled with each inspiration. The Burney-Yeo inhaler (Fig. 99) has a sponge which is saturated with the drug to be inhaled, and in this way the whole of the drug is absorbed in about a quarter of an hour, but great care is necessary in using it, as the mask is so closely applied to the skin that strong drugs which may have been spilt outside the sponge may damage the face of the patient.   In any case it is always compulsory to apply fine paraffin or lanoline to the area of the face in contact with the mask.   In giving amyl nitrite, which is used for all conditions of high blood pressure or of angina pectoris, a special method is employed.   The drug is generally made up in thin glass phials, which are surrounded by thick lint or cotton wool pads, and when the glass is broken by tapping it sharply, or by crushing it with the fingers, the fluid flows out and the fumes quickly rise.   The approved method of giving this drug to patients is to put one of the capsules in a handkerchief and then to break the glass. The handkerchief and its contents are then applied to the patient's mouth and nose until he recovers.

Anaesthetics are dealt with elsewhere (Section VII, Chapter 6). They are rarely given by the old fashioned open mask, and nowadays the art of inducing anaesthesia is one which demands the greatest skill and long experience.

Oxygen Administration

In all hospitals oxygen is available as a stimulant for severe cases of collapse, whether it be the result of a serious operation, of bleeding, of shock or of cardiac failure.   Oxygen is also very useful in the acute stages of pneumonia, when owing to the inflammation of the lung the normal supply of the gas in the air is difficult to absorb.

Oxygen is kept under pressure in cylinders ; these can be obtained much more easily nowadays than formerly.   Most druggists stock small cylinders, for use in private houses or for emergencies and accidents.   No operation theatre is complete without a cylinder of oxygen, which should be kept handy for the anaesthetist as a remedy in the event of the collapse of the patient while under the anaesthetic.

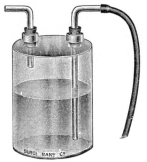

FIG. 100.—WOULFE'S BOTTLE.

*(By courtesy of the Surgical Manu-
facturing Co., Ltd., London.)*

If oxygen were given straight from the cylinder, it would have a very drying effect on the mucous membranes.   To counteract this, it is customary to give oxygen which has been moistened and warmed by passing it first through a Woulfe's bottle (see Fig. 100), which should be half full of warm water.   In cases of great emergency, when there is no time to use a Woulfe's bottle, oxygen must be given straight from the cylinder by rubber tube but a certain amount of risk must be taken regarding the dose.

N. II—11

The oxygen cylinder should be tested daily to see if it is in good order. There is a fine adjustment valve above the tap, which is easily regulated by the hand. The tap opens with a key, an arrow indicating in which direction to turn it. It is always advisable to open the adjustment valve before turning on the tap as the oxygen is under pressure and comes out rather noisily at first. For this reason it should be turned on away from the bedside, so as not to alarm the patients. No vaseline must be used in any adjustment procedures.

On all cylinders nowadays there are gauges which show the amount of pressure within the cylinder; they do not show the speed of flow or amount being used. This is shown by a flow meter measuring the flow in litres per minute.

Methods of Administration.—The method of administration varies ; 3 methods in common use are described below.

Tudor Edwards Frames.—In some cases the Tudor Edwards spectacle frames are used. These are frames with metal tubes attached to the nasal part and fitted with bicycle valve tubing; these are passed up the nostrils. The nose must be cleaned first and the cavity lubricated, preferably with liquid paraffin.

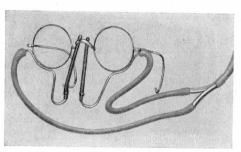

FIG. 101.—TUDOR EDWARDS FRAMES.
(By courtesy of the British Oxygen Co. Ltd., London.)

Y shaped tube.—Another method involves the use of a " Y " shaped tube inverted on a head band; the principle is similar to that mentioned above. The oxygen first passes into the Woulfe's bottle by the longer tube then through the water, and up the delivery tube. The water should be warm, but as the oxygen becomes chilled again as it passes through the delivery tube, it is not necessary to keep it warm.

For the passage of the tubes, a tray is required with boracic swabs, a receiver, liquid paraffin, sinus forceps or orange sticks; sometimes a cocaine spray may be used to ease the discomfort.

B.L.B. Mask.—A third method is based on the use of the Booth-by-Lovelace-Bulbolian ("B.L.B.") Mask. This is a rubber mask which fits over the nose and is fastened round the head with a strap. On either side of the chin is a tube leading from the delivery tube which enters opposite the expiratory valve ; above this is a metal part with perforations called ports, which can be opened or closed by a sliding band. By these ports the oxygen can be diluted with the air as much as is desired. The oxygen enters the bag first and the patient breathes from the bag; if any of the ports are open the gas will be mixed with air. As the patient breathes out, the expired air is mixed with the incoming oxygen, the excess expired air passing out through the valve. The bag when in use should be slightly distended. This method has the advantages of controlling the concentration, and it is also comfortable to the patient after a short time. Another important factor is that nursing treatment can be carried out without handicap. One type of B.L.B. mask has a mouthpiece as well and this has advantages, but it must be removed for feeding and for some kinds of treatment. It is used for patients who cannot breathe through the nose.

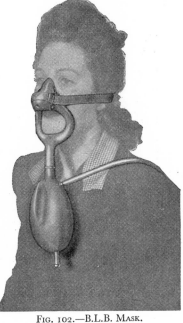

FIG. 102.—B.L.B. MASK.
(*By courtesy of the British Oxygen Co. Ltd., London.*)

Oxygen Tents. — Oxygen tents have been used to much advantage within recent years, but they are cumbersome and very expensive to maintain. There is also danger of fire, therefore the mechanism and working must be fully understood before nursing of a patient in one is attempted. The air inside the tent tends to become hot and humid ; various methods are used to counteract this.

The tent is made of rubber and cellophane or some other thin transparent material ; it hangs over a frame which is mounted on wheels. On one side is a radiator which is packed with ice (this cools and helps to dry the air) and close by is a trough which collects the water which has condensed and which passes to the outside and drains into a bowl. A large cylinder is necessary to keep up the supply of oxygen to the tent ; above the latter is a case of soda lime, which, as the air from the tent leaves, absorbs the carbonic acid gas content; the oxygen from the cylinder joins with this air to return to the tent and so to maintain a constant percentage of oxygen concentration inside.

The structure of the tent allows the sides to be tucked in,

therefore as soon as attention has been given to the patient the sides must be tucked in firmly as otherwise the oxygen content would diminish on account of leakage.

Sleeves are made in the sides to enable minor treatment and attention to be given.

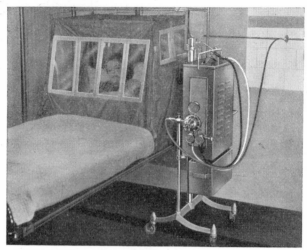

FIG. 103.—OXYGEN TENT.
(By courtesy of the British Oxygen Co. Ltd., London.

The temperature in the oxygen tent should not be more than 65° F. ; this may be checked by reference to the thermometer hung in the tent ; sometimes a Mason's wet and dry bulb thermometer is used.

Fomentations

When we speak of the term, fomentation, we mean an agent which is applied to the surface of the body and which, by the radiation of moist heat, accompanied or not by the action of a drug, has a certain effect on the underlying tissue. The application of fomentations is an everyday occurrence in hospital practice and it is a favourite remedy which has been passed down to us from our grandmothers.

How Heat affects Diseased Tissue.—Underneath the skin is a fine, close network of minute blood vessels running in all directions. These capillaries feed the tissues and keep the skin in a state of health. If there is disease such as inflammation, it may be taken for granted that there is some poisonous element present which the blood is trying to eliminate. Heat has the power to reduce the pain by making more blood reach the surface of the skin and by relieving the pressure in the underlying tissue; it also enables more blood to leave the area, carrying away with it the products of inflammation. We can assume therefore that when constant heat is applied to a certain part of the skin, the area so treated will become red and active looking, because there is increase of blood to the part. It is obvious that a heating agent will maintain the increase of blood supply, and since this allows the liberation of as many leucocytes as possible, there is a complete stimulation of all the powers of repair. In addition to this the muscles are relaxed, and the nerve endings, which have been stimulated by the pressure, are soothed and the pain is reduced to a minimum.

Medical Fomentation.—A medical fomentation (as distinct from a surgical fomentation, details of which are given on p. 348) is an application of moist heat to an unbroken skin surface, made in order to relieve pain and inflammation. Various medicants may be added, but the principle underlying all is the same.

Requisites.—A piece of flannel the required size or a piece of lint doubled to the required size ; jaconet or oiled silk and white wool ; flannelette bandage. The flannel is doubled into a wringer-cloth which is made of strong linen; this is put into a bowl and boiling water is poured over it. It is then wrung out quite dry, given a quick shake (to expel the steam) and applied to the surface. The jaconet and wool are made to cover it and it is bandaged firmly into position. The jaconet square should be a little larger than the fomentation and the wool square still a little larger. The fomentation can be renewed every 2–4 hours.

Turpentine Stupe.—Turpentine stupe may relieve the pain more quickly ; this fomentation is prepared in the same way as is the medical fomentation, with the addition of turpentine (1–4 fluid drachms). The turpentine is sprinkled on the flannel before the boiling water is poured on. The skin must be inspected and usually the stupe can be removed in 20 minutes and warm wool applied. A turpentine stupe is not repeated ; but the warm wool may be reheated when necessary.

Precautions.—Care must be taken, when applying any agent to the skin, that it is not too hot or that the skin is not becoming sodden or the tissues breaking down. The skin must be inspected carefully and any discomfort or pain reported before the next application is made.

Application of Cold

The application of cold is quite as common in medicine as the application of heat. Whereas heat dilates the blood vessels, cold contracts them and causes a local pallor of the skin. Strangely enough, it also has a very soothing effect on any area in which inflammation or acute swelling is present. This is the reason why cold water cloths, or cloths soaked in ice water, are good remedies for sprains and contusions. In a sprain there is sudden bleeding at the part affected, and the swelling is painful owing to great pressure. When a cold compress is applied, the arteries are contracted and the internal bleeding as well as exudation from the blood vessels is controlled. Cold is also applied in various ways viz. by iced compresses, cold compresses, ice poultice or ice bag.

Cold Compress.—The cold compress can be applied to joints in the early stages of sprains and dislocations, since it prevents swelling and relieves the pain.

Requirements.—Two single folds of lint; iced or cold water; cotton bandage. One piece of lint is wrung out lightly and bandaged loosely on the limb, the other piece replacing it as soon as it becomes dry and warm. When a limb is under treatment the bed should be protected with a mackintosh and towel and a cradle put over the part in order to allow the air to reach the affected area. Jaconet will make the cold compress warm very quickly and defeat its own object. A cold compress applied to the eye should be changed every 15 minutes and need not be bandaged unless the patient is restless. One layer of lint is better than a double thickness.

Ice Poultice.—An ice poultice is very soothing and lasts longer than a compress ; it has the advantage of being lighter than an ice bag.

Requirements.—Guttapercha tissue (twice the size required); a thin layer of wood wool, linseed or bran or dressmaker's wadding $\frac{1}{4}$ in. all round smaller than the tissue ; finely chopped ice ; common salt ; turpentine or chloroform ; a paint brush.

The ice is placed on one half of the wood wool, a little salt sprinkled on and the wool folded over it; the edges of the tissue are painted with the paint brush and chloroform which seals it; it is applied to the skin with a piece of lint between it and the poultice and bandaged lightly into position. It should be renewed when the ice melts.

Ice Bag.—An ice bag is a circular rubber bag with a wide screw cap. It is filled with chopped ice which has had common salt sprinkled on it ; the air is expelled and the cap is screwed tightly. If the edges of the ice are sharp, dipping the ice or covering it for a few seconds in hot water will round them off. The bag is placed in a lint or flannel bag or on a piece of lint placed next the skin. The bag should be suspended over the part and must be refilled as soon as the ice has melted.

CHAPTER 9

ENEMAS AND EXCRETA

In this chapter, which is of outstanding importance, the various procedures concerned with the excreta are discussed, including the examination of faeces and urine.

Enemata

The term, giving an enema, is used briefly to describe any procedure in which liquid is introduced by the anal route into the rectum or the bowel above. The enema itself is the bulk of fluid used. Liquids are injected into the rectum for 3 main reasons: 1. to help to empty the rectum; 2. to make replacement of lost fluid; 3. to administer drugs or anaesthetics.

Fundamentals of Enema Action.—The amount to be injected depends upon the conditions for which the enema is given. Thus when a cleansing effect is required and therefore the solution is to be returned in 5–10 minutes, there must be a quantity of the fluid sufficient to distend the bowel and to irritate it enough to cause a reaction on the part of the colon with increased peristalsis and consequent copious evacuation. It is not a question of turning on a hose or of swamping the lower few feet of the bowel, but rather a matter of carefully and slowly adding as much bulk of fluid as may be comfortably retained in the bowel for the necessary period, during which time the faeces are softened, broken up or even liquefied, the result of which is a complete clearance of the mass which it is

319

desired to remove. It has been found that fluid introduced at the anus will travel back to the caecum in 10 minutes, showing that the whole of the large intestine can become flooded in that time.

Sometimes it is desired to inject fluid and let it stay for half an hour or longer ; especially is this so when absorption is necessary.

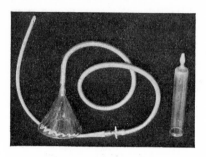

FIG. 104.—FUNNELS AND TUBING FOR ENEMA ADMINISTRATION.

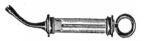

FIG. 105.—VULCANITE AND GLASS SYRINGE.

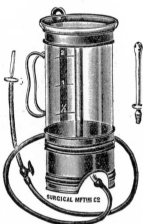

FIG. 107.—METAL AND GLASS DOUCHE CAN WITH RECTAL AND VAGINAL FITTINGS.

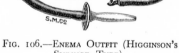

FIG. 106.—ENEMA OUTFIT (HIGGINSON'S SYRINGE TYPE).

(*By courtesy of the Surgical Manufacturing Co., Ltd., London.*)

In such cases the enema is very small in quantity, varying from ½ oz. to 10 oz., and it must be slowly and carefully introduced.

Cleansing Enema.—A cleansing enema usually consists of soap and water and is commonly referred to as *enema saponis*. It is given at a temperature of 100° F. The soap helps to soften the faeces and to expel them. The rectum is emptied by this means before an anaesthetic is given or an operation performed or prior to examination of the rectum. It is also given when there is stubborn constipation which needs to be relieved immediately. In some cases plain water is used (*enema simplex*).

Requisites.—Funnel, rubber tubing, glass connexion and rectal tube fitted with clip; the rectal tube is most suitably kept in a bowl of warm water ; the solution of soap and water (consisting of 2 drachms of soft soap (*sapo mollis*) in 2 pints of water at a temperature of 100° F.) is poured into an enamel jug and the latter should stand in a bowl of hot water to maintain the correct temperature; thermometer; lubricant—soft paraffin on a small square of old linen is best for the lubrication of the end of the catheter and the anus; 2 receivers, one for the soiled swabs and

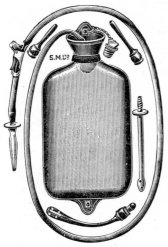

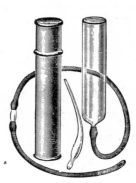

FIG. 108.—FOUNTAIN DOUCHE AND HOT WATER BOTTLE COMBINED.

Note the various Rectal and Vaginal End Pieces.

FIG. 109.—APPARATUS FOR SALINE INFUSION, NASAL FEEDING OR RECTAL FEEDING.

(*By courtesy of the Surgical Manufacturing Co., Ltd., London.*)

the other for the soiled apparatus; a mackintosh and towel to protect the bed. The whole should be placed on a tray and taken to the bedside. The toilet requisites are also prepared beforehand. The bedpan is taken to the bedside. Any nearby window is closed and the screens are placed round the bed to ensure privacy.

Procedure.—The patient is told what is going to be done and is asked to empty the bladder first. The patient lies on the left side as near to the edge of the bed as possible; the clothes are turned back to the minimum extent and a small blanket covers the shoulders.

The air is expelled from the tubing by pouring water through

N. II—11*

the tube until all the air bubbles have passed through. The funnel should be held in the left hand with the tube coiled to shorten it and the end of the rectal tube (catheter) held above the fluid level in the funnel. This should then be lubricated and the swab also applied to the anus. The catheter should then be taken in the right hand between the index finger and the thumb, the catheter eye just level with the end of the finger; the latter presses on the anal sphincter to open it and the catheter is inserted. It must be passed up about 3 inches, after which the funnel is filled and the clip released slowly to allow the fluid to run through. Air should not be allowed to pass in, accordingly the funnel must not become empty; it should not be held too high as the fluid would pass in too quickly. When all the enema has been run in or the patient has had as much as he can take, the end of the catheter is withdrawn. To do this the nurse must nip the tube to the rectum as quickly as possible and withdraw it at once; it should be disconnected and put into the receiver and the remaining tube and funnel should be replaced into the bowl. The patient should be put on the bedpan and asked to retain the enema as long as possible; this may produce a larger result. The nurse must see that the patient is comfortable on the bedpan and must not go too far away as often after an enema the patient feels faint and may collapse or slide off the bedpan. The subsequent toilet consists of seeing that the patient is quite clean and comfortable before the nurse leaves him. The bowel motion (generally referred to as " the result ") should be saved for inspection. The appliances that have been used must be washed thoroughly, first in cold water and then in soapy water and boiled and dried before being put away.

Purgative Enema.—This may take several forms and may consist of olive oil, glycerine or other drugs.

Olive oil.—This is frequently used in very severe cases of constipation with hardened faeces, or in any condition, such as piles or cancer of the rectum, in which there is pain in the movement of the bowel. It is very satisfactory in conditions of severe exhaustion such as are found in prolonged pneumonia, in the later stages of enteric fever and when surgical conditions of the abdomen including operations in the perineum and rectum necessitate the avoidance of all strain in defaecation. To make up the olive oil enema, 5–10 oz. of oil should be carefully heated until it is at a temperature of 105° F.; this can be done by placing the olive oil bottle in hot water; cooling to 100° F. will occur as the oil passes through the apparatus. Often the end of the bed is raised on blocks, in order to ensure complete retention of the enema, which should be run in very slowly, and should be introduced by the funnel and rubber tube method, allowing about half a pint to flow in during half an hour. If smaller quantities are used, the time is naturally shorter. Sometimes the oil is left in for a whole night, but usually after about 4 hours a generous soap and water enema is given to clear out the solution; this relieves the whole of the lower bowel. In some hospitals only 5 oz. of olive oil is given, and the patient is encouraged to retain the amount for 30 minutes, after which a soap and water enema is administered and the bowel thus cleared.

Glycerine.—Another purgative enema is the glycerine enema, which has a certain irritating effect on the bowel wall and therefore has stimulant qualities. The glycerine takes up liquid from the mucous membrane and thus makes the faeces soft or fluid, so that within about half an hour of giving an enema of 4 drachms to an adult or ½ drachm to a child, there is a copious evacuation. In giving this type of enema the solution should be made up by adding from 1 drachm to 1 oz. of glycerine to 2 oz. of warm water. It should be noted that the glycerine suppository has superseded this type of enema.

Other drugs.—Other purgatives can be used to empty the lower bowel, of which the commonest are castor oil, magnesium sulphate and ox bile. The castor oil enema is made by adding 1 oz. of castor oil or more to three times the quantity of olive oil. This is given in the usual way, and about half an hour later an ordinary soap and water enema is introduced. In the magnesium sulphate enema, 6 oz. of warm solution of magnesium sulphate are introduced. The ox bile enema is made by adding 20 grains of purified ox bile to 2 fl. oz. of warm water. This may be injected as it is, or added to about half a pint of soap solution or olive oil.

Flatus Enema.—In some cases of abdominal disease, but particularly after abdominal operations, there is painful retention of fluids which cannot be expelled owing to temporary inactivity of the bowel muscle. The bowel distension can be relieved by giving a flatus enema, which usually consists of turpentine mixed with olive oil and soap solution. Half an ounce of turpentine is added to 2 oz. of olive oil and both are thoroughly mixed by stirring and shaking. Soap and water enema (*enema saponis*) is added until there is a total volume of 8 oz. This is administered in the usual way. The remainder of the soap and water enema is given immediately afterwards, the amount being limited by the ability of the patient to retain it.

Anthelmintic Enema.—The aim in giving an anthelmintic enema is to expel threadworms and other parasites. The simplest anthelmintic enema is salt and water, given cold, in a strength of 1 oz. of salt to 2 pints of water. A more popular remedy is 10 oz. of infusion of quassia, also given cold, and made up by adding 1 oz. of quassia chips to 1 pint of water. Generally 6 to 8 oz. of fluid are quite sufficient to do the work required.

As a preliminary, the bowel should be cleared by giving a simple enema. The longer an anthelmintic enema is retained the better. Turpentine is sometimes also used for this purpose.

Sedative Enema.—In cases of very mild diarrhoea with pain, often associated with an ulcerated or raw condition of the mucous membrane of the colon, some smooth lubricating substance is required, and this can be provided by making up thick solutions of starch, gum or linseed often mixed with opium. The starch and opium enema is made by adding a certain amount of tincture of opium, generally 20–30 minims of tincture of opium to 4 oz. of starch mucilage at a temperature of 100° F. In some cases the starch is slowly introduced first, then the opium and then further starch, a No. 8 catheter being used, or if pressure is necessary a glass syringe.

Retention Enema.—Certain drugs cannot be tolerated by patients, either because they have a dislike for them or because vomiting is the result. A well known sedative and sleeping draught is the drug paraldehyde; this can be given by the rectum either in olive oil or in water, but a good method is to give first ½ oz. of warm water, then the prescribed amount of the drug, then another ½ oz. of warm water.

Stimulating Enema.—In any case of dehydration (excessive loss of water from the tissues) or in the period immediately subsequent to an abdominal operation, this type of enema is usually given. It is more commonly designated as a rectal saline. It can be given continuously over a long period i.e. by the drip method, or an administration of 6 oz. at a time, given 4 or 6 hourly may be more suitable. In some conditions 8 ozs. given once is sufficient. In the majority of cases normal saline (0·9 per cent sodium chloride solution or 80 grains of pure common salt in a pint of hot distilled water) is given with 5 per cent of glucose added. This can be administered by the tube and funnel method or by a Souttar's flask, douche can or glass bottle, but the principle of all methods is the same; the catheter should be small—No. 7 (see Figs. 104, 107, 108 and 110).

The air should be expelled from the tube and the catheter inserted and the funnel held low so that the fluid does not run in quickly; the flow can be regulated by raising or lowering the funnel.

When a continuous saline drip is used, the saline is in a thermos flask and a clip regulates the flow, which is in ideal conditions at the rate of 1 drachm a minute. As the flow is slow the temperature of the saline should be 140° F. When a glass bottle is used, the room temperature is considered to be sufficiently high and warming is unnecessary.

The patient may lie on the back comfortably with the dressing mackintosh and towel placed under the buttocks. The bladder should be emptied first and the rectum too if the bowels are known not to have been opened that day.

Black coffee is also given in cases of shock and collapse. In the first method one ounce of ground coffee is put into a jug and 10 oz. of boiling water is poured over it. The coffee should stand for 5 minutes and then it should be carefully strained so

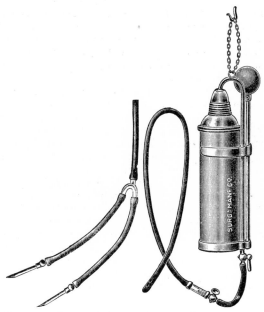

FIG. 110.—SOUTTAR'S SALINE INFUSION APPARATUS FOR BOTH RECTAL AND SUBCUTANEOUS ROUTES.
(By courtesy of the Surgical Manufacturing Co., Ltd., London.)

that no grounds are left (these act as irritants). The second method is that of giving the concentrated coffee enema, made as follows: 4–6 oz. of coffee are boiled in 10 oz. of water with ½ oz. of salt to form a concentrated solution; this is strained through muslin and introduced at a temperature of 105° F.

Care of Enema Apparatus

There is a considerable amount of wear and tear so far as enema apparatus is concerned: this may be unavoidable.

The chief things to remember about the care of enema apparatus is that olive oil has a deleterious effect on rubber, and that it should never be allowed to remain a minute longer than necessary in contact with tubing, mackintosh sheets and similar fabrics.

Catheters should be rinsed out very carefully, especially the eye portions. All rubber should be boiled for about 5 minutes in salt and water. Glass should also be washed in soap and water, and then placed in boiling water for a few minutes. All oils should be carefully removed from every part of the apparatus by boiling in soap and water and then thoroughly rinsing in warm water. The Higginson syringe should have the nurse's special attention. She should make sure that it is carefully cleaned and dried, especially the nozzle, and it should be hung with the nozzle pointing downwards. Rubber perishes very easily if it is folded in any way.

It is advisable before giving an olive oil enema to place the funnel and tubing in a hot solution of soap, contained in an enamelled basin set at the side of the bed. This solution prevents the rubber from being affected by the oil and also assists in the lubrication. Drops of oil on mackintosh sheets should at once be mopped up, otherwise they will cause rotting of the rubber.

Enema Rashes

An alarming looking eruption may be found sometimes at any period between 12 and 24 hours after an enema has been given. The distribution varies ; sometimes there is a general rash like scarlet fever, but more usually very small patches of red rash arise prominently on the knees and elbows, on the hips and on the cheeks. There is no discomfort, nor is the temperature raised, but the appearance is alarming to the patient and sometimes infectious disease is suspected. The rash usually passes off on the second day.

Excreta

Excretion takes place chiefly through the bowel and the bladder, although there is a considerable amount of disposal of waste products through the skin and by the breath. In the following pages only the faeces (or bowel excretions) and the urine (or bladder excretions) are discussed.

The Faeces

The physiology of defaecation has already been discussed in Vol. I, p. 222, and the hygiene of bowel regularity in pp. 66, 68 and 79 of this volume. Constipation and diarrhoea are dealt with later in Section VIII, Chapter 4.

The Normal Specimen.—The discarded products of digestion, known as faeces or stools, vary according to the individual,
to his food and to his general health.

Normally the daily stool should amount to about 6 oz. in
an adult, and about half that quantity in a young child. If
digestion is perfect there should be no evidence of undigested
food, although the latter may be present in many conditions
compatible with normal health. An analysis of an ordinary
stool shows it to contain quantities of cellulose, mucus, epithelium,
some fibrous and elastic tissue, stercobilin, masses of bacteria in
various stages of activity (many of them dead) and also water,
which forms the major portion of the stool.

The amount passed per day depends upon the activity of the
peristalsis and upon the quantity of food which is taken. A
normal stool may be described as being slightly acid or slightly
alkaline, light brown in colour owing to the bile pigment present,
solid but yet soft and preserving the mould of the rectum from
which it has been passed. Owing to the large amount of end
products of protein digestion there is a considerable odour,
which is characteristic of these substances.

The Abnormal Stool.—Stools may vary in character as
mentioned below.

Colour.—A clay coloured or pale yellow stool indicates that
there is a deficiency of bile; it is characteristic of all jaundiced
conditions. If there is considerable bleeding in the lower part
of the small intestine, the stool is reddish brown or chocolate
coloured. This is typical of a certain stage of enteric fever.
When the colour is definitely as black as tar, the condition is
known as melaena and is always found when there is bleeding
high up in the alimentary canal e.g. in the stomach or duodenum.
It must also be remembered that this condition may be the result
of swallowing blood from the socket of a recently extracted tooth.
Again, certain drugs cause a greyish brown colour of varying
degrees; this dark pigmentation is not of the tone associated with
melaena nor is there any sign of the gloss or sheen typical of this
condition. Common drugs in this category are bismuth, iron
and senna. The stool may be bright red owing to fresh blood
coming from the lower part of the bowel or it may be very pale
yellow, especially in children who are on a milk diet. Green
stools result from large doses of calomel, and they also indicate
alimentary disturbance in infants.

Odour.—If the odour is stronger than usual, it may mean, apart
from the effect of purgatives, that there is some disease of the
alimentary tract. In ulceration of the bowel, accompanied by
melaena, the stools are very offensive. If there is much bacterial
fermentation a sour character is added to the odour.

Shape.—If the stool is not normally spindle shaped or cylin drical in outline, it may indicate that there is an increased amount of bowel irritation, causing the formation of a semi-solid stool. In some cases the stool is passed as a ribbon, which frequently means that there is a condition of internal piles or that some growth is pressing the contents of the rectum ; occasionally the stool is grooved on one side.

Amount.—It is very difficult to assess what is the normal and what is an abnormal amount of the daily evacuation; every individual has a different standard. In feverish conditions most of the fluid which forms the bulk of normal faeces is absorbed and therefore the stool is very small and hard; the same applies to chronic constipation. The quantity is increased when the peristaltic movements of the bowel are more active, when foreign bodies or " roughage " causes irritation of the bowel wall or when there is catarrh of the lining of the bowel, due to germs or other inflammatory agents.

Consistence.—In all cases in which water has been extracted from the faecal mass before evacuation, the consistence is hard and the motion takes the form of pellet-like masses known as scybala. On the contrary, very fluid stools, loose and watery and often most offensive, result from summer diarrhoea, colitis, dysentery, cholera and typhoid fever; the last has a character-istic stool very like pea soup. Meat is apt to produce a dry small motion, while vegetables, since they consist of a great amount of residue containing cellulose, result in increase of faeces.

Other Unnatural Constituents of Stools.—The abnor-malities described below are to be found in certain circumstances in the stools.

Undigested food.—This should always be reported upon, although the presence of various seeds of fruits, pips, green vegetables and so on need not be regarded with any alarm.

Mucus.—When there is much mucus it appears as threads of slime, and may be the result of colitis ; in dysentery, however, considerable masses of slightly blood-stained mucus may be passed at intervals.

Shreds of membrane.—These indicate that there is ulceration of some part of the bowel. In cholera the epithelium of the bowel comes off in flakes, which float among the watery motion and which give it the characteristic title of " rice-water " stool.

Fat.—If the stools are rather loose and frothy, with numerous small bubbles of fat, it is an indication that there is a deficiency of the bile or of the pancreatic juice. In the somewhat un-common disease of children known as coeliac disease a very bulky stool of this type is to be found.

Gallstones.—Gallstones and other foreign bodies may be found, and it is especially important to filter out the small faceted calculi after a previous attack of suspected gallbladder colic, since their discovery proves the diagnosis to be accurate.

Pus.—Various quantities of purulent matter may be passed when there is much inflammation, as in dysentery, or if there is any abscess or fistula in the neighbourhood of the rectum. Sometimes an abscess of the appendix discharges through the bowel.

Curdy stools.—These are sometimes found in children in whom the digestion in the stomach is unsatisfactory.

Blood.—Blood is one of the commonest unnatural constituents, and it appears in various forms. It may be bright red, showing that it comes from the lower bowel ; it may be black as a result of gastric or duodenal ulcer. If it is mixed with mucus, it may indicate obstruction of the bowel or dysentery; again, it may be associated with certain blood diseases such as purpura.

Parasites.—From the tiny threadworm, frequently found in children, to the large roundworm, often the cause of trouble to adults, intestinal parasites are represented constantly in the stool. Roundworms are usually passed one at a time, but threadworms are well known as occurring in crops, and they are a great source of annoyance to children. The tapeworm evacuates its flat proglottides, so many inches at a time. Often it is the nurse's duty to search for the head of the tapeworm after special treatment has been employed to evacuate it.

Examination of the Faeces.—The routine adopted in most hospitals is that the first motion passed by a patient after his admission to a ward is inspected by the sister, or at least by the senior nurse. If the doctor wishes any particular examination to be carried out, there are special facilities for this. In such cases it is not advisable to retain the motion in the bedpan, but it should be carefully transferred to a glass jar provided with a tightly fitted or overlapping lid ; a square of lint soaked in strong phenol may be tied over the top of the jar, which is left in a special place in the lavatory or in the open air cupboard until the examination has been made.

Often it is necessary to have the faeces examined bacteriologically, although a negative result of such examination e.g. in dysentery or enteric fever does not prove that these diseases do not exist; a positive result clinches the diagnosis. All bacteriological laboratories send out special glass tubes with corks to which are fitted small spoons, dipping into the tube. In selecting a specimen of faeces for examination the nurse should take a small spoonful of the last portion of the motion as soon as it is passed, then the cork should be tightly fitted into the tube and the whole should be sent, accompanied by full particulars, to the laboratory as soon as possible. (See also p. 227.)

Bedpans.—There are various types of bedpan, some of which are illustrated overleaf. They may be made of enamel ware or earthenware, preferably the latter, which are more easily cleaned and much more hygienic. At any time a bedpan is an unwelcome contraption, as those who have had to suffer from its peculiarities have learned to their cost. Nevertheless, it is the only method of ensuring sanitary efficiency, and the nurse should make a point of helping the patient as much as possible to overcome his discomfort in the use of this appliance. The selection of a suitable pattern depends upon the nurse and the patient. The slipper bedpan is more easily applied but it is more uncomfortable than the circular bedpan. In placing a patient on the bedpan, the nurse should steady the body with her left hand at the base of the spine, and should gently raise the patient up,

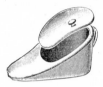 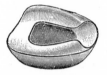 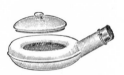

Fig. 111.—Slipper Bedpan.   Fig. 112.—The " Perfection " Bedpan.   Fig. 113.—Ordinary Type of Bedpan.

(By courtesy of the Surgical Manufacturing Co., Ltd., London.)

while he draws his heels up almost to his hips, thus helping to make a modified form of the " human bridge." With her right hand, the nurse then places the bedpan in position and carefully lowers the patient. Wnen the time comes to remove the bedpan, there should be no attempt made to drag it away forcibly; even if it means getting extra assistance, the patient should be lifted clear of it. It should then be rapidly taken away, covered with a cloth, and carried to the sluice room, where its contents should be immediately flushed out by the special apparatus installed, unless the specimen has to be retained for inspection. As a routine, it is generally necessary to rinse bedpans out once a day with strong disinfectant, and then to wash carefully with soap and hot water (see Figs. 111, 112 and 113).

Urine

The liquid excretion which comes from the bladder is called urine and the passage of urine from the bladder is known as micturition. This function is one of the most important guides in the assessment of the patient's general condition, and nurses must at all times be able to discuss with their seniors the amount of urine passed, the characters and anything unusual associated with micturition. The nurse is recommended to revise pp. 231–233 of Vol I, before going on with the study of abnormal conditions of the urine.

Abnormal Micturition.—Frequency is the term used to describe the passage of small quantities of urine at very short intervals. It occurs in any condition in which there is some irritation of the bladder—stone, inflammation or ulceration of the bladder wall; enlargement of the prostate gland; or the presence of " gravel, " the popular name given to the fine crystals of oxalate of calcium insoluble in the urine. It may also be the result of pus in the kidney, tuberculous disease and small or large stones. In a certain group of cases there is a reflex irritability due to prolapse of one or more of the pelvic organs; the pressure on the bladder carries considerable irritation. In this category are included prolapse of the rectum, displacement of the uterus and the effects of certain tumours. In children, frequency may be associated with threadworms, with irritation of the genital organs (especially phimosis) and sometimes merely with apprehension.

It is generally possible to retain urine for about 4 hours without discomfort, but in many cases patients can tolerate collection of urine in the bladder only for half that time. It is a point of great importance that nurses should not object to the provision of urinals when they are demanded by patients, no matter how unreasonable the request may seem to the nurse or how busy she may be. Many patients are nervous, highly strung and even hysterical, and in conditions such as these, the control of the bladder is one of the first powers to weaken. Apart from ordinary frequency, there may be increase in the actual amount of urine; this is called polyuria and is found in diabetes, in many kidney diseases, in those suffering from the effects of alcohol and occasionally when certain drugs have been given which cause increased action of the kidney filters and therefore of the bladder. The normal daily output for an adult is about $2\frac{1}{2}$ pints daily, but it varies in different states and conditions. Oliguria is a state in which the urine is diminished in amount; it occurs in some kidney diseases and some heart conditions.

Incontinence.—Incontinence of urine may or may not be accompanied by incontinence of faeces. It is a sign of loss of bladder control and it is a very trying condition for the patient especially in cases in which the urine constantly leaks e.g. in senile people and in those who have some spinal cord affliction; it is almost impossible to maintain sanitary or hygienic conditions in such circumstances. There are various degrees of incontinence; the bladder may fill up and then suddenly expel its contents without the patient's knowledge; this is known as reflex incontinence. On the other hand the bladder may become very much over-distended so that only the surplus urine is passed. This is called overflow incontinence.

Enuresis, especially during the night, is one of the great problems of childhood. In this condition there may be slight inflammation of the bladder or some external irritative factor, or threadworms in the lower part of the intestine which cause incontinence during sleep; in the majority of cases, it is due to some psychological defect, and it is often found to be the most difficult condition to cure. Experience has shown that the psychologist is often successful in apparently hopeless cases.

Suppression of urine.—Suppression of urine is also known as anuria. If this is prolonged for any period it usually ends fatally. It means that the mechanism of the kidneys has completely broken down and that the urine is being stored up in the blood (uraemia), instead of being extracted by the kidneys and passed into the bladder. Uraemia, which is characterized by convulsions, delirium and coma, and which may end fatally, must be carefully distinguished from oliguria (see above) the condition of partial suppression which may be due to an acute but transitory breakdown of the kidneys.

Retention.—Retention of urine means that the kidneys are probably acting quite normally, but that there is some obstruction of the outlet from the bladder, which fills up as usual and which may become very distended and painful. It is a common condition in certain types of paralysis and often demands the use of a catheter, which has to be passed by the urethral route every few hours. On the other hand, there may be narrowing of the urethra, owing to disease, causing a stricture. In some cases it is the result of nervousness, there being a sort of spasm which prevents the normal act of voiding the urine from being carried out. This is especially noticeable after operations in the pelvis or lower parts of the abdomen, and retention of urine is one of the many important things to be wary of in cases of severe accident accompanied by shock.

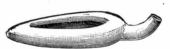

FIG. 114.—SPOONBILL URINAL.
(By courtesy of the Surgical Manufacturing Co., Ltd., London.)

Collection of Urine.—Numerous appliances have been devised for both sexes for the collection of urine from patients confined to bed. Some of these are illustrated here.

For male patients a glass, earthenware or enamel urinal is most popular; it should be kept clean and should be disinfected exactly in the same manner as the bedpan and on no account should a urinal be left at a patient's bedside, underneath the bed or in a cupboard, but immediately the patient has passed urine, the nurse should cover the urinal with a cloth provided for the purpose and should then dispose of the urine in the sluice room.

For female patients there is greater difficulty as bedpans are not entirely satisfactory. There are many patterns of specially devised earthenware urinals and bowls, which are illustrated, and which can be used if the bedpan is not suitable, and also when a special specimen is required (Figs. 114 and 116).

In cases of nervousness and inability to pass urine, the application of hot cloths to the lower part of the abdomen or sponging

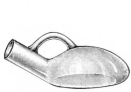

FIG. 115.—GLASS MALE   FIG. 116.—GLASS FEMALE URINAL
URINAL, WITH HANDLE.   WITH HANDLE.

(*By courtesy of the Surgical Manufacturing Co., Ltd., London.*)

the perineum with hot water should be tried.   Usually it is found that if the patient is left to himself without fuss and is not made nervous by people offering suggestions and gratuitously giving old wives' tips, everything passes off successfully.

Saving a Specimen of Urine.—No matter what the condition of the patient may be, all those newly admitted to hospital must have the urine examined within 24 hours.   At first it is necessary to collect only the morning specimen, this being put up in a special standard urine glass, which should be covered with a plug of cotton wool and set on a shelf in the doctor's room, with the name of the patient affixed to the glass.   The nurse should therefore make sure that the specimen she saves is one which has not been contaminated in any way.   Occasionally the doctor wishes to know how much urine has been passed during 24 hours, and this is done by setting aside a glass jar with a tightly fitting cover in the sluice room, and adding to it the various amounts passed during the 24 hours, care being taken that the bladder is empty at the beginning of the test and that micturition takes place at the end of the period.   If the nurse is aware of any unavoidable loss of urine, she should report it. On a test day such as that mentioned above, it must be ensured that none of the urine is passed into the bedpan during defaecation. The normal amount passed during 24 hours is about 50 oz.

When there is a special type of micro-organism under suspicion causing disease of the bladder or kidneys, the urine must be withdrawn with all sterile precautions from the bladder by a catheter, so that there is no question of the introduction of other organisms to the specimen from outside.   The urine is carefully sealed up in a sterile tube and sent to the laboratory.   Normal urine contains a certain number of bacteria, but urine which has been allowed to stand in the open air swarms with all types of bacterium.

Testing of Urine

Assuming that the specimen of urine to be tested is in front of the nurse, and that it has been allowed to cool and settle for a few hours, a routine must be adopted in carrying out the tests.

The stand shown in Fig. 117 contains the apparatus required. In the drawers are litmus and filter papers, notepaper and

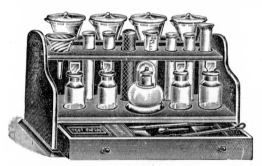

FIG. 117.—URINE TESTING SET.
(By courtesy of the Surgical Manufacturing Co., Ltd., London.)

pencil. The bottles contains various reagents in common use A small spirit lamp is also provided, a number of test tubes and a measuring glass. There is also a glass instrument known as a urinometer. This is weighted by a certain amount of mercury in a bulb, and when it is placed in a jar of water it registers 0, but in another fluid it does not sink so deeply, therefore it may float at a level indicated by one of the degrees marked on the stem, which is graduated from 0 to 60. The reading at the point of steady flotation added to 1,000 gives the specific gravity of the fluid ; thus if the stem remains fixed at a level of 28, the specific gravity is 1,028. The following are the essential tests approved by most authorities.

1. **Quantity.**—This does not come actually under the present system, as it depends upon observation of 24 hours. Nevertheless, when necessary, it should be included in the urine report.

Urine is increased in diabetes, chronic kidney disease, hysteria, alcoholism and after diuretic drugs have been taken to increase the output of urine. Urine is diminished in acute inflammation of the kidney, fevers, valvular heart disease, after severe diarrhoea vomiting or sickness, by narcotic drugs and in injury of the brain.

2. **Appearance.**—A small cloud of mucus at the bottom of the glass is of no significance.

Normal urine should be pale amber in colour, but when there is diminution in the amount the colour may be much darker. If a great quantity of urine has been passed, the urine may look like water ; this suggests chronic kidney disease or diabetes. On the other hand, after certain drugs have been taken and in certain forms of poisoning (e.g. phenol) the colour may be almost black. A smoky urine indicates the presence of blood, while dark green colour indicates bile. Acute kidney disease or any of the fevers cause very highly coloured urine.

In addition to, or replacing, the deposit described above, urine may contain considerable quantities of pink urates or white phosphates. Pus may also settle down as a yellowish deposit at the bottom of the glass. To distinguish between pink urates and white phosphates, heat a little urine in a test tube ; if urates are present they will disappear ; phosphates can be dissolved by adding a small quantity of weak acetic acid. Pus can be tested for by the method described below.

3. **Odour.**—It is always advisable to smell the urine, and the odour may be best appreciated immediately after the plug of cotton wool has been removed. Urine which contains acetone is supposed to resemble the scent of new mown hay or of very ripe fruit and may indicate diabetes. When there is much pus present in urine, there is the characteristic smell of decomposition.

4. **Reaction.**—Urine is either acid or alkaline. Normally it is acid except immediately after meals, but as the specimen is usually collected first thing in the morning before any food has been taken the normal specimen should therefore be acid. The blue litmus test paper is turned red while the red paper remains red. An alkaline urine behaves in exactly the opposite way. When the urine stands for any time it decomposes, turns alkaline and gives rise to a strong odour of ammonia. For this reason specimens of urine should always be examined in the fresh state. If urine is found to be alkaline it must be made acid by adding a small quantity of acetic acid which does not affect other tests. Occasionally urine is said to be amphoteric i.e. it has a positive reaction to litmus paper of both colours.

5. **Specific Gravity.**—This is carried out by using the urinometer described above. Care should be taken that when this instrument is placed in the specimen glass it does not touch the sides of the glass or rest on the bottom. The eye should be brought down to the level of the surface of the urine in order to get a correct reading. Usually the reading is about 1,020 ; if it is as low as 1,008 it may be due to increase of fluid intake,

diabetes insipidis or chronic nephritis.   When the urine is very pale and registers anything above 1,035, sugar is probably present and diabetes mellitus should be suspected.

6. **Tests.**—The following tests should be carried out in order to prove the presence or absence of abnormal constituents which are important in certain diseases.

Albumin.—The first test is the heat test.   Put about 4 inches of urine into a test tube and hold it at an angle over the flame so that the upper portion only is boiled.   If a cloudiness is produced, the indication is albumin or phosphates.   One drop of nitric acid or a few drops of acetic acid will clear up the phosphates but will not affect the albumin.   As a confirmatory test for albumin, about 1 inch of nitric acid should be put into a clean test tube.   A small quantity of urine should then be very carefully run down the side of the test tube, which is held at an angle of 45°.   At the point of junction of the two fluids a definite white ring indicates that albumin is present.   This is known as the cold test.   The presence of albumin generally indicates inflammation of the kidneys, but it may also be found in anaemia, heart disease and various other diseases.   The white cloud formed by heating is exactly the same as the white substance which appears when an egg is poached; naturally in urine testing the amount of albumin is minute.   Albumin can also be tested quantitatively by using picric acid in a special test tube called Esbach's albuminometer, but nurses are very rarely expected to do this test, which should be carried out by a doctor.

Blood.—About ½ inch of urine is placed in a test tube and a few drops of tincture of guaiacum are added, then the thumb is placed over the end of the tube, and the contents are vigorously shaken.   In another test tube should be placed about 1 inch of ozonic ether; then a little of the first mixture is carefully added.   If blood is present, a distinct blue ring will develop at the meeting place of the two fluids.

Bile.—Bile in urine indicates liver affections.   The test for this is as follows: a white glazed tile is obtained and a few drops of urine are put on one part, while a few drops of strong nitric acid are put about 1 inch from it.   When the two run together, there is usually produced a rainbow effect which quickly passes off, but if green is found to predominate it is a proof of bile. Another test for bile is the addition of a few drops of liquor iodi mitis (B.P. 1932); a green reaction indicates the presence of bile.

Sugar.—Two test tubes are taken, one containing 1 inch of urine and the other 1 inch of Fehling's solution ; each should be boiled.   Then the urine is poured carefully into the blue solution.   A yellow reaction indicates a moderate amount of sugar, but if it becomes orange or brown it means that there is a large quantity of sugar, and quantitative tests may be required.   Sometimes a faint green reaction is obtained which is quite compatible with good health. An alternative test is made by putting 5 c.cm. of Benedict's solution into a test tube and adding 8 drops of urine; after boiling for 2 minutes the colour will change from blue to bright orange if sugar is present. As in the case of albumin, nurses are not expected to be able to estimate the quantity of sugar present.

Acetone and Diacetic Acid (the Ketones).—The ketones are found in people who are starving, especially in those who have not been taking enough starchy food. It is also an evidence of diabetes and it may also prove chloroform poisoning of a delayed type.

The test for acetone consists in adding about a teaspoonful of ammonium sulphate to a small amount of urine in a test tube, and after this has been shaken vigorously, 2–5 drops of freshly prepared solution of sodium nitroprusside (2 per cent) is added, and following this about $\frac{1}{2}$ inch of concentrated ammonia. The mixture is agitated slightly and left to stand for half an hour, when a deep violet-red colour develops (Rothera's test).

Gerhardt's test.—For diacetic acid, the test is the addition of a little ferric chloride (10 per cent) to about 1 inch of urine in a test tube. There may be a slight precipitation of phosphates, in which case the ferric chloride should be added drop by drop. A port wine colour indicates diacetic acid.

Before operations involving the giving of chloroform, the patient's urine should be tested for ketones.

Pus.—The test for pus consists in taking a small portion of the deposit and examining it by the microscope. Other well known tests are the addition of a little liquor potassae to the deposit. A ropy precipitate is obtained.

CHAPTER 10

WARD DRESSINGS AND INSTRUMENTS

EQUIPMENT FOR WARD DRESSINGS. FURNITURE. UTENSILS.
WARD INSTRUMENTS. DRESSING OF WOUNDS. STERILIZA-
TION. CARE OF GLOVES. SURGICALLY CLEAN HANDS.
MATERIALS FOR DRESSINGS. PREPARATION OF THE
TROLLEY. ROUTINE OF DRESSING. SURGICAL FOMENTA-
TION. ASSISTANCE. DISPOSAL OF TOWELS AND MASKS. LINEN
BAG ENVELOPES. PREVENTIVE MEASURES. CLEANING
AND STERILIZING INSTRUMENTS. THE STERILIZER. STER-
ILIZATION OF EQUIPMENT. CATHETERS.

THE dangers of pathogenic bacteria are obvious, and before doing even the simplest surgical dressing the nurse should be clear in her mind with regard to all the possibilities of microbic action (see Sections III and IV). This chapter is concerned with the routine daily dressing as carried out in the ward. Further consideration is given to surgical cleanliness and other subjects akin to it later on.

Equipment for Ward Dressings

The following is a brief outline of the equipment usually provided for surgical wards. It is obvious that every hospital has its own methods and its own list of instruments and dressings, but the articles mentioned below can be added to as circumstances require.

Furniture.—The first essential in ward furniture is a dressing wagon (universally referred to as a trolley) which usually consists of a framework of steel, plated or painted white, and provided with two plate glass shelves. It also has rubber tyred castors, so that it can be moved about easily and noiselessly (see Fig. 119). There are numerous types of wagon, depending on the kind of work that is being done.

Secondly, a sterilizer on a stand (Fig. 118) of a capacity suitable to take most of the utensils and instruments used in the ordinary surgical dressing. This sterilizer may be 18 inches × 14 inches × 12 inches, but the sizes are graded, the biggest type being 27 inches × 20 inches × 16 inches. (See also p. 350.)

Utensils.—On the lower shelf of the trolley is usually placed a drum, square or round, made of copper and heavily nickel plated (Fig. 120). Many have neither seams nor orners. Inside this drum are all the dressings required for one patient; these

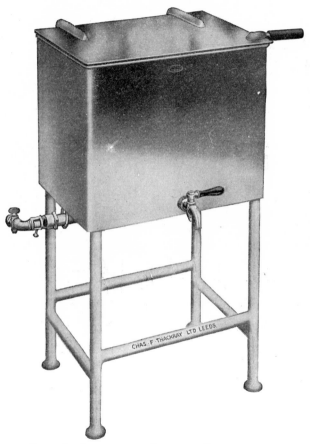

FIG. 118.—STERILIZER ON STAND FOR BOWLS AND OTHER WARD UTENSILS.

(By courtesy of Messrs. Chas. F. Thackray, Ltd., Leeds.)

have been sterilized within the previous 24 hours, and the drum must not be opened until immediately before use. A small square enamelled tray may also be included ; on this is placed a pair of sterilized rubber gloves and a mackintosh square. There are also one or two circular enamelled basins or glass bowls containing the lotions in common use and a tray of instruments in an antiseptic lotion. A glass jar is usually provided, into which will be placed dirty instruments ; this should be about half full of 5 per cent phenol. Another fairly tall glass jar should be

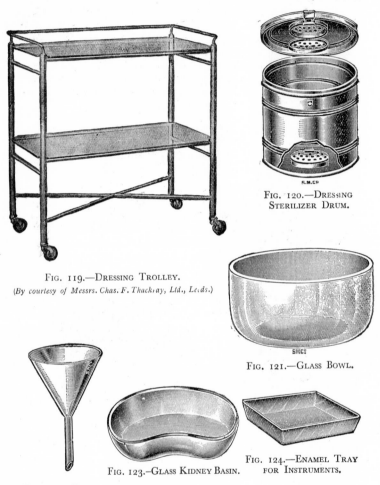

FIG. 120.—DRESSING
STERILIZER DRUM.

FIG. 119.—DRESSING TROLLEY.
(By courtesy of Messrs. Chas. F. Thackray, Ltd., Leeds.)

FIG. 121.—GLASS BOWL.

FIG. 124.—ENAMEL TRAY
FOR INSTRUMENTS.

FIG. 123.—GLASS KIDNEY BASIN.

FIG. 122.—ENAMEL
FUNNEL.   *(By courtesy of the Surgical Manufacturing Co., Ltd., London)*

three-quarters full of strong disinfectant ; in this are placed the blades of a pair of large forceps (Cheatle's pattern) used for the removal of the dressings from the drum. There should also be a tray for dirty dressings, and a kidney shaped tray for the reception of any discharges, rubber tuning or plugs which may be removed from a septic wound. A supply of bandages and safety pins should also form part of the furniture of the wagon.

An enamel bucket with cover is usually provided for soiled dressings.

If hot water is laid on in a ward, there is no necessity to introduce facilities for sterilization of the hands before or between dressings. In the absence of this, however, there is usually a table provided with a plate glass top on which are several large enamelled basins, a supply of hot water in an enamelled jug,

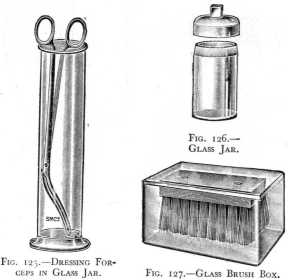

Fig. 126.—
Glass Jar.

Fig. 125.—Dressing Forceps in Glass Jar.

Fig. 127.—Glass Brush Box.

(*By courtesy of the Surgical Manufacturing Co., Ltd., London.*)

stoppered bottles containing various antiseptic lotions, ethereal soap and a scrubbing brush which is kept in 5 per cent phenol lotion in a glass jar (see Fig. 127).

Whenever possible, all the above appliances must be thoroughly sterilized immediately before use.

Ward Instruments.—The instruments in common use are illustrated in the following pages and usually consist of the following items.

Surgical Scissors.—There are scores of patterns but the most useful type for doing ward dressings is Mayo's scissors, nickel-plated and with rounded blades.

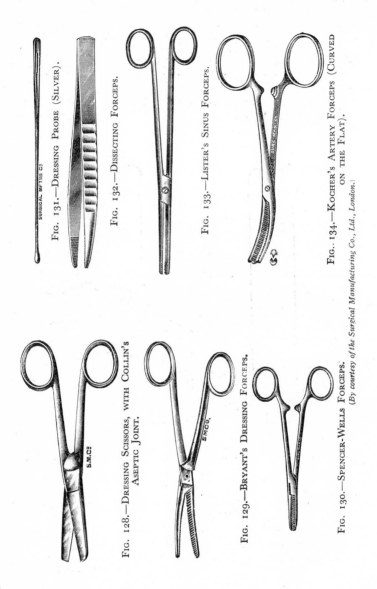

Fig. 131.—Dressing Probe (Silver).

Fig. 132.—Dissecting Forceps.

Fig. 133.—Lister's Sinus Forceps.

Fig. 134.—Kocher's Artery Forceps (Curved on the Flat).

Fig. 128.—Dressing Scissors, with Collin's Aseptic Joint.

Fig. 129.—Bryant's Dressing Forceps.

Fig. 130.—Spencer-Wells Forceps.

(By courtesy of the Surgical Manufacturing Co., Ltd., London.)

Dressing Probe.—This is made of silver or of white metal, one end blunt and rounded, the other end slightly flattened and with an eye (Fig. 131).

Dissecting Forceps.—These are of stainless steel, and are made also in many varieties. Probably the type illustrated is the most useful (Fig. 132).

Dressing Forceps.—These are for removing dressings, and may be provided with or without a catch (Fig. 129).

Sinus Forceps.—These are also made of stainless steel with straight or curved blades which can easily be introduced into a deep wound (Fig. 133).

Artery Forceps.—Numerous varieties are available for selection,

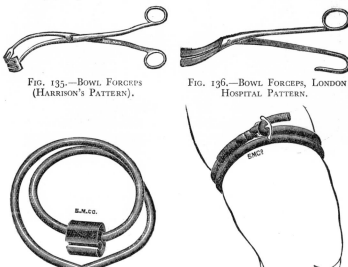

FIG. 135.—BOWL FORCEPS
(HARRISON'S PATTERN).

FIG. 136.—BOWL FORCEPS, LONDON
HOSPITAL PATTERN.

FIG. 137.—FOULIS'S TOURNIQUET.   FIG. 138.—SAMWAY'S TOURNIQUET.
(By courtesy of the Surgical Manufacturing Co., Ltd., London.)

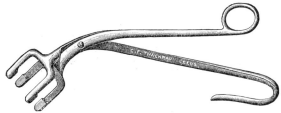

FIG. 139.—HARRISON'S STERILIZER FORCEPS.
(By courtesy of Messrs. Chas. F. Thackray, Ltd., Leeds.)

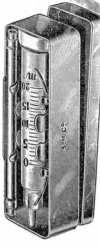

Fig. 141.—3-piece All-Glass Hypodermic Syringe

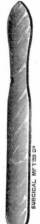

Fig. 143.—Metal Spatula.
(May be used for examination of the throat.)

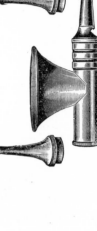
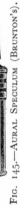

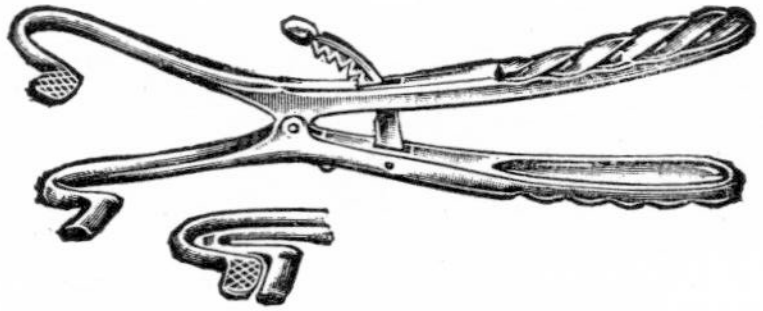

Fig. 145.—Aural Speculum (Brunton's).

(By courtesy of the Surgical Manufacturing Co., Ltd., London.)

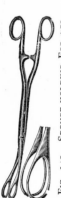

Fig. 140.—Sponge-holding Forceps.

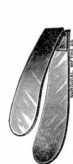

Fig. 142.—Tobold's Tongue Depressor.

Fig. 144.—Ackland's Mouth Gag.

but the favourites are Spencer-Wells's and Kocher's (Figs. 130 and 134).

Bowl Forceps.—See Figs. 135 and 136.

Tourniquets.—These are used in emergencies when sudden bleeding occurs, and therefore they should be as simple as possible. The patterns recommended are Foulis's, Esmarch's or Samway's (Figs. 137 and 138).

Sponge Holders.—These are made either with wire loop handle or, as illustrated, as forceps with wide open blades (Fig. 140).

Syringes.—Hypodermic syringesofvarious sizes, 1 c.cm., 5 c.cm., 20 c.cm., and 50 c.cm., should all be provided and should preferably be of the all glass variety (Fig. 141).

Tongue Depressor, of glass or of nickel steel (Figs. 142 and 143).

Mouth Gag.—See Fig. 144.

Aural Specula.—A selection of these should be kept in readiness for ear examination (Fig. 145).

Laryngeal Mirror and Headlight.—For the examination of the throat when necessary (Fig. 146).

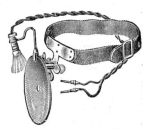

FIG. 146.—ELECTRICAL HEAD-LAMP.

(By courtesy of the Surgical Manufacturing Co., Ltd. London.)

Additional Equipment.—As already mentioned, there are many other instruments available and the inclusion of one or another is a matter for the decision of the surgeon in charge or of the sister of the ward.

Dressing of Wounds

In the preparation for and assistance in surgical dressings, surgical cleanliness is an absolute necessity. A student nurse must realize that surgical cleanliness means infinitely more than mechanical freedom from dirt. Asepsis aims at the destruction of bacteria which are ever present on the surface of the body, in the mouth and in other parts of the alimentary tract. Some of these are indeed harmless—but many are poisonous and if the skin surface be cut or injured by an abrasion they may enter the tissues and set up suppuration. The modern idea is that special dressing rooms should be set aside in each ward.

Sterilization.—There are various ways of destroying organisms. General consideration has already been given to them in Sections III and IV, but methods may now be studied in greater detail.

Steam is used in the autoclave for dressings, towels, gowns and masks ; the steam passes through them at a pressure of 15 lb. for 20 minutes, the garments being packed in a drum or special tin which is furnished with slots which can be opened to allow the steam to pass through.

With regard to boiling, bowls, instruments and receivers and indeed almost any appliance can be boiled. Boiling should be allowed to go on for 20 minutes, a small amount of sodium carbonate being added in order to raise its boiling point. These appliances may be used at once or stored on a sterile tray and covered with a sterile towel. The instruments should be specially dealt with, being put in a tray and covered with a solution of dettol or methylated spirit (which is clean and transparent) when it is available ; a sheet of glass put over the tray prevents rapid evaporation.

Sharp instruments such as scissors and scalpels can be placed in one of the sterilizing solutions in common use, or in pure lysol. They must be rinsed in saline or plain sterile water before being used.

Rubber gloves may be steam sterilized or boiled for 5 minutes. The gloves must be examined first for flaws, then powdered inside and out with talcum powder ; the wrists should be turned back and a small square of old linen tucked inside, by which to hold the glove when it is being pulled on. A small puff made of 2 layers of gauze containing talcum is placed between the gloves and the old linen folded over so that the gloves do not touch each other during the sterilization process. They are then folded double and placed inside the drum. The gloves should be paired and their size recorded on the outside of the packet.

Care of Gloves.—After use gloves are soaked in cold water in order that any blood or discharge may be got rid of ; then the gloves are washed in warm soapy water until they are quite clean. In the next stage they are rinsed thoroughly and hung up to dry on one surface ; later they are turned inside out so that they may dry on the other surface. They are examined for holes and if necessary repaired with a small piece of rubber cut from a discarded glove. As in mending a bicycle tube, special rubber solution is used to seal the patch over the hole. The patch should be rubbed over with a little French chalk.

Surgically Clean Hands.—A nail brush, which has been boiled, should be in a jar or bowl (see p. 341) at the scrubbing up basin—and there should be provided also antiseptic lotion, a packet of sterilized hand swabs, a bowl of biniodide of mercury (1 in 5000), ether soap and toilet soap. The nurse's sleeves should be fastened up above the elbows. The hands, fingers and nails must be scrubbed thoroughly under running water ; the fingers are then rubbed with ether soap with a swab and immersed in the lotion. After scrubbing up, the nurse should touch nothing that is not sterile until the dressing is completed.

Materials for Dressings.—The various dressings commonly in use are as follows.

Plain Gauze.—This is cut into squares varying in area. 4 inches by 4 inches is a very useful size.

Cotton Wool.—This is dry and fluffy, and therefore takes up a great deal of moisture, at the same time allowing the wound to be aired. It is best applied in several thin layers over the gauze. In some cases non-absorbent wool is put on as a last protective layer.

Gamgee Tissue.—Gamgee tissue is a composition in the form of a " sandwich," made by putting a layer of cotton wool between two squares of gauze.

Plain or White Lint.—Plain lint is sometimes used for fomentations.

Antiseptic Dressings.—Boric lint is always coloured pink, and is so much saturated with boric acid that it is always very powdery, It is a dressing applied in certain septic conditions and is well known in the moist dressing which is made by a square of boric lint, applied hot and moist, and then covered over with gutta-percha tissue.

Double cyanide gauze is usually tinted faintly purple and has well known antiseptic properties due to the presence of mercury and zinc cyanide.

Picric acid gauze is made by soaking gauze in picric acid solution and allowing it to dry. It is very useful for burns and in many septic conditions.

Iodoform gauze is very powerful, but its odour is so strong that many patients cannot stand it, and relatives very often object to it. It is used in tuberculous cases especially when there are chronic discharges.

Salicylic wool is impregnated with salicylic acid and is slightly pink in colour. It is a very well known remedy used in parts of the body where the skin lies in folds and where there is much perspiration.

Other Types of Dressing.—With the advent of sulphonamide powder and penicillin, many of the above dressings are not now in use. Liquid paraffin is used for septic dressings where there is local inflammation. Sphagnum moss, *tulle gras* and wood wool may be employed when certain conditions demand them.

Preparation of the Trolley.—The trolley is scrubbed and wiped all over with 1 in 20 phenol lotion. A mackintosh and sterile towel may be placed over the top. The instruments are put in a sterile tray containing some fluid, either water or weak antiseptic solution. Any bowls, gallipots or receivers that are required are placed with forceps on the top shelf.

On the under shelf of the trolley is a tray with bandages, strapping, pins, mackintoshes and bowl for soiled bandages.

The lotions and ointments that are required are placed on the lower shelf and the drum and Cheatle forceps in a jar.   A bucket with a lid, or a special soiled dressing bin should be kept apart and taken separately to the bedside.   The best type is one with a lid which lifts with a foot pedal ; the inner container can be taken out and thoroughly immersed in disinfectant lotion afterwards (see Fig. 147).

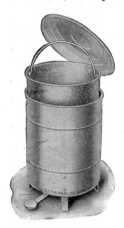

FIG.   147.—CONTAINER FOR SOILED DRESSINGS. (*By courtesy of Messrs. Chas. F. Thackray, Ltd., Leeds.*)

Routine of Dressing.—In ideal circumstances and in order to save time 2 nurses should be present at each dressing. The " no touch " technique which was talked of so much during World War II is not by any means new ; it has been in existence many years and is very simple and easy.   If a knowledge of the technique is built up from the beginning and if complete understanding is gained, it can be performed quite competently by one nurse.

The following essentials should however be established.

1. The trolley must be prepared with the greatest attention to detail and accuracy; the nurse should wear a mask.

2. Screens are put round the patient; the bedclothes are turned back and only the part to be dressed exposed.   The patient is given a mask to wear.

3. For protective purposes, a mackintosh is placed over the bedding and clothes.   The bandage is unfastened and removed ; it is rolled up or put away.

4. The necessary dressings, swabs and towels are placed in one bowl ; the lotions are in another.

5. The nurse scrubs up, returns and places her towels and with one pair of forceps removes the top dressing.   This may be quite clean and can be placed on the sterile towel ; if it should be in the slightest way soiled, it must be put in the bucket.

6. The soiled dressing next the skin dressing is removed with forceps ; if it should be stuck to the part it must be swabbed with lotion.   This is done by taking another pair of forceps in the left hand and these are used to take out clean swabs which are moistened and applied to the gauze.

7. It is with the second pair of forceps that the wound is cleaned, the soiled forceps being returned to a receiver.   If necessary another pair may be used but on no account are the fingers to touch the wound or dressing—sterile or dirty.

8. When the wound is clean or the stitches removed, clean

gauze, or gauze soaked in a lotion, is applied, this being covered with cotton wool ; finally the bandage is applied.

9. Any towels which may not have been soiled are folded and placed in a bag hanging beside the trolley ; the mackintosh may also go with them. The mask which was worn by the patient is put into another bag hanging on the other side of the trolley.

10. The bed is tidied and the patient made comfortable ; the screens are taken away and put round the bed of the next patient to be dressed.

11. The trolley is taken back to the sluice room and the top shelf is completely emptied. Fresh bowls, receivers and instruments required for the next dressing are prepared.

Surgical Fomentation.—This is a procedure which requires skill and forethought, since the fomentation is applied to an open wound and the risk of adding infection must be avoided. A piece of lint, doubled to the size required, is placed in a wringer and is boiled, the ends of the wringer being protected. There are various methods of doing this ; a special saucepan may be kept for it or a bowl with a handle. The fomentation should boil for 10 minutes and when ready to apply should be transferred to a sterile bowl and taken to the trolley. The trolley is set as for a dressing with 3 pairs of forceps—one to remove the soiled dressing, one to clean the wound and the remaining pair to remove the clean fomentation from the wringer after it has been wrung out. The fomentation should be shaken to remove the steam, applied over the wound and covered with jaconet. The latter is made antiseptic by immersing it in dettol and wiping it dry with a cotton wool swab. It is finally covered with white sterile cotton wool and bandaged in position.

Assistance.—In these days of scarcity of nurses it is advisable that all nurses should know how to perform these duties aseptically without needing the assistance of another nurse who can be spared only with great difficulty.

It is impossible to discuss the individual peculiarities of every case so far as actual dressing is concerned. There are various methods but they are all based on the same principles. When a patient has a wound in a place difficult to be exposed, a second nurse must be present to support the limb or hold the patient. This nurse should also wear a mask.

Disposal of Towels and Masks.—The towels which have been used and are not soiled may be sterilized again. Soiled towels should be put into phenol solution (1 in 40) and all stains removed before they are sent to the laundry. The face masks are washed and can be boiled and sterilized in drums in the ward annex.

Linen Bag Envelopes.—A very clean method of dressing is to use linen bags as envelopes ; in these are two dressing towels, a piece of cotton wool, 2 or 3 pieces of folded gauze and some cotton wool swabs.　When there is need of it, a mackintosh may be included.　These bags are put into a drum and sterilized and when the trolley or tray is being prepared one bag is taken out and put on the top shelf.　Such a method saves the using of a bowl ; it is tidy and there is no fear of the dressings becoming contaminated before use.　There is not any waste—and there is no need to take the drum round the ward on the trolley.

Preventive Measures.—Dressings, or preparations for them, must not be carried out while the ward sweeping and cleaning are being done ; there should not be any visitors in the room or ward.　As little movement as possible is the maxim, especially with regard to walking about.

The nurse herself must bear in mind that her hands may not be the only source of infection to a patient.　She must make certain that she is not suffering from boils, septic fingers, sore throat or other infectious conditions.　Certain diseases are very virulent and the usual custom is that nurses who are in charge of these cases do not dress those wounds which are clean and progressive and likely to be infected and upset if any risks are taken.

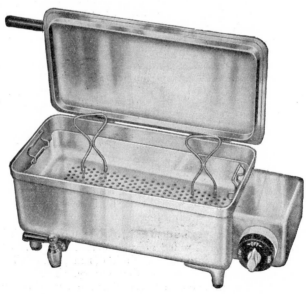

Fig. 148.—Instrument Sterilizer for Ward Use.

(By courtesy of Messrs. Chas. F. Thackray, Ltd., Leeds.)

Cleaning and Sterilizing Instruments

With few exceptions, instruments can be made sterile by boiling water. For this purpose sterilizers of various types are in use (Fig. 148).

The Sterilizer.—The tray, which is removable, should be covered by a layer of white lint or several layers of gauze, since the instruments become tarnished when metal is in contact with metal. The sterilizer is half filled with water to which washing soda is added in the strength of one teaspoonful to the pint and the solution is allowed to boil for about 5 minutes. Then the tray can be taken out and placed across the body of the sterilizer while all the instruments, with the exception of scissors, knives and needles, are placed on it. The tray is replaced, the cover is put on the sterilizer, and the whole is allowed to boil for a period up to 20 minutes. The instruments are then removed and placed in antiseptic solution.

Sterilization of Equipment.—With regard to knives and scissors, since the cutting edges are quickly blunted by boiling, it is better to wash them carefully, after which they are put in methylated spirit or in pure lysol. Needles may also require to have special treatment, and it is customary to pin them into a piece of lint and store them in methylated spirit. It should be noted that aluminium is damaged by soda, therefore when dealing with instruments made with this metal plain water should be used. Mackintosh material must be washed with 5 per cent phenol solution. All towels and similar linen articles should be sent to the laundry. Soiled dressings and similar articles are deposited in the waste bucket which is covered with a closely fitting lid and stored in the sluice room until it is taken to the incinerator. Enamelled basins, porringers, kidney basins and dressing trays should all be boiled for 20 minutes after careful washing.

Catheters.—A catheter is an instrument which is passed through the urethra (male or female) into the bladder for the purpose of drawing off urine. Catheters may be made of metal, gum-elastic, glass or rubber; the one most commonly used is made of the last mentioned material and is known as Jacques's catheter. In Great Britain, the sizes of catheters range from No. 1 to No. 16; as a rule Nos. 3–5 are the most suitable (Fig. 149). It should be kept in mind that there is also a French gauge, with a

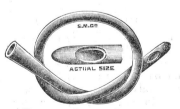

FIG. 149.—RUBBER CATHETER.
(*By courtesy of the Surgical Manufacturing Co., Ltd., London.*)

range of 30 sizes, and here the usual size for most purposes is 6–8.   Nowadays catheters are used in parts of the body other than the bladder.

Varieties.—A brief review of the various types of catheter in use may help the nurse to understand clearly how each catheter is used and how it is sterilized before it is passed and afterwards ; a very important point to remember about catheters in general is that they must be preserved carefully when not in use and they must be ready for speedy application when the need arises— often suddenly.

Glass Catheters.—These are used almost exclusively for female patients and it is essential that they should not be cracked or chipped ; careful examination before the operation is therefore

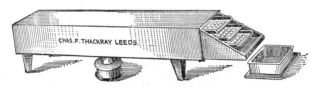

FIG. 150.—CATHETER STERILIZER.
(*By courtesy of Messrs. Chas. F. Thackray, Ltd., Leeds.*)

required. Sterilization is effected by boiling for 20 minutes, the catheter being first wrapped up in several layers of gauze, placed in warm water in the sterilizer and quickly brought to the boil.

After use, the glass catheter should be carefully washed in running water to make sure that the eye end and all other parts are freed from foreign material ; a thorough rinsing should follow in which soap and hot water are used.   Finally the catheter is again boiled for 20 minutes, then put into store ; sometimes catheters are merely dried and packed in the container in cotton wool, at other times they are left immersed in a solution of boric acid or perchloride of mercury (1 in 500).

Metal Catheters.—Silver was at one time the common metal used but nowadays various alloys are available.   They are treated before and after use by boiling, as described above, and then they may be polished and put away dry.

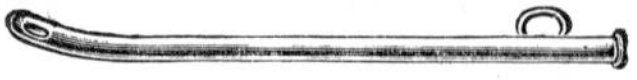

FIG. 151.—METAL (FEMALE) CATHETER.
(*By courtesy of the Surgical Manufacturing C.., Ltd., London.*)

Indiarubber Catheters.—An indiarubber catheter is easy to pass on both sexes and is the catheter of choice when there is no urethral obstruction.   Sterilization follows the same lines as those mentioned above, but one very important fact about rubber is that it tends to perish with age, therefore the nurse should always inspect the rubber catheter carefully before allowing it to be used.

Gum-elastic Catheters.—These require to be treated in a manner different from that already described. What is stated here also applies to silk web catheters. These types do not stand boiling ; the methods of sterilization before use are therefore soaking in a solution of perchloride of mercury (1 in 500) for 30 minutes, boiling in paraffin or fumigation by formalin generated by speci-

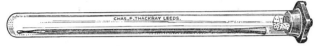

FIG. 152.—CATHETER IN HOLDER.
(*By courtesy of Messrs. Chas. F. Thackray, Ltd., Leeds.*)

ally prepared tablets in a closed jar. After use the usual washing is done, then the gum-elastic or silk web catheter is put into a solution of mercury perchloride (1 in 500) for 30 minutes, then taken out, wiped, and left to dry before being put away. In some cases the catheter can be left in the formalin atmosphere for 12 hours, and then rinsed in normal saline or boric acid solution.

Use of Stilettes.—A stilette is a piece of fine pliable wire which can be left in the lumen of the catheter when the latter is not in use. Glass and rubber catheters do not require stilettes, bu gum-elastic, silk web and metal catheters should always be put away with the stilette in position.

Shapes.—As illustrated in Fig. 153, catheters vary in shape ;

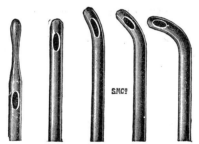

FIG. 153.—VARIOUS TYPES OF CATHETER.
Left to right.—Olive headed ; cylindrical;
semi-coudé; coudé; bi-coudé.
(*By courtesy of the Surgical Manufacturing Co., Ltd.,
London.*)

the ends may be cylindrical or round, olive headed (bulbous), slightly bent (semi-coudé), moderately bent (coudé) or bent as much as is practicable (bi-coudé).

Storage of Urinary Catheters.—Nurses are reminded that as catheters are used for introducing fluids into the body (e.g. in

N. II—12*

giving enemas), those employed for bladder purposes should be kept separately and used only in the genito-urinary region.

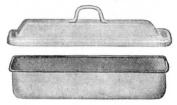

FIG. 154.—TRAY FOR CATHETERS WITH LID.
(*By courtesy of Messrs. Chas. F. Thackray, Ltd., Leeds.*)

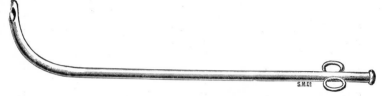

FIG. 155.—METAL CATHETER.

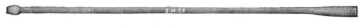

FIG. 156.—ACORN-TIP BOUGIE.

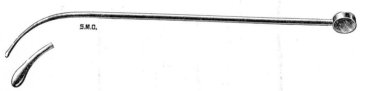

FIG. 157.—LISTER'S URETHRAL SOUND.
(*By courtesy of the Surgical Manufacturing Co., Ltd., London.*)

Bougies.—These are usually made of silver or of stout gum elastic, and are used to dilate strictures of the urethra (Fig. 156). They are sterilized in exactly the same way as catheters.

CHAPTER 11

PREPARING AND SERVING MEALS

PREPARING MEALS. FOOD PORTIONS: QUANTITY AND TYPE. SETTING OF TRAYS AND ARRANGEMENT OF FOOD. THE DISTRIBUTION OF FOOD. FEEDING HELPLESS PATIENTS AND CHILDREN. MAKING TEA.

FOOD is the fuel of the body. A sick person is in such a depressed state of health that his machinery is entirely out of gear and he may have reached the stage at which his whole being revolts at the idea of any stoking of his fire. To a certain extent loss of appetite is salutary, as it removes all congestion of the cells and ensures the disposal of the waste products. There is a strong mental element in all disease, however, and the influence of the will has much to do with the recovery of the patient so that all those in attendance on the sick should endeavour to stimulate the patient's mind towards his belief in quick recuperation. As soon as the acute stages of a disease have passed off, therefore, it is a vital point to aim at the institution of a condition of willingness on the part of the patient to take nourishment.

It is not to be expected that a sick person, labouring under the disadvantages of a tired body or of an incompetent system, should be able to take or to digest the average amount of protein, carbohydrate and fat required by the normal healthy individual (see Vol. I, Chapter 16, and pp. 124–140 in this Vol.). Nevertheless, according to the conditions of each case, the maximum amount of these essential elements should be ingested, and a capable nurse who understands the situation will see to it that her patients are each made the subject of a special dietetic study, for indeed each one provides an individual problem and much of the success of the treatment depends not upon the medicines given but on the adjustment of the constituents of the diet to the patient's powers of assimilating to the full their very necessary reinforcing material.

Preparing Meals

The subject of invalid cookery has already been discussed (see pp. 151–159). The nurse in her preliminary course is concerned only with the way in which to prepare the meals when they arrive from the kitchen, and with the method of serving them in the most attractive manner.

Food Portions : Quantity and Type.—The food for the ward is ordered by the sister in charge, who sends an order to the main kitchen to say how many patients there are and what diet they can take. Many patients can take a full diet ; this includes meat, potatoes, vegetables, milk or steamed pudding, bread and butter, jam and cake. A light diet usually comprises steamed or boiled fish, mashed or creamed potatoes, thin bread and butter, custards and jellies. The fluid diet is made up of milk, lucozade and any of the patent foods e.g. Benger's Food, Horlicks Malted Milk and Ovaltine.

Setting of Trays and Arrangement of Food.—Assuming that the food which has arrived from the kitchen on an insulated food trolley conforms to the standards of first class cooking, heat

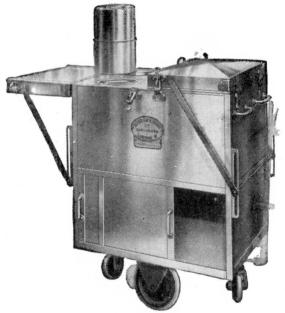

Fig. 158.—INSULATED FOOD TROLLEY.
(By courtesy of Messrs. Benham & Sons, Ltd., London.)

and palatability, it is the nurse's duty to make sure that none of its good qualities are lost in the service. The trays should be attractively laid out with knives, forks and spoons, clean and shining. The glass for the water should be polished carefully, and should be little more than half full of water so that there is no possibility of a small pool on the patient's tray which is trans-ferred to the bedclothes when he takes the first drink. The con-diments should be provided for those who want them. Bread should be neatly cut and should not be hard as the result of being left in the open air for several hours. It is quite an easy matter for a nurse to enlist the services of one or two convalescent patients as waiters, and then she can concentrate on the serving of the food. Food should not be " dished " out. It should be neatly and carefully arranged, with considerable art, on the centre of the plate, so that the patient will feel he wants to eat it and will develop a further appetite for it. Plates should be hot ; only one course should be served at a time.

The Distribution of Food.—If possible, all meals should be distributed at one time. It is irksome to patients to have to sit and watch their neighbours eat. The nurse must remember that a watchful eye must be kept on those who are apathetic over their food, but at the same time, sensitive patients do not like to feel that they are being observed like animals in the zoological gardens at feeding time.

In a surgical ward, where patients have to adopt all sorts of unusual attitudes, it may be necessary for the nurse to assist at the feeding, this being fully described below, but there are many cases of patients who are not helpless but who require certain adjustments to be made e.g. the provision of a bed-table or a pillow or some other extra support. A meal may be spoilt by the fact that the patient has to strain his muscles in order to support an unsteady tray, which may indeed upset his food over the bed and ruin his repast.

As soon as the patient has finished his meal, the tray should be removed and crumbs carefully brushed from the bed, especially those which may have found their way to the drawsheet. Milk, bread or other types of food must never be left at the patient's bedside, unless specially ordered. If a patient is not taking his usual amount of food or is otherwise abnormal with his diet, the matter should be reported to the sister. Water in a covered glass, syphons of soda water and clean tumblers or mugs may be allowed to remain on the locker or bedside table.

Feeding Helpless Patients and Children.—People who are very ill require to be fed at frequent intervals with small quanti-ties of nourishment, generally of a liquid nature. These patients are in a different category altogether from those who may take their food at the normal times, but yet may be in such a position, owing to accident or to paralysis, that they are not able to feed themselves. Such disabled people and young children, therefore, must be helped by the nurse, and careful spoon feeding is indicated during which the nurse should see that small quantities are given at a time, and that the patients have a long enough period between each spoonful to allow them to masticate the food and swallow it carefully. It may be necessary to provide two very small portions of the same course and leave one on the hot plate in order that the whole meal may be given hot.

The best method of feeding a helpless patient is as follows.

The nurse should stand at the right side of the bed, and should make sure first of all that the head of the patient is well supported by pillows. There should be no constriction about the head and neck. A napkin should be tied under the patient's chin, after which the nurse should support the head on her left hand and offer the food in small spoonfuls, without fuss or hurry. For children, a teaspoonful at a time is sufficient, but an adult may require a dessertspoon. If beef tea is given, it should be supplied in a feeding cup which is half full. The contents must not be too hot otherwise the patient will scald his mouth and tongue. After the nourishment has been given, the mouth should be washed out.

Children are always capricious about meals when they are ill, and they do not always fancy the things that are good for them; therefore, the nurse must demonstrate her tact, combined with firmness, in persuading the child to take what is prescribed for him. Children should have plenty of soups, mince and potatoes, and milk pudding and fruit. They may be allowed mineral water or plain water after meals, and fruit and sweets may be given. Unless there is a good reason for it, children should not be helped at meals ; they should be encouraged to feed themselves. Bibs should be worn and the beds should be protected by coverings. When parents visit their children a watch should be kept so that sweet cakes or pastry and other fancy articles of diet are not smuggled in to the patients.

Making Tea.—Tea is often spoilt when large quantities are made, and care and thought must go into this important item. The teapot or urn must be first heated and then the tea put in (in a muslin bag) ; boiling water must be poured over it and the infusion should stand for 3 minutes before any attempt is made to pour the tea out. It should be stirred first. The milk, which usually comes to the wards in bottles, should be taken round the ward in a jug; this is cleaner and nicer, also it mixes the milk, so that each patient gets a share of the cream in the milk. Sugar should not be added to the urn; it should be put in a basin and taken to the patient, so that as far as possible each may have his tea to his liking. If a patient is especially ordered to have weak tea, a small pot should be made for him separately.

CHAPTER 12

BANDAGING AND SPLINTING

TYPES OF BANDAGE. THE TRIANGULAR BANDAGE. THE
ROLLER BANDAGE : DESCRIPTION AND USES. PARTS
OF THE ROLLER BANDAGE. BANDAGING METHODS. RULES
OF BANDAGING. SHAPES OF REGIONS TO BE BANDAGED.
HOW THE BANDAGE IS APPLIED. CONVENTIONAL TURNS.
BANDAGES FOR VARIOUS AREAS. HEAD AND NECK
REGION. THE BREAST. THE SHOULDER. THE ELBOW.
WRIST AND PALM. THE CLOSED FIST. THE FINGERS.
THE THUMB. THE ABDOMEN. THE PERINEUM. HIP
AND GROIN. THIGH AND LEG. KNEE. ANKLE. FOOT.
TRIANGULAR BANDAGES FOR THE LOWER LIMB.
AMPUTATION STUMPS. SLINGS. THE LARGE ARM SLING.
THE SMALL ARM SLING. SPLINTS IN COMMON USE. SIMPLE
SPLINTS. PADDING OF SPLINTS. APPLICATION OF SPLINTS.
SPECIAL SPLINTS. LISTON'S LEG AND THIGH SPLINT.
CARR'S SPLINT. GORDON'S SPLINT. COCK-UP SPLINTS.
CLINE'S LEG SPLINTS. JOINTED ARM SPLINTS. FIXED
ANGULAR WOODEN SPLINTS. MIDDLEDORPF'S TRIANGLE.
NEVILLE'S SPLINT. JONES'S GUTTER SPLINT. MACINTYRE'S
SPLINT. BRYANT'S SPLINT. PHELPS'S BOX. HODGEN'S
SPLINT. SCOTT'S SPLINT. JONES'S ABDUCTION FRAME.
THOMAS'S SPLINT. BALKAN FRAME. SALTER'S CRADLE.
SANDBAGS.

BANDAGES are applied to various parts of the body for the following reasons : 1. to affix dressings ; 2. to give support ; 3. to
correct deformity ; 4. to check and reduce swelling ; 5. to
check haemorrhage.

There are various kinds of bandage and they are made from
different materials according to the use to which they may be
put. Bandages are named mostly after their shape e.g. triangular, roller, many-tailed, four-tailed, T-bandage. Triangular
bandages are usually made of linen or calico and are used for
applying splints and making slings. Roller bandages have
many uses and can be made of gauze, cotton, muslin, linen,
flannelette and flannel; they are of varying widths—from $\frac{3}{4}$ inch
to 6 inch or 8 inch.

359

Types of Bandage

The Triangular Bandage.—The bandage which has proved of most value in this category is one made of linen or calico, with two equal sides measuring about 40 inches, and a base measuring roughly 57 inches. The angle at the point (or apex) of the bandage is 90°. The angles at the ends are considerably less (see Fig. 159). The triangular bandage can be used as a covering, as a support for an injured part or as a sling. It can be folded as follows:

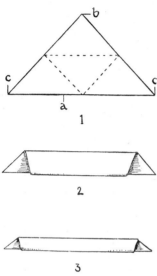

FIG. 159.—METHODS OF MAKING THE BROAD BANDAGE (2) AND THE NARROW BANDAGE (3) FROM THE TRIANGULAR BANDAGE (1).

The bandage is first folded by bringing the point (*b*) to the middle of the base (*a*).

1. *The Broad Bandage.*—This is made by bringing the point to the middle of the base as shown in Fig. 159, 2, then by folding the bandage again on itself vertically.

2. *The Narrow Bandage.*—This is half the width of the broad bandage ; it is made by turning the upper half oₗ the broad bandage on itself (Fig. 159, 3).

Triangular bandages are almost invariably fixed by tying the ends in reef knots; all loose ends should be neatly tucked in. Their use as slings is described on p. 376.

The Roller Bandage.—The fabric of a roller bandage varies according to its use; the following list describes each in brief.

1. *Domette.*—A species of flannel, open wove so as to allow the maximum amount of elasticity, makes the most comfortable bandage known. For all serious and extensive cases, domette is the material of choice. It has the advantage that it can be adjusted easily at each turn and so moulded to the part, but it can give its maximum support without being too tight. The result is a contented, comfortable patient, and a lasting demonstration of neat bandaging, which is satisfactory to all concerned. Up to a certain point, domette can be washed like a blanket and used several times. The criticisms made of it are that it is a very expensive bandage and somewhat heavy.

2. *Cotton.*—Bleached cotton bandages, open wove and some-times impregnated with phenol or other strong disinfectant, are used for dressings of less serious type and also in cases in which it may be necessary to destroy the old bandage at each dressing. Sometimes calico, muslin or other cotton mixtures are used. In the application of the plaster of Paris bandage, a coarse, open wove muslin bandage, previously impregnated with the plaster, is kept dry in a tin and wetted before use ; it dries as a hard mould or cast.

3. *Linen.*—Bandages made of this material are durable and strong, but they have very little elasticity. They are the most economical for long-standing cases.

4. *Crêpe velpeau* bandages are like domette with elastic strands, and are often used in early varicose veins and other conditions in which much support is required. Elastic webbing is much heavier and stronger.

5. *Rubber.*—Two kinds of rubber bandage are available, the plain variety and the perforated variety. They are expensive and perish easily, and while they give support and even act as efficient tourniquets, they are employed much less frequently than they used to be, owing to the adoption of better methods. Elastoplast and similar types of bandages, medicated and non-medicated, are now extensively used.

The Roller Bandage : Description and Uses

Roller bandages vary in length and width ; the commonest size is 6 yards by 3 inches, but all widths, from $\frac{1}{2}$ inch to 6 inches, are in use ; occasionally a short bandage, about 4 yards long, is employed. Everything depends upon the area to be dressed ; it is better to avoid cutting bandages short, especially domettes.

Parts of the Roller Bandage.—The rolled part of the bandage is called the head, whereas the loose portion is conventionally known as the tail. We speak of the head rolling up on the inside or anterior aspect of the bandage ; the reverse is the outside, or posterior aspect.

Bandaging Methods

Rules of Bandaging.—The following general rules may be termed the 10 commandments of bandaging.

1. Stand in front of the patient except when putting on a capeline bandage.

2. Choose a suitable bandage for the part to be bandaged.

3. Begin with an oblique turn and always fix the first turn.

4. Begin below and work upwards and bandage from within outwards.

5. Use firm and even pressure.

6. Reverse on the outside of the limb.

7. Two skin surfaces must not be brought into approximation and thus fixed by the bandage.

8. The axilla and groin must be padded when a bandage is being applied around these parts.

9. Two-thirds of the preceding turn must be covered by the next turn.

10. Finish with a special turn and put a safety pin through twice, with the point uppermost. In some cases application of adhesive plaster, light stitching or knotting of split ends may be desirable.

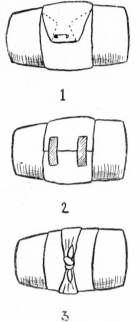

1

2

3

FIG. 160.—THREE WAYS OF FINISHING A BANDAGE.

1. By safety pin. 2. By adhesive plaster. 3. By knotting.

Shapes of Regions to be Bandaged.—The topography of the body roughly consists of a series of cones, cylinders and junctions of cones. Examples of the first are the thigh, leg, forearm and upper arm; of the second, the upper part of the neck and the areas just above the wrist and ankle; of the third, the elbow and knee joints. Padding is always used to make the region suitable for the fixation of a bandage, but it should never be clumsy or unwieldy. Over-padding will not neutralize the effect of unskilled bandaging.

How the Bandage is Applied.—
With the above outlines, the methods of putting on the bandage must be adjusted so that the essential functions are made full use of. Apart from the usual types of circular turns, special bandages may be made as follows.

1. *The Double Roller Bandage.*—This is made either by sewing together two bandages at their tails, or by rolling up one-third or one-half of the bandage from the tail end and thus producing a two-headed bandage (see Fig. 161).

2. *The Many-tailed Bandage.*—This is much in use for bandag-

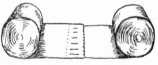

FIG. 161.—HOW TO MAKE A DOUBLE ROLLER BANDAGE.

ing the abdomen.   To make a many-tailed bandage, cut about half a dozen lengths of domette, 4 inches wide, each length being about 5 feet long.   Lay them out on a table, with each one over-lapping the other, like shutters or Venetian blinds, for two-thirds of the width.

Then take another 5-foot length, preferably in duplicate, and lay it, as shown in the illus-tration (Fig. 162) like the vertical part of a **T**, down the middle of the other strips.   Now stitch the vertical por-tion carefully to the overlapping strips. The result is the many-tailed bandage. Its uses are described later.

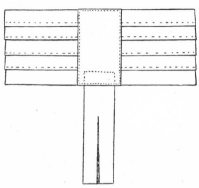

FIG. 162.—THE MANY-TAILED BANDAGE.

3.   *The* **T**-*bandage*.— This is not unlike the above.   There is, however, only one 3-inch or 4-inch strip representing the horizontal part of the **T**, its length being about 2 yards i.e. 1 yard on either side of a double strip of similar length, which is sewn to the middle of the horizontal strip and thus forms a **T**.   The two vertical strands are used to pass round the perineum and to become fixed into the horizontal strand which is tied round the waist.

4.   *The Four-tailed Bandage.*—This is especially useful for frac-tures of the lower jaw.   To make the bandage, a strip of domette 3 inches by 36 inches is taken, and it is slit up into two equal tags at either end, leaving a central portion about 4 inches long or slightly more.   In this a small diamond is cut out at the centre. The method of application is described on p. 368.

Conventional Turns.—Other special types of bandage may be devised according to the needs of the case.   In the ordinary way, there are 6 conventional turns employed regularly in using the roller bandage, as follows.

1.   *Circular.*—The turns completely cover each other ; this is used in fixing the bandage at the start and finish.

2.   *Spiral.*—As its name implies, this bandage is wound round the limb in spiral fashion, each turn overlapping its predecessor by two-thirds, and so forming the typical " shuttered " pattern (Fig. 163).   It is used for cylinders.

3.   *Reversed Spiral.*—This is very commonly used for covering cones e.g. the leg, thigh and forearm.   At every turn the band-age is folded over on itself.   To make a reverse, about 3 inches

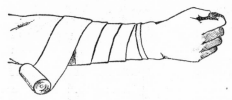

FIG. 163.—SIMPLE SPIRAL BANDAGE, AS APPLIED
TO THE ARM.

of bandage should be unrolled ; place the right thumb at
the lower edge of the previous turn (Fig. 164), and then, using the
left hand, allow the upper edge of the bandage to fall naturally
over by twisting round the head of the bandage. Gently but
firmly pull the margin into position. A tight diagonal line
should mark the fold. Continue similarly up the limb until the
pattern shown in Fig. p164 is produced. By this method it is
ensured that no space is left uncovered.

4. *Figure-of-Eight.*—This is used for joints, one circle passing
above and the other below the joint ; the middle point of the 8 is
just over the joint. The two circles are equal. When one circle
is greater than the other, the
special name of spica is given;
this is used in the large joints
such as the shoulder and
elbow, knee and hip.

Various patterns of this
bandage may be formed ac-
cording to whether the spica
is convergent or divergent,
ascending or descending. Examples of each are demon-
strated in the following pages.

5. *Recurrent.*—This bandage
is commonly used for stumps
or for cylindrical regions with
a free end such as a finger.
The bandage is passed longi-
tudinally on the cylinder,
backwards and forwards

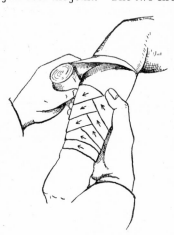

FIG. 164.—REVERSED SPIRAL.

several times, the left hand
keeping the loose loops fixed until circular turns fix the whole
system in position. The end of the stump shows the turns
gradually diverging outwards, except in the case of a finger,
where the bandage is often slightly broader than the finger.

6. *Oblique.*—Now and then large areas require to have preliminary fixation. This is done by passing the bandage in the

way it naturally runs; if spaces are left they are cov‑ ered later after the cotton wool has been roughly fixed.

For cylinders, the spiral bandage is used; for cones, the reverse spiral; for joints, the figure-of-eight, or spica, bandage. In nearly every case combinations of

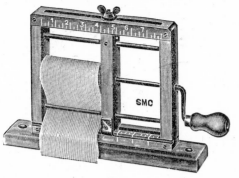

FIG. 165.—BANDAGE MACHINE.
(*By courtesy of the Surgical Manufacturing Co., Ltd. London.*)

these must be used, and there are no hard and fast rules, so long as the bandage is neat, comfortable and efficient. Many surgeons believe in using the largest single bandage known—the binder— when they are dealing with abdominal wounds, as it acts like a corset. The tail should be laid just over the right border of the abdomen, then the bandage is carried once round and finishes up at the left edge, where it is fixed with a series of safety pins; a double fold thus covers the front of the abdomen. In order to obtain the best results bandages should be rolled tightly on the special machine provided for the purpose (Fig. 165).

Bandages for Various Areas

The only way to become proficient in bandaging is to practise. Textbook descriptions cannot compete with actual experience of going through the process. In the following pages the common established methods are described ; many however are omitted. It must be understood that nothing can be laid down definitely; each patient is an individual with his own peculiarities, and his disability requires applied science and not theoretical patterns. The triangular bandage is described in conditions for which it is most suitable. In all cases of sepsis and in other diseases requiring frequent changes, the triangular bandage is most suitable as it is quickly removed and quickly replaced.

Head and Neck Region.—1. *Triangular Bandage for the Head.* —The triangular bandage can be used in various ways for the head, but the commonest example of its use is found in the bandage which covers the scalp completely. For this we take an ordinary triangular bandage, and the base is folded into a 2-inch hem; the centre of the base is then placed on the centre of the forehead as close to the eyebrows as possible. The point is somewhere in the region of the nape of the neck.   The nurse stands behind her patient, and taking the two ends pulls them firmly and ties them in a knot after they have encircled the head

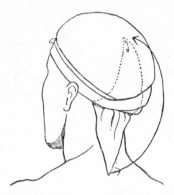

once, crossing below the occiput; there should be just enough material to make a neat knot in the centre of the forehead.   The long point now lies below the band so formed.   It is pulled tightly downwards, then brought forward over the crown, where it is fixed by a safety pin, as shown in the illustration (Fig. 166). The ears should be left uncovered.

2. *The Knotted Bandage.*—This is also called the spica for the head.   It can be used to cover either the anterior or the posterior half of the head.   The nurse should stand behind the patient.   With the right hand place the tail of a bandage just above the left ear; pull down about 8 inches of the tail behind the ear with the left hand, and use the latter to hold the tail in position. Then with the right hand roll the bandage round the forehead, carrying it above the right ear, below the occiput, and back to the starting point.   Keeping the tail taut with the left hand, pass

FIG. 166.—TRIANGULAR BANDAGE AS APPLIED TO THE HEAD.

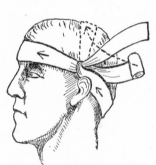

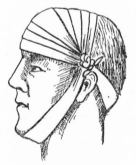

FIG. 167.—KNOTTED BANDAGE. FIRST TURNS.

FIG. 168.—KNOTTED BANDAGE.

the head of the bandage under it and run the next turn right up across the middle of the scalp, thus making a half knot at the starting point.   Carry the turn down behind the right ear under the chin, but not too tightly, and back to the starting point, where another half knot is made. This divides the scalp into two main areas, anterior and posterior. Either or both can be filled in, but it will be sufficient to describe the anterior space. The first and second turns are repeated alternately, but while the first type forms a series of circular bandages below the occiput, the second type consists of a divergent spica, each turn overlapping the predecessor by two-thirds. Finally the original surplus tail and end of the bandage are tied in a reef knot behind the ear (Figs. 167 and 168).

3. *The Capeline Bandage.*—Although the bandage to be described is noted chiefly for its historic interest and not for its efficiency, it must be mentioned. Nurses are warned, however, that unless they are very proficient at the application of it they should leave it alone, as it brings nothing but complaints from the patient and from critics if it is not properly put on. Make a double roller bandage; one roller, used for the horizontal turns, should be bigger than the other by about one-third; the remaining roller may be termed the " vertical " roller. The nurse should stand behind the patient, a roller in each hand, the vertical in the right and the horizontal in the left; the centre of the bandage should be put over the root of the nose, and the rollers carried round, one on each side to the nape of the neck. The vertical bandage is transferred to the left hand, and the horizontal to the right, a crossing being made. The next stage is the passing of the vertical bandage over the vertex to the root of the nose; while traction is put on the vertical head of the bandage, the horizontal head is carried round the skull, passing above the ear, and then round to the front of the head to take in the vertical portion and fix it. By taking turns backwards and forwards over the crown, making them gradually diverge, and fixing them by horizontal turns at the forehead and occiput each time, the whole scalp can be tightly covered in. Finish with a horizontal turn which is pinned securely.

4. *Bandage for the Eye.*—A single or double eye bandage may be required. Two-inch bandages are best. The double eye bandage consists of alternate turns passing over each eye, and will be easily understood when the method of the single eye bandage has been learned. The procedure is as follows. Suppose the right eye to be affected. Place the tail of the bandage on the forehead over the left (sound) eye ; pass a turn to the left, round the head above the left ear, below the occiput, and back above the right ear to the starting point; this fixes the bandage. The next turn follows the same route until the occipital region is reached, after which the bandage passes below the right ear, and sweeps obliquely across the middle of the dressing over the affected eye, across the side of the crown of the head, and down again below the right ear and so on over the eye. Continue with overlapping

edges as usual until the eye is completely covered in. Finish by making a horizontal turn round the forehead. Put a safety pin in above the root of the nose (Fig. 169).

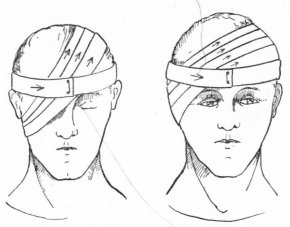

FIG. 169.—BANDAGE FOR THE EYE.　　FIG. 170.—METHOD OF BANDAGING ONE EAR.

5. *Bandage for the Mastoid Region.*—There are several ways of doing this ; only one need be described. To fix a bandage, a horizontal turn should be taken as usual passing round away from the affected ear, round the head above the ears, and below the occiput. This fixes the upper part of the dressing on the affected side. Continue the turns, covering the dressing lower down each time, and making reverses before taking the turn horizontally round the forehead and sound side. The last turn should be horizontal and should be fixed by a safety pin at the middle of the forehead or above the sound ear (Fig. 170).

6. *Bandage for the Lower Jaw.*—For a fractured jaw apply the special four-tailed bandage described above (p. 363). The point of the chin should protrude through the diamond shaped space. The upper tags are then tied behind, *above* the occipital process; the two lower ones are tied over the crown of the head, passing in front of the ears (Fig. 171). All 4 ends should be tied together.

7. *The Figure-of-Eight.*—This is a very useful bandage for the head and neck, and is employed in mastoid disease, in various gland affections and in other similar conditions; it can be varied to suit the different circumstances. Generally speaking, 3 main turns are applied viz. horizontally round the head, horizontally round the neck and vertically over the head. It is thus easy to fill up the

space to be covered, indeed a form of Balaclava helmet may be made.   It is very useful for children.   The first turn is begun behind the left ear, then the head of the bandage is rolled forward

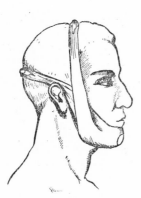

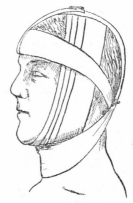

Fig. 171.—Bandage for Lower Jaw.

Fig. 172.—Bandage for Ear and Mastoid Regions.

round the forehead, passing above the right ear, round below the occiput and so to starting point.   The next turn passes as above, except that it runs down the left side of the neck, round the chin, up the right cheek in front of the ear, over the crown of the head, down the left cheek, under the chin and round to the nape of the neck.   This can be repeated until the whole area is covered in. Fix the bandage at the back of the neck.   Note that at no point

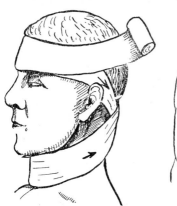

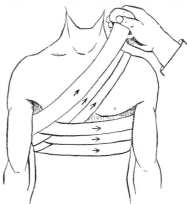

Fig. 173.—Figure-of-Eight Bandage round Head and Neck.

Fig. 174.—Ascending Spica of the Breast.

is a complete circular turn made round the neck (Fig. 172). In some cases, a simple figure-of-eight bandage can be made round the neck and forehead (Fig. 173). If the bandage is applied low down on the neck it may be securely fixed by making a few turns round the axilla.

The Breast.—The best type of bandage for this region is the ascending spica. The tail of the bandage is placed just below the affected breast, and two turns are made passing towards the opposite side. At the end of the second turn, the third turn is passed over the lowest part of the dressing and allowed to run over the opposite shoulder. It then runs obliquely across the back of the chest to the starting point, then round the waist again at one-third of the width higher level, and similarly in the oblique direction across the breast. Ultimately, the whole breast should be covered in as shown in the illustration (Fig. 174). When both breasts are affected, it is better to use two separate single bandages, so that each breast is supported in an upward direction.

The Shoulder.—A 2½-inch bandage is to be preferred. The ascending spica is again used. The axillae should be padded with cotton wool after being well powdered. The upper part of the arm should be covered by reverse spirals until the armpit is

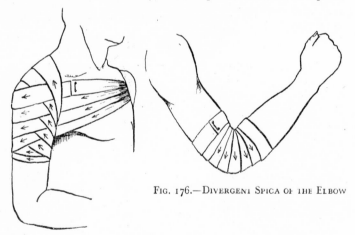

FIG. 176.—DIVERGENT SPICA OF THE ELBOW

FIG. 175.—SPICA OF SHOULDER.

reached. The next turn passes under the armpit, over the front of the shoulder, down the back obliquely to the lower part of the opposite armpit, then obliquely across the chest to the point of the shoulder, and so under the armpit and over the front of the shoulder again. Continue until the area is covered (Fig. 175).

The Elbow.—The divergent spica is used for the elbow. The procedure is typical of that carried out for all hinge joints. The best result is obtained when the forearm is at right angles to the upper arm. To begin, pass two ordinary turns round the middle of the joint, running over the olecranon process. Then gradually diverge the figure-of-eight turns so that the overlapping edges steadily recede from the central point. One spiral turn should be made on the upper arm to finish (Fig. 176).

Wrist and Palm.—For this area, a figure-of-eight bandage is used (Fig. 177). First the bandage should be fixed as usual by taking two turns round the wrist, then the bandage is passed across the back of the hand to the base of the little finger, turned across the palm, round the index finger, across the back of the hand and again round the wrist. Several turns like this make a complete covering for the wrist and hand, leaving out the thumb and fingers. Finish either by continuing a spiral bandage up the forearm or by a circular turn round the wrist.

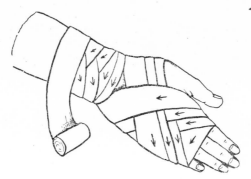

FIG. 177.—METHOD OF BANDAGING HAND, WRIST AND ARM, BY FIGURE-OF-EIGHT AND SUBSEQUENT REVERSED SPIRAL.

A triangular bandage can also be used to cover the whole extended hand (Fig. 178). The usual hem is made on the base. On this the wrist is placed, palm downwards, and the tips of the fingers towards the point. Cover the hand by folding back the point as far as it will go. Tie the ends after passing them several times round the wrist to include the surplus peak. Make a pull on the point, and draw it forward again over the back of the hand where it is pinned.

The Closed Fist.—In many cases of fracture of the metacarpus, the hand has to be bandaged with the fist closed. For this condition, the descending spica is used. The first turn passes from without inwards round the wrist. The tail having been

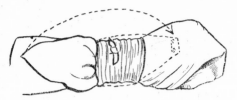

FIG. 178.—TRIANGULAR BANDAGE AS APPLIED TO
THE HAND.

fixed, the next turn is taken over the back of the wrist to the web
of the thumb; then it passes over the knuckles close to the thumb
and back to the wrist, the turns
descending on the arm and going
inwards away from the thumb by
$\frac{3}{4}$ inch each time until the area is
covered. The bandage should be
finished by making a circular turn
round the hand. It is not an
easy bandage to adjust properly
(Fig. 179).

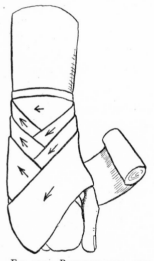

FIG. 179.—BANDAGE FOR THE
CLOSED FIST.

The Fingers.—If two or three
fingers are injured or diseased, it
is best to treat the injury as a
whole and not to bandage each
finger separately. In this case
proceed as described under the
heading of " Wrist and Palm,"
extending the figure-of-eight to
cover the affected area. Plenty of
padding should be put between
the fingers. In dealing with individual fingers, a spiral bandage
should be used, the ends being
carried back over the back of the
hand to be tied round the wrist. In some cases, the recurrent
method is used, finishing off with a series of spirals and tying the
ends at the base of the fingers. Here a finger-stall is usually
necessary in order to keep the dressing fixed.

The Thumb.—A spica is the simplest way of treatment. It
begins by the usual turns round the wrist, then passes as a loop
through the web of the thumb, as far up the thumb as is required,
and back to the wrist. The spica is worked towards the wrist as
shown in the illustration (Fig. 180). In all single finger and in
thumb dressings, narrow bandages (1 inch to $1\frac{1}{2}$ inches) are
commonly used.

The Abdomen.—For the abdomen, the binder may be used as described in Vol. IV. But the most popular bandage is the many-tailed bandage (p. 363). The bandage is carefully smoothed out and adjusted so that the patient lies evenly on the middle of the vertical portion. The slips are then passed upwards and inwards, from below upwards, until the whole of the abdomen is covered, the points of crossing being kept neatly in line.

The Perineum.—The T-bandage is used for this area (see p. 363). The horizontal and vertical parts are applied as already described, the latter passing one on each side of the genital organs and being tied to the horizontal portion. This allows rapid, frequent and easy changes.

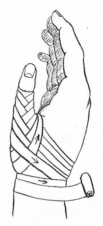

Fig. 180.—Spica of the Thumb.

Hip and Groin.—Two classical methods are in use here—the ascending spica, and the descending spica. The main difference is that in the former the successive turns continue to mount higher, whereas in the latter they descend at each turn. The ascending spica should begin at the middle of the inner aspect of the thigh; it then passes obliquely over the front of the

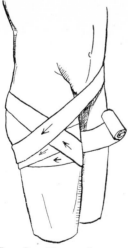

Fig. 181.—How to Start Ascending Spica of Groin.

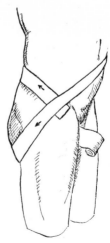

Fig. 182.—Descending Spica of the Groin.

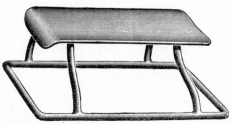

Fig. 184.—Pelvic Rest.

(*By courtesy of the Surgical Manufacturing Co., Ltd., London.*)

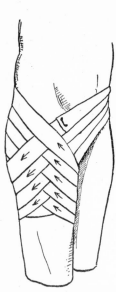

Fig. 183.—Spica for the Groin and the Upper Part of the Thigh (completed).

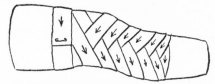

Fig. 185.—Figure-of-Eight Bandage as Applied to the Leg.

The reversed spiral may also be used.

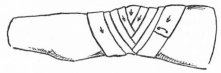

Fig. 186.—Spica of the Knee.

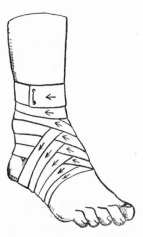

Fig. 187.—Figure-of-Eight round the Ankle.

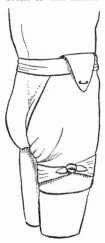

Fig. 188.—Dressing for the Hip, using Two Triangular Bandages.

thigh, round the back of the abdomen at the level of the pelvic
crests, forward over the front of the abdomen, round the back of
the thigh about its middle and so back to the start. Make the successive turns cover the one below by two-thirds, and thus continue to ascend, and the routine presents no difficulty. Fix the
bandage by a few circular turns round the waist. Use a pelvic
rest to support the patient (Fig. 184). So far as the descending
spica is concerned, the bandage should be placed with the tail on
the lateral and upper side of the thigh; it runs inwards round the
back of the thigh close to the lower fold of the buttock, appears at
the fork of the thigh and goes obliquely outwards to cross the
back over the lower ribs ; then it passes downwards and inwards
to the outer side of the thigh again. In this way the area is
covered from above downwards, the opposite of the process
described above (Figs. 182 and 183).

Thigh and Leg.—Remembering always that these are cones,
treat them by reverse spirals or by figure-of-eight bandages.

Knee.—Make a divergent spica over the patella (Fig. 186),
in a manner similar to the spica of the elbow, already described
on p. 370.

Ankle.—The heel can be covered in by a divergent spica
exactly the same as in bandaging the elbow or knee. As shown
in the diagram (Fig. 187), a figure-of-eight can also be used.

Foot.—After two fixation turns round the ankle, a figure-of-
eight bandage is made round the instep. To bandage the foot
farther forward, apply spirals and reverse spirals as necessary.
When the toes are affected, treat the injury as a whole, and
bandage as described for the fingers. Very often the whole of the
anterior portion of the foot is best covered in by recurrent
bandaging. The great toe can be dealt with separately by using
convergent spicas.

Triangular Bandages for the Lower Limb.—At the hip,
two triangular bandages may be used. One is folded into a
narrow bandage, and tied round the waist, being knotted above
the affected hip. The other is applied by drawing the point
through the circular bandage at the knot, and making a hem on
the base as far up as necessary, and according to the size of the
thigh ; the hem should be folded inwards. The ends are then
circled round the thigh and tied, while the point is drawn downwards and fixed with a safety pin (see Fig. 188).

At the knee the base of the bandage, turned up as usual into a
suitable hem, is passed round the leg below the patella. The
point is well up on the thigh. The ends are crossed behind the
knee, and then tied above the patella. The point is pulled downwards and fixed with safety pins (Fig. 189).

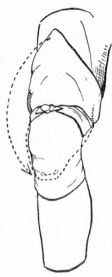

FIG. 189. — TRIANGULAR
BANDAGE AS APPLIED
TO THE KNEE.

The foot can also be dealt with by the triangular bandage. It should occupy an area roughly in the centre of the bandage, the toes towards the point. Pull the point back over the toes to the instep, and bring the ends round from the back of the ankle to be tied over the point on the instep. The point may then be pulled forward and fixed with a safety pin.

Amputation Stumps.—When dealing with these, the best method to use is the recurrent method; if the end of the stump is fairly wide, the turns may be made to overlap. The loops should be fixed securely by circular turns round the base of the stump, and long pieces of adhesive plaster, fixed to the joint above or to the abdomen or chest as the case may be, help to retain the dressing in position.

Slings

The triangular bandage is used for slings. These are necessary to take the strain off any area (chiefly the upper extremity) which is painful, or which requires support during the healing processes of bone, muscle or other tissues. Always apply the base of the sling towards the part requiring support (see Figs. 190 and 191).

The Large Arm Sling.—This is used to take the strain off the forearm and, to a certain extent, the upper arm. The bandage is spread out on the same side of the chest as the injured limb, the point towards the elbow. One end is pulled round the shoulder of the sound side, behind the neck, and is allowed to hang down for a few inches over the shoulder of the affected side. The arm is carefully laid on the sling, the base passing over the wrist, and the second end drawn up to be tied just in front of the shoulder of the affected side. The point is pulled out, then folded neatly over the point of the elbow and fixed by a safety pin in front or behind. If more flexion is required, the " reefing " method should be adopted by tucking up the bandage with safety pins as shown in Fig. 192.

The Small Arm Sling.—This supports the wrist only. A broad bandage is made from a triangular bandage, as already described. The end is pulled round to the affected shoulder as detailed above, and the wrist and half of the hand are laid over

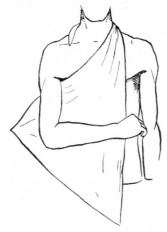

FIG. 190.—APPLICATION OF SLING (Part 1).

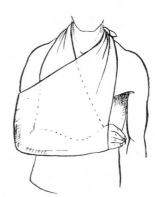

FIG. 191.—LARGE ARM SLING.

the middle of the bandage. The other end is then taken up in front and tied over the shoulder of the affected side (Fig. 193).

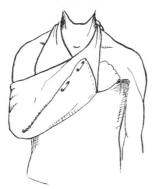

FIG. 192.—" REEFING " OF A SLING.

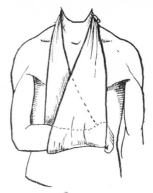

FIG. 193.—SMALL ARM SLING.

Splints in Common Use

Many splints today are really complicated pieces of machinery, and the nurse is not expected to understand the intricacies of such apparatus, unless she is working for a length of time with a particular surgeon. But all nurses must know the commoner varieties of splint, the simple types of which are briefly outlined

N II—13

below, and illustrated in the following pages. It must be stressed that splinting is essentially a practical subject, and furthermore, each patient has individual peculiarities ; alterations must be made to suit everybody.

A splint may be defined as an artificial support to take the place of a bone when the latter loses its supporting power owing to injury or disease. Many splints combine manipulative properties with support. Extension and plaster methods have in many cases taken the place of even the most perfect types of splinting. This is due in some measure to the experience of surgeons in World War II in which far reaching advances were made in immobilization of injured parts. These are discussed in Vols. III and IV. Meanwhile, since splints are of service in emergencies, for first aid purposes and in certain routine types of treatment, a brief review is necessary.

Simple Splints.—These are also called fixation splints. They are made of boards of various lengths and widths, planed flat with rounded ends and bevelled edges. A splint should always be longer and wider than the fractured bone ; indeed, in most cases it is as wide as the broadest part of the limb. Metal splints, shaped into " gutters," and made of aluminium, tin, zinc and other light metals, are much in use because they are light and rigid. Gooch splinting can be cut to various shapes and sizes; it is made by gluing on thin strips of wood to washleather or American cloth, the result being a sheet of closely applied spars,

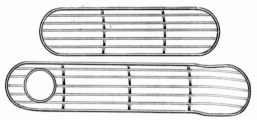

FIG. 194.—WIRE SPLINTS.
(*By courtesy of the Surgical Manufacturing Co., Ltd., London.*)

similar to the top of a rolltop desk. Felt soaked in resin (poroplastic felt) is also useful ; it can be softened, moulded to the part, then dried to hardness and employed as a support (Figs. 194, 195 and 196). There is no limit to the ingenuity of the surgeon in altering a splint to suit the purposes of the case. The material may be wire netting, pasteboard, iron, zinc, leather and so on, in addition to that mentioned above. It may be perforated, adapted with " windows " for dressing the wounds of compound fractures, shaped into angles, hinged and provided with large holes for protruding points like the ankle, or with special portions for gripping.

Padding of Splints.—Before we apply a splint, we must

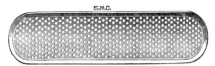

FIG. 195.—PERFORATED ZINC SPLINT.
(By courtesy of the Surgical Manufacturing Co., Ltd. London.)

make sure that the hard material does not press on the tissues and cause an ulcer or other serious sore. The limb can be prepared by careful washing, thorough drying, copious powdering with boric acid and talcum powder or application of boric lint.

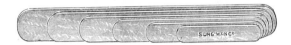

FIG. 196.—SET OF DURALUMIN SPLINTS.
(By courtesy of the Surgical Manufacturing Co., Ltd., London.)

Splint wool, containing oily matter, is best. Care should be taken that all the limb is well padded with it and that bony prominences are cushioned.

The splints themselves may be treated by laying on strips of cotton wool, and sometimes the splint is actually padded in a permanent way by making a layer of tow, well teased out, and covered with splint wool. Over this is put a covering of linen, muslin or calico, drawn tightly by cross stitching with splint thread passed across the back of the splint.

Application of Splints.—Splints must be applied carefully to the area involved ; this is the doctor's province, but the nurse may have to adjust the splint. The usual fixing agent is a piece of webbing with buckle ; adhesive plaster, split bands, sheeting or bandages (triangular or domette) are also employed. The utmost care should be taken to ensure that all splints are comfortable; thus the addition of various small pads or cushions, of various shapes, but usually about 2 inches in diameter, and always in readiness as a ward stock, makes all the difference to the welfare of the patient.

Special Splints

Liston's Leg and Thigh Splint.—This is a very simple splint (Fig. 205). Made of wood, it stretches from the axilla to beyond

N. II—13*

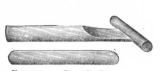

FIG. 197.—CARR'S SPLINTS.

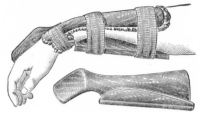

FIG. 198.—GORDON'S RADIUS SPLINTS.

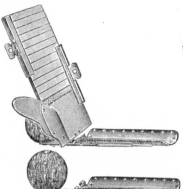

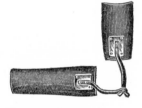

FIG. 200.—CLINE'S LEG SPLINTS.

FIG. 199.—SINCLAIR'S COCK-UP HAND
SPLINTS.

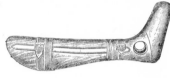

FIG. 201.—JOINTED ANGULAR
ARM SPLINT.

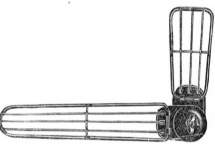

FIG. 202.—JOINTED ARM SPLINTS (WIRE).

FIG. 203.—RIGHT-
ANGLED WOODEN
ARM SPLINT.

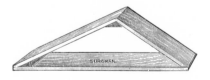

FIG. 204.—MIDDLEDORPF'S TRIANGLE.

(By courtesy of the Surgical Manufacturing Co., Ltd., London.)

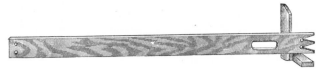

FIG. 205.—LISTON'S SPLINT.
(By courtesy of the Surgical Manufacturing Co., Ltd., London.)

the foot. It is less used than formerly, but is sometimes employed as a means of immobilizing the sound limb when the other is being treated by extension.

Carr's Splint.—This splint is of wood, and has been devised to treat the condition of Colles's fracture of the radius at the wrist (Fig. 197). There are two constituents. The first is the anterior portion, on which the forearm is placed. The lower part is planed into a groove to take the wrist, while an oblique cross-piece allows the fingers to form a firm grip over it. The second is a short thin back splint.

Gordon's Splint.—As illustrated (Fig. 198), this splint is of light metal and is a development of Carr's splint.

Cock-up Splints.—These are made in various forms, and are used for the wrist and hand. Common types are Jones's and Sinclair's (Fig. 199).

Cline's Leg Splints.—Various modifications of these are now in use based on the original pattern, which consists of a pair of wooden splints, carefully moulded and shaped to the leg and foot with circular openings over the area of the malleoli, and provided with straps. They may also be obtained in metal (Fig. 200).

Jointed Arm Splints are used when there is injury of the elbow e.g. excision. They are made in wood with iron joints (Fig. 201), or all-metal (Fig. 202), and usually have a butterfly screw for adjustment of the two portions.

Fixed Angular Wooden Splints for the arm are plain or shaped, the latter akin to the Cline's leg splint (Fig. 203).

Middledorpf's Triangle.—This may be fixed or adjustable. The base lies vertically on the side of the chest and abdomen, while the upper and lower arms lie on the sides. It is rather clumsy to fix, requiring a cumbersome harness to attach it to the body, but it is useful in fractures of the upper part of the humerus (Fig. 204).

Neville's Splint.—This is a stout metal posterior splint and footpiece, used in fractures of the tibia and fibula. It is representative of a large group devised to immobilize the ankle and keep the whole of the leg below the hip at rest (Fig. 207).

Jones's Gutter Splint.—Jones's universal gutter splint is often used in treatment of fractures of the humerus and femur, either as a temporary measure or as a local splint, when fixed traction is used.

MacIntyre's Splint is a more elaborate type of the above. It can be used for the knee as well as the leg. A special type of screw allows the knee angle to be adjusted, while a butterfly nut permits the movement of the footpiece through a wide angle. The framework is of iron, pieces fitted on being made of carefully planed and moulded wood. There are numerous modifications (Fig. 208).

Bryant's Splint.—This splint is used on both sides, and is very like a Liston's splint, with footpiece which is adjustable. Bryant's splint is valuable in hip disease of children (Fig. 209).

Phelps's Box.—A complete wooden encasement for the whole body is provided by this splint, which might better be described as a special cot. Each leg is fixed in its respective compartment, while the arms hang over in special grooves. The bottom is well padded by a mattress, the child being securely immobilized by splint sheeting and domette bandages. This apparatus is used for spinal or hip disease (Fig. 210).

Hodgen's Splint.—When the femur is fractured near the trochanter, and we wish to keep the knee partially flexed, Hod-

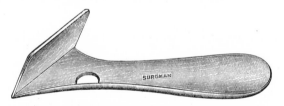

Fig. 206.—Scott's Leg Splint.
(By courtesy of the Surgical Manufacturing Co., Ltd. London.)

gen's splint is used. It is a stout iron framework, fitted with hooks and protective arches. The hooks are intended for the fixation of suspensory cords. At the top of the thigh, the wide end of the framework arches over the limb, and the two side bars terminate in another and narrower and more rectangular arch well beyond the foot (Fig. 211). The two side bars support a trough of strong flannel, and the whole limb thus lies suspended in a cradle. Extension is applied also, as described later.

Scott's Splint.—A wooden leg splint with attached lateral footpiece useful in fractures of the ankle (Fig. 206).

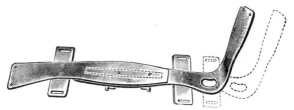

FIG. 207.—NEVILLE'S ADJUSTING SPLINT FOR LEG AND THIGH.

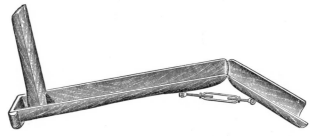

FIG. 208.—BACK LEG SPLINT, WITH ADJUSTABLE FOOTPIECE AND
HINGED THIGH PIECE.

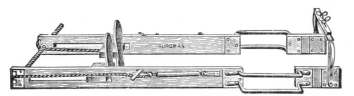

FIG. 209.—BRYANT'S DOUBLE LEG SPLINTS.

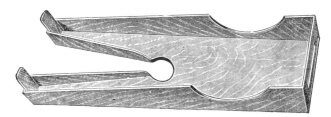

FIG. 210.—PHELPS'S BOX.

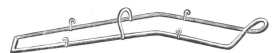

FIG. 211.—HODGEN'S SUSPENSION SPLINT.

(By courtesy of the Surgical Manufacturing Co., Ltd., London.

383

Jones's Abduction Frame (Fig. 212).—This is a " skeleton " of Phelps's box, and its framework is more adjustable. Strong iron supports are provided to form a cage for the immobilization

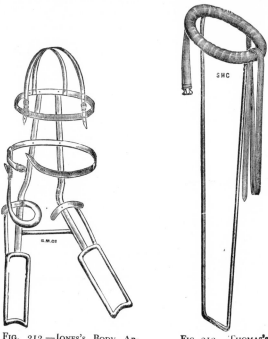

FIG. 212.—JONES'S BODY AB-
DUCTION SPLINT.

FIG. 213.—THOMAS'S
LEG SPLINT.

(*By courtesy of the Surgical Manufacturing Co., Ltd., London.*)

of the body in hip disease or fracture of the femur. Ample padding is provided by the " saddle " below. The patient is well strapped in, and because of the provision of a joint on the splint on the affected side, the limb under treatment can be gradually abducted or otherwise moved at the discretion of the surgeon. A strap also passes round the perineum to

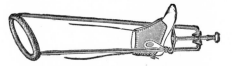

FIG. 214.—JONES-THOMAS KNEE SPLINT.
(*By courtesy of the Surgical Manufacturing Co., Ltd., London.*)

give counter extension, since extension is required for the injured limb.

Thomas's Splint.—The name of Thomas is immutably connected with the fractured femur of warfare. The adoption of this splint for various serious wounds with fractures has saved thousands of lives. Several varieties are used, differing according to the limb under treatment. Many modifications have been devised.

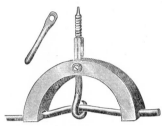

FIG. 215.—BENDING APPARATUS FOR THOMAS'S SPLINTS.

(By courtesy of the Surgical Manufacturing Co., Ltd., London.)

Thomas's Hip Splint.—The double hip splint is very like Jones's abduction frame described above, except for the absence of the mobile and extensory parts. The single bar type, which is not much used nowadays, consists of a long, flat, soft iron bar, moulded to the body, and extending from the scapula to the calf. It is suspended from the shoulders, and strapped to the chest, waist, thigh and calf. The patient wears a patten on the sound side, going about on crutches. He is not able to sit. The padding of the body must be carefully done. This was formerly the method of treating hip joint disease.

Thomas's Knee Splint.—This also requires a patten on the sound side (Fig. 214). A padded iron ring fits close to the groin; on either side there runs down two strong iron bars, terminating in an oval patten above which is a transverse bar on which the foot rests. The back of the leg rests on a soft leather sling between the bars. The splint is suspended from the opposite shoulder. Bandages pass round the thigh above the knee and below the knee round the leg.

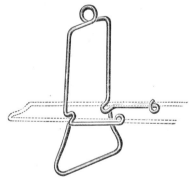

FIG. 216.—FOOTPIECE SUPPORT FOR USE WITH LEG SPLINT.

(By courtesy of the Surgical Manufacturing Co., Ltd., London.)

A patten is provided for the other boot. A modification is the " caliper " splint, which fits into the thickened heel of a special boot; the splint in this case keeps the heel of the foot about an inch from the sole of the boot.

Thomas's Fracture Splint.—This is used for fractures of the upper as well as the lower extremity. The original model was very

much like the knee splint, except that the side bars terminated in
a very narrow U with a shallow notch for extension apparatus.
The routine of application of the Thomas's fracture splint is fully
described later on in this work.   It will suffice at this point to
say that it has revolutionised the treatment of serious fractures of
the femur and humerus, especially when the added effects of the
modifications of men like Sinclair, Jones and all the orthopaedic
experts of World War II are carefully considered one by one.

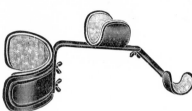

Jones's humerus exten-
sion splint is simply a
modification   of   the
straight Thomas's splint,
the bars being bent and
shaped   to   form   two
cradles at right angles to
each other.   Many other
varieties of splint have
been devised to allow the
arm and forearm to be
carried about comfort-

FIG. 217.—JONES'S ARM ABDUCTION SPLINT
*By courtesy of the Surgical Manufacturing Co., Ltd.
London.)*

ably in any position.

Balkan Frame.—This and various other types, chiefly in-
vented by Sinclair, form a framework at the sides and above the
bed, so that suspension and extension may be carried out.

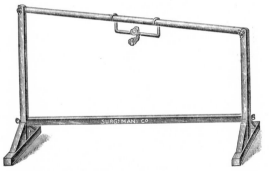

FIG. 218.—BALKAN FRAME.
(By courtesy of the Surgical Manufacturing Co., Ltd., London.)

Especially is this important in the case of Thomas's splint and
Hodgen's splint work.   Pulleys, cords and other adjustments are
provided (Fig. 218).

Salter's Cradle is like the Balkan frame, but used when there
is no need to fix the injured limb to the bed.   The cradle runs on

pulleys along a central bar. It is often used in cases of excitability and delirium (Fig. 219).

Sandbags are useful splints, reinforcing the wooden splints and preventing the limb from being moved. By fixing one on each side of the neck the head may be kept rigid.

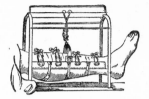

Fig. 219.—Salter's Cradle.

(By courtesy of the Surgical Manufacturing Co., Ltd., London.)

INDEX

Beds and pillows—*continued*
air pillows and rings, 276
circular air ring, 277
rubber mattresses, 278
rubber mattresses, aerated type, 278
rubber mattresses, Dunlopillo, 278
water beds and pillows, 277
See also Special beds
Bedside locker, modern pattern, 244
Bedsores, 273
causes, 273
general causes, 274
irritation and rubbing of susceptible part, 274
local causes, 274
moving patients for, 276
progress of, 274
symptoms and signs, 275
treatment, 275
trophic sore, 274
Beef tea, recipe for, 154
Beetroot, nutritional value of, 136
Benham access trap for sinks, 61
Berkefeld aseptic irrigator for purification of water, 38
Berkefeld filter, for sterilization or destruction of bacteria in liquids, 221
Beverages, 137
cocoa, nutritive value of, 138
coffee, nutritive value of, 138
tea, nutritive value of, 138
Beverages for invalids, 159
appleade, 159
blackcurrant tea, 159
cocoa, 159
coffee, 159
lemonade, 159
Bi-coudé catheter, 353
Bile, tests for (urine), 336
Bin, soiled dressings, 347
Bioaeration treatment (sewage dis-
posal), 54
Blackcurrant tea, recipe for, 159
Bladder evacuation, 79
Blanket bath, 257
Blankets, care of, 246
Bleaching powder for sterilization or
destruction of bacteria, 224
Blood agar, cultivation of bacteria, 176
Blood circulation and clothing, 84
Blood culture for investigating vari-
ous fevers, 231
Blood fluke, 98
Blood in stools, 329
specimen, apparatus for collecting
(*see* Apparatus for collection of
blood specimen)
tests for (urine), 336

Body louse (pediculus corporis), 88
Cox's vaccine for protection agains
typhus when delousing, 89
D.D.T. for use against, 88
powder, use of, to destroy, 89
pustular dermatitis caused by, 89
relapsing fever caused by, 89
removing, 88
Thresh disinfector, 88
trench fever caused by, 89
Boiled blood agar, media for cultiva-
tion of bacteria, 176
Boiling (disinfection), 105
Boiling food, 151
Boiling water for purification, 39
Bonney's blue paint (aniline), 222
Boothby-Lovelace-Bulbolian (B.L.B.)
mask for oxygen administration, 314
Bordet-Gengou medium for cultiva-
tion of bacteria, 178
Botulism, caused by bacillus botu-
linus, 169
Bougies, catheter, 354
Bouillon broth for cultivation of bac-
teria, 175
Bowel evacuation, 78
Bowl forceps, 345
Harrison's pattern (illustration), 343
London Hospital pattern (illustra-
tion), 343
Boyle's ventilators, 23, 24
Bradycardia, 295
Braising food, 152
Breast bandaging, 370
Breathing, correct, 79
rate of, 298
varieties of, 299
Brilliant green dyes, aniline, 222
British College of Nurses, formation
of, 237
British gauge catheters, 351
British Pharmaceutical Codex
(B.P.C.), 302
British Pharmacopoea, 302
Broad bandage (triangular), 360
Broiling food, 153
Bronchitis kettle, 311
Bronchitis (respiration), 300
Brucella abortus, 205
Brucella melitensis, 204
Brunton's aural speculum, 344
Bryant's dressing forceps, 342
Bryant's splint, 382
Bubonic plague, rat flea as carrier of, 89
Buchan trap, 59
Buchner's tube for extraction of
oxygen from a medium, 179

Echinococcus granulosis cestode, 95

Edinburgh University solution for sterilization or destruction of bacteria, 224

Egg dishes, 158
baked custard, 158
battered egg, 158
cup custard, 158
egg flip, 158
poached egg, 158
savoury omelette, 159
scrambled egg, 159

Egg flip recipe, 158

Eggs, nutritive value of, 133
preservation of, 133

Elbow bandaging, 371

Electric heaters, 111

Electric kitchen, care of, 248

Electric radiator, Electrovex hospital type, 112

Electric vacuum cleaner, use of, for dust removal, 25

Electrical devices for heating beds, 278

Electrically heated pads for heating beds, 278

Electricity, 112
for lighting, 121
for sterilization or destruction of bacteria, 222
hospitals, heating of (*see* Heating of hospitals)

Electrolux water softener, 40

Electrolytic hypochlorite for sterilization or destruction of bacteria, 224

Electrovex hospital electric radiator, 112

Ellison's conical bricks (ventilation), 23

Endocarditis, blood culture for investigating, 232

Enema apparatus, care of, 325

Enema outfit, 320

Enema rashes, 326

Enema saponis, 320

Enema simplex, 320

Enemas and excreta, 319
care of enema apparatus, 325
enema rashes, 326
enemata (*see* Enemata)
excreta, 326
faeces, the (*see* Faeces, the)
requisites for (*see* Requisites for enemas and excreta)
urine (*see* Urine)
urine, testing of (*see* Urine, testing of)

Enemata, 319
anthelmintic enema, 323
cleansing enema, 320
enema action, fundamentals of, 319
enema saponis, 320
enema simplex, 320
flatus enema, 323
procedure for cleansing enema, 321
purgative enema, 322
requisites for cleansing enema, 321
retention enema, 324
sedative enema, 324
Soutter's saline infusion apparatus for rectal and subcutaneous routes, 325
stimulating enema, Soutter's flask for, 324

England and Wales, designated milk in, 146

Enterobius vermicularis, removal of, 96

Envelopes, linen bag (dressing of wounds), 349

Equatorial spores, 166

Equipment, sterilizing, 350
for ward dressing (*see* Ward dressings, equipment for)

Esmarch's tourniquets, 345

Ether for sterilization or destruction of bacteria, 225

Ethical aspects of modern nursing, 238
management of patient, 239
nurse herself, 239
private nurse, ethics for, 240
professional secrecy, 240
recreation for nurse, 239
value of charm, 239

Ethics of nursing, 233
ethical aspects of modern nursing (*see* Ethical aspects of modern nursing)
evolution of nursing (*see* Evolution of nursing)
hospital etiquette, 241

Eusol for sterilization or destruction of bacteria, 224

Evacuation of bowel, 78

Evaporated milk, 150

Evolution of nursing, 233
British College of Nursing, formation of, 237
College of Nursing, 237
early history, 234
General and Supplementary Register of Nurses, 238
General Nursing Council, establishment of, 237
Middle Ages, 234

[]

Evolution of nursing—*continued*
 modern days, 237
 Nightingale, Florence, 237
 Nurses' Registration Acts, 237
 nursing in the nineteenth century, 235
 Royal British Nurses' Association, formation of, 237
 Royal Nursing Services, formation of, 237
 Sisters of Charity, 234
 Victorian era in nursing, 236
Excrement, removal of, in the country, 47
Excrements (sickroom disinfection), 106
Excreta and enemas (*see* Enemas and excreta)
Excreta (*see* Enemas and excreta)
Excreta, destruction of, in town and country, 49
 removal of, in towns, 47
 See also Disposal of refuse *and* Inland sewage disposal
Excreta removal, 47
 combined system, 47
 conservancy system (town), 47
 country, 47
 deep trench latrines (country), 48
 middens (country), 47
 pail closets (country), 48
 privies (country), 47
 separate system (town), 47
 See also Disposal of refuse *and* Inland sewage disposal
Exercise, importance of, to health, 67
External acarus, 91
External parasites, 86
 bugs (cimex lectularius), 90
 fleas (*see* Fleas)
 lice on persons (*see* Lice)
 ringworm (*see* Ringworm)
Extraction system of artificial ventilation, 15
Eye, bandage for, 367
Eyesight and lighting, 122

Fabrics, clothing for hygiene, 82
 artificial silk, 84
 cotton, 83
 flannelette, 83
 linen, 83
 other materials, 84
 plastic clothing, 84
 silk, 83
 wool, 82
Factories, workrooms, standards of air space for, 18

Faeces, the, 326
 abnormal stool, 328
 bedpans, various types, 329
 blood in stools, 329
 collection of specimen, 227
 curdy stools, 329
 examination of, 329
 fat in stools, 328
 gallstones, 328
 normal specimen, 327
 parasites in stools, 329
 pus in stools, 329
 unnatural stools, constituents of (*see* Stools, unnatural, constituents of)
 See also Stools
Fahrenheit thermometer, 286
Fasciola hepatica, 98
Fat in stools, 328
Fat soluble vitamins, 129
Fats, 126
Febrile states summarized, 292
Feeding helpless patients and children, 357
Feet, care of patient's, 261
 toilet of, 75
Felt treated splints, 378
Female patient, long hair, treatment of, 261
Fermentation of bacteria, 167
Fever, 290
 chart showing three common varieties (temperature), 291
 crisis of, 293
 termination of (temperature), 293
 types of, 290
Figure of eight bandaging, 364, 368
Filaria, 97
Filtration for sterilization or destruction of bacteria in liquids, 221
Filtration, mechanical, for purifying water, 38
 slow sand method for purifying water, 37
Fingers, bandaging, 372
Fires, briskly burning for ventilation, 23
 coal, 108
 gas, 110
 ventilation of room with gas fire, 111
Fish, nutritive value of, 134
 shell, nutritive value of, 134
Fist, closed, bandaging of, 371
Fixation splints, 378
Fixed angular wooden splints, 381
Flagella of bacteria, 166
Flannelette (hygiene of), 83
Flatus enema, 323

Milk—*continued*
  spread of infection by, 6
  storage and preservation of (*see*
    Storage and preservation of milk)
  tuberculin tested, 146
Milk, diseases spread by, 163
  abortus fever, 169
  diphtheria, 169
  paratyphoid fever, 168
  streptococcal infections, 168
  tuberculosis, 168
  typhoid fever, 168
Milk contamination, 142
  clean milk, 142
  dirt in milk, in dairy and in transit,
    143
  sources of contamination, 142
Minerals, food sources of, 130
  calcium, 130
  copper, 131
  iodine, 131
  iron, 131
  magnesium, 132
  phosphorus, 130
  potassium, 131
  sodium chloride, 131
Moderate temperature, 292
Moist method of inhalation, 309
Moisture, factor of bacterial growth,
  165
Monilia albicans, causing " thrush,"
  211
Monilia and odium (fungi), 211
Monsol, 223
Mosquitoes, 99
  anophelini, or malaria spreading
    type, 99
  culicini, or harmless type, 99
Motility of bacteria, 166
Moulds, 181, 211
Mouth, daily cleaning of patient's,
  263
  hygiene of the, teeth cleaning, 77
  hygiene of the, throat gargling, 78
  temperature of, 288
Mouth gag, 345
  Ackland's, 344
Mouth washing, tray for patient's, 264
Musca domestica (house fly), 101
Mustard, nutritive value of, 138
Mycobacteria, 189, 190
Mycobacterium leprae, 189
Mycobacterium smegmatis, 190
Mycobacterium tuberculosis, 189

N.P.L., thermometers marked, 287
Narrow bandage, triangular, 360
Nasal discharges (sickroom disinfec-
  tion), 106

Nasal feeding, apparatus for, 321
National Institute of Psychology,
  66
National Physical Laboratory
  (N.P.L.), thermometers marked,
  287
Natural immunity, 215
  age (individual immunity), 216
  habits (individual immunity), 216
  immunity of the species, 216
  individual immunity, 216
  occupation (individual immunity),
    216
  racial immunity, 215
Natural lighting, 116
  analysis of light, 117
  heliotherapy treatment, benefits of,
    118
  Holviglass, benefits of, 119
  houses, of, 119
  insolation, 117
  sunlight, 116
  ultra-violet rays, 117
  Vita-glass, benefits of, 119
  window space, 119
  windows, position of, 119
Natural ventilation, 14
  adjuncts to, 20
  aspiration, 15
  convection, 14
  diffusion, 14
  perflation, 14
  propulsion, 14
Neisser's stain, 174
Neisseria catarrhalis, 188
Neisseria gonorrhoeae, 187
Neisseria meningitidis, 188
Nelson's inhaler, 310
Nematodes, 95
  anchylostoma duodenale (hook-
    worm), 97
  ascaris lumbricoides, 95
  dracunculus medinensis (guinea-
    worm), 98
  enterobius vermicularis, 96
  filaria, 97
  trichinella spinalis, 97
  trichuris trichiura, 98
  wucheraria bancrofti, 97
Neville's splint, 381
New York, constituents of air in, 9
Nicotinic acid, 128
Nightingale, Florence, 237
Nineteenth century, nursing to, 235
Non-pathogenic organisms, 164
Normal temperature, 289
Nurses, Register of, 237
Nurses' Registration Acts, 237
Nursing, College of, 237

Poultice, ice, 318
Powder to destroy body lice, 89
Practice and theory of nursing (*see* Theory and practice of nursing)
Precipitins (antibodies), 215
Preparation and serving of food, 151
 cooking, methods of (*see* Cooking, methods of)
 meals, serving of, 154
 recipes for sickroom cookery (*see* Recipes for sickroom cookery)
Preparing and serving meals, 355
 distribution of food, 357
 feeding helpless patients and children, 357
 food portions, quantity and type, 356
 insulated food trolley for, 356
 making of tea, 358
 preparing meals, 355
 setting of trays and arrangement of food, 356
Prescription writing, 302
 common abbreviations in, 304
 form of, 303
 typical, 304
Privies, excreta removal (country), 47
Probe, dressing 343
Proflavine dye, 222
Proprietary preparations, value and dangers, 140
Propulsion, method of artificial ventilation, 15
Propulsion, natural ventilation, 14
Proteins, 124
 biological value of, 125
 use of, 125
Protozoa, 4
Pseudomonas pyocyanea, 203
Pubic lice, destroying, 89
Pugh's stain, 174
Pulex cheopis, 89
Pulex irritans, 89
Pulse, 294
 capillary pulsation, 297
 collapsible, 297
 compressible, 297
 Corrigan's pulse, 297
 estimate, how to, 294
 heart block pulse, 298
 other types of, 297
 rate (*see* Pulse rate)
 ratio of to respiration, 298
 rhythm, 297
 tension, 296
 volume, 296
 water hammer (or collapsible), 297

Pulse—*continued*
 See also Records, temperature, pulse, respiration
Pulse rate, 295
 bradycardia, 295
 frequent, 295
 rapid, 295
 running, 295
 temperature and pulse rate, 296
Pulverization, refuse disposal, 47
Pumpkins, nutritive value of, 136
Pure air, 9
Purgative enemas, 322
Purification and delivery of water, 35
 Berkefeld aseptic irrigator for, 38
 chlorination method of, 38
 domestic purification, 39
 large scale methods of, 37
 mechanical filtration, 38
 ozone method of, 39
 slow sand filtration method, 37
 treating hardness, 37
 ultra-violet ray treatment, 39
Purification of London water, 39
Purity, essentials of, in water, 34
Pus, collection of specimens, 227
 in stools, 329
 tests for, in urine, 337
Pustular dermatitis caused by body louse, 89
Putrefaction of bacteria, 167
Pyogenic cocci, 182
Pyrexia, high, 292
 low, 292
Pyridoxin, 128

Racial immunity, 215
Radiation, for sterilization or destruction of bacteria, 220
Radiation heating, 108
Radiator, Electrovex hospital type, 112
Rainfall, 28
Rainwater, 28
Rainwater pipes, 61
Rapid pulse, 295
Rat flea, 89
Rat week, importance of to health, 89
Ratio of pulse to respiration, 289
Raw beef tea, recipe for, 155
Reaction (urine), 335
Réaumur thermometer, 286
Recipes for sickroom cookery, 154
 albumen water, 158
 arrowroot, 157
 barley water, 158
 beef tea, 154

Royal Nursing Services, forming of, 237
Rubber bandage, 361
Rubber catheter, 351
Rubber gloves (sickroom disinfection), 106
Rubber hot water bottle (heating of beds), 279
Rubber mattresses, 278
Running pulse, 295

'S trap, 59
Sabouraud's medium, bacteria cultivation, 177
Saccharin, 126
Sack disinfector, for steaming, 105
Saffranin aniline dye, 222
Salad vegetables, nutritive value of, 135
Salicylic wool for dressings, 347
Saline infusion, apparatus, 321
Salmonella group of bacilli, 200
Salt, nutritive value of, 138
Salter's cradle, 386
Samway's tourniquets, 345
Sandbags (splints), 387
Sarcinae, 182, 185
Sassafras, oil of, for hair treatment for vermin, 262
Savoury omelette, recipe for, 159
Scabies, treatment for, 91
Scalp, treatment for vermin, 262
Scalp ringworm, 211
Scarlet fever, 231
  Dick test for diagnosis, 231
  Schultz-Charlton reaction for diagnosis of, 231
Schick reaction for diphtheria diagnosis, 230
Schistosoma haematobium (blood fluke), 98
Schools, standards of air space for, 18
Schultz-Charlton reaction for diagnosis of scarlet fever, 231
Scissors, dressing, with Collins's aseptic joint, 342
  surgical, 341
  surgical, Mayo's, 341
Scotland, designated milk in, 147
  certified, 147
  pasteurized, 147
  standard, 147
  tuberculin tested, 147
Scott's splint, 382
Scrambled egg, recipe for, 158
Screening (sewage treatment), 51
Sea air, 12
Sea disposal of refuse, 46
Sedative enema, 324

Selective media for cultivation of bacteria, 177
Semi-coudé catheters, 353
Separate system of excreta removal (town), 47
Septic tanks, use of for sewage disposal, 51
Septicaemia, blood culture for investigating, 231
Serum agar, cultivation of bacteria, 176
Serum sickness (immunity), 218
Serum therapy (immunity), 217
" Settlement tanks," sewage disposal, 55
Sewage, sterilization of, 55
Sewage disposal, 50. *See also* Disposal of refuse *and* Inland sewage disposal
" Sewage farm," 52
" Sewage sick," 52
Sewers, 49
Shallots, nutritive value of, 136
Shallow wells, 31
Shell fish, nutritive value of, 134
Sheringham's valve (ventilation), 23
Sherry whey, 157
Shiga type dysentery bacillus, 199
Short hopper in wash-down closet, 56
Shoulder bandaging, 370
Sickroom cookery, recipes for (*see* Recipes for sickroom cookery)
Sickroom disinfection, 106
  air and light, 106
  excrements, 106
  fabrics, 106
  hand lotions, 106
  nasal discharges, 106
  rubber gloves and overalls, 106
  sputum, 106
  thermometer, 106
Sickroom hygiene, 160
  choice of sickroom, 161
  cleaning sickroom, 161
  disinfection of sickroom, 106
  heating of sickroom, 161
  temperature of sickroom, 161
  ventilation of sickroom, 162
Sigma reaction for syphilis, 230
Silk, for clothing, 83
Sinclair's cock-up splints, 381
Sinks, Benham access trap for, 61
Sinus forceps, 343
Sisters of Charity, 234
Skimmed milk, 150
Skin, cleanliness of the, 73
  hardening of patient's, 260

Temperature—*continued*
acute pneumonia, daily chart showing crisis, 284
axilla, temperature of, 288
Centigrade thermometer, 286
cleaning the thermometer, 289
clinical thermometer, 286
collapse, state of, 292
diurnal variations of, 290
Fahrenheit scale, 287
Fahrenheit thermometer, 286
febrile states, summarized, 292
fever, crisis of, 293
fever, termination of, 293
fever, types of, 290
groin, temperature of, 288
high pyrexia, 292
how to take temperature, 287
hyperpyrexia, 290
intermittent temperature, 291
inverse temperature, 292
low pyrexia, 292
lysis of fever, 294
moderate, 292
mouth, temperature of, 288
National Physical Laboratory (N.P.L.), thermometers marked, 287
normal, 289
pneumonia, typical four-hourly chart of, 285
pyrexia, 290
Réaumur thermometer, 286
rectum, temperature of, 289
remittent, 291
rigors, 292
sub-febrile state, 290
subnormal temperature, 291
three common variations of fever, chart showing, 291
times at which temperature should be taken, 294
typhoid fever, typical temperature chart of, 293
See also Records, temperature, pulse, respiration
Temperature and pulse rate, 296
Temperature as factor of bacterial growth, 166
Temperature of sickroom, 161
Tension (pulse), 296
Terminal spores, 166
Testing of drains, 62
Tests for hard water, 34
Tetanus bacillus, 191
Theory and practice o nursing, 233
bandaging and splinting (*see* Bandaging and splinting)

Theory and practice of nursing—*continued*
beds and making of beds (*see* Beds and making of beds)
bedsores, special types of beds and pillows, heating of beds (*see* Bedsores ; Beds and pillows, special types ; Special beds ; Heating of beds)
domestic ward management (*see* Domestic ward management)
enemas and excreta (*see* Enemas and excreta)
ethics of nursing (*see* Ethics of nursing)
general care of patient (*see* General care of patient)
giving of drugs, the (*see* Giving of drugs)
hospital etiquette, 241
preparing and serving meals (*see* Preparing and serving meals)
records ; temperature ; pulse ; respiration (*see* Records, temperature, pulse, respiration ; *also* Temperature ; Pulse ; Respiration
special applications and methods of giving drugs (*see* Special applications and methods of giving drugs)
ward dressings and instruments (*see* Ward dressings *and* Ward instruments)
Thermometers, bath, 256
Centigrade, 286
clinical, 286
Fahrenheit, 286
N.P.L. marked, 287
Réaumur, 286
sickroom disinfection, 106
wet and dry, 13
Thiamin, 128
Thigh bandaging, 375
Thigh splint, Liston's, 379
Thomas's caliper splint, 385
Thomas's fracture splint, 385
Thomas's hip splint, 385
Thomas's knee splint, 385
Thomas's splint, 385
Thresh disinfector, for steaming, 105
Throat, gargling, 78
" Thrush " caused by fungi, 211
Thumb bandaging, 372
Tinea cruris, 211
Tissue, diseased, how heat affects, 316
Tissue, for collection of specimens, 229

INDEX

421

Utensils for ward dressings (*see* Ward
dressings, utensils for)

Vaccination, 217
Vacuum cleaner, electric, use of for
dust removing, 25
Vacuum system of artificial ventilation, 15
Valve closet, 58
Varieties of bacteria, 181
bacilli, 181
bacteriological tables, 184
cocci (*see* Cocci)
fungi, 181
organisms, description of, 182
spirilla, 181
spirochaetes, 181
vibrios, 181
viruses, 181
yeasts and moulds, 181
Vegetables, nutritive value of, 135
asparagus, 136
beans, 136
beetroot, 136
carrots, 136
celery, 136
cucumbers, 136
dried and canned vegetables, 136
groups, 135
leeks, 136
lentils, 136
marrows, 136
onions, 136
parsnips, 136
peas, 136
potatoes, 136
pumpkins, 136
salad vegetables, 135
shallots, 136
swedes, 136
turnips, 136
Ventilation, 13
adjuncts to (*see* Adjuncts to ventilation)
air allowance, how to calculate,
18
amount required, 17
artificial (*see* Artificial ventilation)
Cooper's disc, 20
definition of 14
efficient, essentials of, 17
efficient methods, 20
gas fires, ventilation of room with,
111
how methods are employed, 24
" ideal allowance limit," 18
louvre method, 20
natural (*see* Natural ventilation)
sickroom, 162

Ventilation—*continued*
standards of air space for variou
buildings, 18
Ventilators, wall (*see* Wall ventilators)
Vibrio cholerae, 207
Vibrio class of bacteria, 207
Koch's comma bacillus, 207
vibrio cholerae, 207
Vibrios, 181
Victoria era in nursing, 236
Vincent's angina, bacilli and spiro
chaetes of, 209
Vinegar, nutritive value of, 138
Viruses, 4, 181
Vita-glass, benefits of, 119
Vitamins, 126
A, 129
B, 127, 128
C, 127
D 129
E, 130
P, 127
Volume of pulse. 296
Von Pirquet's reaction for tubercu-
losis detection, 231

Wagon, for ward dressings, 338
Wales, and England, designated milk
in, 146
Wall ventilators, 23
Ellison's conical bricks, 23
Sheringham's valve, 23
Tobin's tubes, 23
Ward, work in, 245
Ward dressings, equipment for, 338
furniture, 338
utensils (*see* Ward dressings, utensils for)
Ward dressings, utensils for, 339
dressings sterilizer drum, 339
enamel bucket, 341
enamel funnel, 340
enamel tray for instruments, 340
glass bowl, 340
glass brush box, 341
glass jars, 341
glass kidney basin, 340
Ward hygiene. 160
Ward instruments, 341
Ackland's mouth gag. 344
additional equipment, 345
artery forceps, 343
aural-speculum, 345
bowl forceps, 345
bowl forceps (Harrison's pattern),
343
bowl forceps (London Hospita
pattern), 343
Brunton's aural speculum, 344